THE CORE OF
GERIATRIC MEDICINE

A guide for students and practitioners

THE CORE OF GERIATRIC MEDICINE

A guide for students and practitioners

Edited by

LESLIE S. LIBOW, M.D.

Medical Director, Jewish Institute for Geriatric Care, and Chief of
Geriatric Medicine, Long Island Jewish–Hillside Medical Center,
New Hyde Park, New York; Professor of Medicine, School of Medicine,
State University of New York at Stony Brook, Stony Brook, New York

FREDRICK T. SHERMAN, M.D.

Chief, Division of Geriatric Medicine, Mount Sinai Hospital, and
Assistant Professor of Clinical Medicine, Mount Sinai School of Medicine
of the City University of New York, New York, New York; formerly
Physician-in-Charge, Division of Geriatric Medical Education,
Jewish Institute for Geriatric Care, New Hyde Park, New York;
Assistant Professor of Medicine, School of Medicine, State University of
New York at Stony Brook, Stony Brook, New York

with **81** illustrations

The C. V. Mosby Company

ST. LOUIS • TORONTO • LONDON   1981

This book was made possible by a grant from the Administration
on Aging, Office of Human Development, U.S. Department of Health,
Education, and Welfare (Public Health Service) to the Jewish
Institute for Geriatric Care, New Hyde Park, New York (Grant
Number 90A-1172).

Printed in the United States of America

The C. V. Mosby Company
11830 Westline Industrial Drive, St. Louis, Missouri   63141

Library of Congress Cataloging in Publication Data

Main entry under title:

The Core of geriatric medicine.

  Bibliography: p.
  Includes index.
  1. Geriatrics. I. Libow, Leslie S., 1933-
II. Sherman, Fredrick T. [DNLM: 1. Geriatrics.
WT 100 C797]
RC952.C595   618.97   80-24704
ISBN 0-8016-3096-7

C/CB/B 9 8 7 6 5 4 3 2 1   05/A/600

Contributors

FRED B. CHARATAN, M.D.

Chief of Psychiatry, Jewish Institute for Geriatric Care, New Hyde Park, New York; Associate Professor of Psychiatry, School of Medicine, State University of New York at Stony Brook, Stony Brook, New York

CORNELIUS J. FOLEY, M.D., M.R.C.P.

Physician-in-Charge, Division of Medical Education, Jewish Institute for Geriatric Care, New Hyde Park, New York; Instructor, School of Medicine, State University of New York at Stony Brook, Stony Brook, New York

PAUL D. GILBERT, M.D.

Chief, Thyroid Clinic, Mount Sinai Hospital, and Associate Professor of Clinical Medicine, Mount Sinai School of Medicine of the City University of New York, New York, New York; Consultant in Thyroid Disease, Jewish Institute for Geriatric Care, New Hyde Park, New York

ARTHUR E. HELFAND, D.P.M.

Professor and Chairman, Department of Community Health, Pennsylvania College of Podiatric Medicine, Philadelphia, Pennsylvania

CYRUS KAHN, M.D.

Consultant in Ophthalmology, Jewish Institute for Geriatric Care, New Hyde Park, New York

SAUL KAMEN, D.D.S.

Chief of Dentistry, Jewish Institute for Geriatric Care, New Hyde Park, New York; Professor of Dental Health, School of Dentistry, State University of New York at Stony Brook, Stony Brook, New York

BARBARA LEVY, M.S., C.C.C./A.

Audiologist, Jewish Institute for Geriatric Care, New Hyde Park, New York

LESLIE S. LIBOW, M.D.

Medical Director, Jewish Institute for Geriatric Care, and Chief of Geriatric Medicine, Long Island Jewish–Hillside Medical Center, New Hyde Park, New York; Professor of Medicine, School of Medicine, State University of New York at Stony Brook, Stony Brook, New York

SARA MARCHBEIN MEISELLS, M.S., C.C.C.

Speech Pathologist, Jewish Institute for Geriatric Care, New Hyde Park, New York

EMMANUEL MARGOLIS, M.D.

Assistant to Chief, Department of Medicine, Coler Hospital, New York, New York; formerly Staff Physician, Administration on Aging Curriculum Development Grant, Jewish Institute for Geriatric Care, New Hyde Park, New York

ZENA SCHECHTER, M.Ed.

Associate Project Director, Administration on Aging Curriculum Development Grant, Jewish Institute for Geriatric Care, New Hyde Park, New York

v

FREDRICK T. SHERMAN, M.D.

Chief, Division of Geriatric Medicine, Mount Sinai Hospital, and Assistant Professor of Clinical Medicine, Mount Sinai School of Medicine of the City University of New York, New York, New York; formerly Physician-in-Charge, Division of Geriatric Medical Education, Jewish Institute for Geriatric Care, New Hyde Park, New York; Physician Coordinator, Administration on Aging Curriculum Development Grant; Assistant Professor of Medicine, School of Medicine, State University of New York at Stony Brook, Stony Brook, New York

RAMON VALLARINO, M.D.

Chief of Geriatric Physiatry, Jewish Institute for Geriatric Care, New Hyde Park, New York

HOWARD WERTER, D.P.M.

Chief of Podiatry, Jewish Institute for Geriatric Care, New Hyde Park, New York

LARRY D. WRIGHT, M.D.

Internist-Geriatrician, Rogers Medical Center, Rogers, Arkansas; formerly Resident Physician in Geriatric Medicine, Jewish Institute for Geriatric Care, New Hyde Park, New York

To all of the older persons who have contributed to the
knowledge that makes this book possible,
to our children
Adam, Alana, Rachel, and William,
and to our wives
Linda and **Susan**

Foreword

Equal opportunity to "the best possible physical and mental health that science can make available" is identified by the Older Americans Act as one of the objectives that the federal government, in partnership with state and local government, should help older people to secure.

Responsibility for a national manpower policy and concern for personal needs in the field of aging are also given special emphasis in the 1978 Amendments to the Older Americans Act. In view of these purposes and responsibilities, the Administration on Aging has in recent years taken several initiatives, including the long-term care gerontology centers program and the geriatric fellowship program. Supportive of these efforts are several initiatives to improve the quality and increase the accessibility of curriculum materials for educational programs dealing with health care for the elderly. Notable among these is the project that has produced the present excellent volume. It is with great pleasure and pride that I take part in introducing it to the clinical and educational community.

The education of those in medicine and other health professions will be significantly enhanced by *The Core of Geriatric Medicine: A Guide for Students and Practitioners*, edited by Leslie S. Libow, M.D., and Fredrick T. Sherman, M.D. This material, which serves as a curriculum and text for students of geriatric medicine, has been developed with the support of a grant from the Administration on Aging to the Jewish Institute for Geriatric Care in New Hyde Park, New York (Leslie S. Libow, M.D., Principal Investigator).

It is my belief that the training programs developed at the Jewish Institute for Geriatric Care provide an excellent source of materials for adaptation into a written guide for students, practitioners, and teachers. Few programs, to my knowledge, have comparable experience in training students and practitioners in geriatric medicine. Students of medicine, nursing, physical therapy, occupational therapy, and social work as well as nurse practitioners and physician assistants are the beneficiaries of pioneer work by the institute.

A particular quality of this book is the manner in which it reflects the bringing together of related or traditionally distinct programs of the institute. The material developed focuses on aspects of health care that are central to the care of the elderly but often overlooked in standard educational and training experiences. The modular approach lends a distinct strength to this book. Each chapter clearly sets down objectives; provides a practical, clinical body of knowledge;

and is accompanied by test questions and problem-solving case histories. The clinician is presented with the core of interviewing and history taking; economic aspects of health care affecting the elderly; speech and hearing difficulties; oral, dental, podiatric, and visual problems; rehabilitative issues (focusing on stroke, fracture, amputation, decubitus ulcers, and incontinence); and pharmacology. Also presented is the geriatric medical aspect of hypertension and thyroid disease.

The Administration on Aging is pleased to have supported the development by this group of clinicians of a videotape,

The Rehabilitation of the Elderly Patient, as well as an audio-slide combination presenting materials on oral and dental disease in the elderly. These audiovisual materials serve as an elective supplement to the book.

I am confident that this material will enhance the education of students and practitioners and enable instructors in this field to develop more rapidly, appropriate courses in geriatric medicine and gerontology.

Robert Benedict, M.P.H.
Commissioner, Administration on Aging, Washington, D.C.

Dr. Leslie S. Libow and Dr. Fredrick T. Sherman and their collaborators have developed a most valuable guide for students and practitioners who wish to acquire the basics of geriatric medicine.

As a result of this book, *The Core of Geriatric Medicine: A Guide for Students and Practitioners,* we now have clinical insights that have advanced the body of knowledge that constitutes geriatric medicine. Readers will enjoy firsthand, presentation of the basic concepts of geriatric medicine, especially the intricacies of diagnosis, and the special features of treatment and rehabilitation. They will learn how inapplicable the notion is that one should find one explanation for as many symptoms as possible. This simplistic application of Ockham's razor is so out of keeping with the realities of the increasing complexity, multiple pathology, and polypharmacy that are associated with advancing years. Readers will also learn how critical social and economic factors are to older persons. I would hope that readers would emulate

the emphasis on prompt, effective diagnosis and treatment, for example, in the response to "pseudosenility." They will note how salient communicative skills are to older patients. Not least, they will become familiar with the importance of podiatry with advancing age.

It has been my very great pleasure to have accompanied Dr. Libow on his medical rounds, both in person and through the literature, since 1960. Most recently, I visited Drs. Libow and Sherman and colleagues at the "teaching-nursing home" at the Jewish Institute for Geriatric Care (JIGC). During these twenty years I have profited enormously from Dr. Libow's compassionate use of his clinical skills and comprehensive knowledge as a teacher and investigator. Many others have gained from their association with Drs. Libow and Sherman and colleagues: medical students who have traveled great distances from all over the country to take electives at the JIGC, geriatricians-to-be who have been the first to obtain recognized residencies in geriatric medicine in the United States, and, perhaps most of all, patients who have improved or recovered through their care.

Drs. Libow and Sherman and colleagues would be the first to say that this book is just the beginning: a first effort to create a guideline for all of us concerning selected topics of geriatrics. There is still so much to be learned.

Robert N. Butler, M.D.

Director, National Institute on Aging,
National Institutes of Health,
Bethesda, Md.

Preface

This book presents aspects of care of the elderly patient that usually are not dealt with in standard medical textbooks or classical educational courses for students or clinicians. Topics covered include interviewing the elderly patient; medication; rehabilitation techniques following stroke, hip fracture, and amputation; psychogeriatrics; and an approach to differential diagnosis and classification of disorders of mentation ("organic brain syndrome—dementia"), ambulation, speech, hearing, vision, and nutrition. Podiatric and dental problems of the elderly are also discussed. The chapter on demography, economics, and legislation and regulations (Medicare and Medicaid) is directed at issues affecting patients and practitioners on a daily basis. Organ-type illnesses are not the emphasis of the book. However, two common illnesses, hypertension and thyroid disease, are presented with full exposition of the body of knowledge of geriatric medicine for these areas.

The material was developed under an Administration on Aging grant (Leslie S. Libow, M.D., Principal Investigator) at the Jewish Institute for Geriatric Care (JIGC). The entire book emanates from one program's approach to this particular aspect of geriatric medicine, developed over several years at JIGC.

JIGC is professionally integrated with and physically linked to the Long Island Jewish–Hillside Medical Center (LIJ-HMC), a major clinical campus of the School of Medicine and other health professional schools of the Health Sciences Center at the State University of New York at Stony Brook. JIGC serves as a major focus of LIJ-HMC's and Stony Brook's efforts in geriatric education, training, and research.

The education and training of students and graduate physicians in geriatric medicine has been a central theme at JIGC. Specific programs include a residency/fellowship program that has served as a model for other medical centers and long-term care facilities, a "selective" clinical clerkship for senior medical students at Stony Brook, an elective clinical clerkship in geriatric medicine for third- and fourth-year medical students, a mandatory subinternship for "Fifth Pathway" students, and a clerkship for physician assistant students. These programs feature supervised clinical responsibilities, daily teaching rounds, special rehabilitation and geropsychiatry rounds, weekly seminars on geriatric and gerontological topics, didactic teaching sessions, home care visits, and ambulatory care programs.

Three years ago we decided to formalize one key aspect of our clinical clerkship approaches and materials and make them available to other health professional schools. A grant from the Administration on Aging (AOA) enabled us to refine our clerkship by producing a formal curriculum.

The curriculum consists of 15 instructional units, presented in this book as separate chapters. Together, these units constitute a basic "core" approach to the practice of geriatric medicine. Although common themes regarding the management of the geriatric patient appear throughout the book, each chapter, or unit, is designed to stand on its own, leaving the instructor and the student the latitude to focus only on those aspects of geriatric care germane to their educational program.

Each chapter contains the following components:

1. A statement of educational objectives (attitudinal, cognitive, and skill)
2. A pretest to establish the student's current knowledge
3. Basic text (including references)
4. Problem-solving exercises (usually involving case histories)
5. Posttest (same as pretest)
6. Answers to pretest and posttest and problem-solving exercises

The material in this book can be read by students as a complete text, or individual chapters can be used in instruction as part of a formal curriculum in geriatric medicine. Although the chapters are ordered to build on a base of geriatric medicine, their sequence of presentation is not critical.

We have found, in pilot testing individual units, that the seminar is a valuable teaching method. Several days before the seminar, students receive the objectives, pretest, text, and problem-solving exercises. Students are asked to complete the pretest, read the text, and then complete the problem-solving exercises. At the seminar session, which usually lasts about 2 hours, the instructor (usually an attending physician or resident) attempts to guide the students through the problem-solving exercises, always keeping in mind the objectives for the unit.

Instructors in other institutions may want to vary the teaching approach, depending on the students' backgrounds. The results of the pretest may assist the instructor in evaluating each student and obtaining a profile of the class as a whole. Among the teaching techniques to be considered are discussions carried on in a lecture-seminar form, with the instructor clarifying points; problem-solving case history exercises, which tend to introduce the multiple problems frequently encountered in caring for the elderly; role-playing exercises; and audiovisual presentations.

With respect to evaluation, the pretest and posttest questions provide an opportunity for the instructor and the student to assess the ideas, concepts, and facts learned.

There are two audiovisual presentations that could be used in a course based on this material. One, a videotape (available from The C. V. Mosby Co.), *The Rehabilitation of the Elderly Patient*, focuses on the phases of rehabilitation for stroke, fracture of the hip, and amputation. The other is an audio-slide presentation on oral and dental disease in the elderly (available from Douglas Fogarty and Associates, P.O. Box 1324, Iowa City, Iowa 52244). While complementing the text, these audiovisual materials could also be used independently.

The following specialists critically reviewed individual chapters and made valuable suggestions for improvement:

Kenneth Freedman, D.M.D.
Assistant Professor of Prosthodontics,
University of Illinois College of Dentistry,
Chicago, Illinois

Edward D. Fries, M.D.
Senior Medical Investigator,
Veterans Administration Medical Center,
Washington, D.C.

Norman Geschwind, M.D.
James Jackson Putnam Professor of
    Neurology,
Harvard Medical School,
Cambridge, Massachusetts;
Director, Neurological Unit,
Beth Israel Hospital,
Boston, Massachusetts

Merrill Goodman, M.D.
Medical Director,
Hearing and Speech Center,
Long Island Jewish – Hillside Medical
    Center,
New Hyde Park, New York

A. L. Kornzweig, M.D., F.A.C.S.
Chief of Eye Research,
Jewish Home and Hospital – New York
    City, and
Emeritus Clinical Professor,
Mount Sinai School of Medicine of the
    City University of New York,
New York, New York

Alvin J. Levenson, M.D.
Assistant Professor of Psychiatry and
Chief, Section on Geriatric Psychiatry,
University of Texas Medical School at
    Houston,
Houston, Texas

Simon Parisier, M.D.
Professor of Clinical Otolaryngology,
Mount Sinai School of Medicine of the
    City University of New York,
New York, New York

Manuel Rodstein, M.D.
Professor of Clinical Medicine,
Mount Sinai School of Medicine of the
    City University of New York, and
Chief of Medical Services,
Jewish Home and Hospital for the Aged,
New York, New York

Anne R. Somers, D.Sc. (Hon.)
Professor of Environmental and Community
    Medicine,
College of Medicine,
Rutgers Medical School,
Princeton, New Jersey

Howard G. Thistle, M.D.
Associate Professor of Clinical
    Rehabilitation Medicine,
New York University School of Medicine,
New York, New York

Robert E. Vestal, M.D.
Coordinator for Research and
    Development,
Veterans Administration Medical Center,
Boise, Idaho;
Assistant Professor of Medicine,
University of Washington School of
    Medicine,
Seattle, Washington

Special thanks are due to Howard Spierer, Director of the Office of Grants, Research, and Education at JIGC, who managed the AOA grant and contributed to the editing of this book. Thanks are also due to Zena Schechter, Associate Project Director, who attended to many of the details required in a project of this scope and played a key role in preparing the manuscript for publication. We are appreciative of Susan Sherman for reading, editing, and rereading many of the chapters. Isabel Vader and Joan Roth did excellent work in typing the manuscript. For assistance in delineating the com-

ponents of the curriculum and for applying accepted pedagogical and evaluation
techniques to a geriatric medical curriculum, we thank David Harmon, Adult
Education Specialist, and Marilyn Felt,
Curriculum Specialist.

We wish to express our appreciation to
Sidney Feinberg, Executive Director of
JIGC, and to the Board of Trustees of
JIGC for their support of the growth of
geriatric medicine at this institute.

We wish to express our gratitude to
AOA for awarding this grant, which allowed us to develop the curriculum,
train students, and prepare this book. In
particular, we are grateful to Byron Gold,
Richard Schloss, Jeanette Pelcovits, Ber-
nice Harris, Barbara Fallon, and Terry
Wetle for their support during all phases
of the project.

We thank our wives, Linda and Susan,
and our children, Adam, Alana, Rachel,
and William, for bearing with us through
the many long evenings and weekends
when we worked on this material.

Leslie S. Libow
Fredrick T. Sherman

How to use this book

Each chapter has the following six components:

1. Educational objectives (what should be achieved in terms of attitudes, cognitive information, and skills at the completion of each chapter)
2. A pretest to assess the reader's knowledge prior to reading the text
3. The text with references
4. Problem-solving exercises requiring application of the newly acquired knowledge to typical cases
5. A posttest (same test as the pretest) to measure the knowledge that has been acquired
6. Answers to the pretest and posttest and problem-solving exercises

The chapters have been designed as comprehensive learning experiences for groups of students taking a course in geriatric medicine or for the individual student who is studying the subject on his own. If the book is used in a course, the student is asked to do the following prior to a discussion session with the instructor:

1. Complete the pretest
2. Read the educational objectives
3. Read the text
4. Complete the problem-solving exercises

During the 1- to 2-hour discussion session, the problem-solving exercises and any questions raised by the students are discussed. Finally, the posttest is completed. The instructor may want to use the pretest and posttest as evaluation instruments to determine changes in the student's knowledge. Although the chapters are arranged so as to build on a foundation of basic concepts in geriatric medicine, the order of presentation of the chapters is not critical.

The individual student may want to read the text and use some or none of the other components. This is perfectly satisfactory, because each chapter has been designed so that the text can be read by itself.

Contents

THE CORE OF
GERIATRIC MEDICINE

A guide for students and practitioners

Chapter 1

General concepts of geriatric medicine

LESLIE S. LIBOW

EDUCATIONAL OBJECTIVES
Attitudinal

The student should:
1. Understand that geriatric medicine is a specific body of knowledge and set of approaches
2. Know that the geriatrician serves as teacher, researcher, consultant, primary care physician, and health planner
3. Know the history of geriatric medicine and note its obvious correlation with changing demographic patterns
4. Have some understanding of demographic and epidemiological patterns of the elderly
5. Separate, as well as integrate, the effects of aging and of disease
6. Realize the importance of the team approach in clinical care
7. Understand that "ageism" can potentially interfere with health care
8. Explore the ethical issues that frequently occur in care of the elderly

Cognitive

The student should:
1. Know the key demographic and epidemiological factors about the elderly that directly affect health care
2. Know the "normal" aging changes of various organs and systems and their possible linkage to health changes
3. Know the components and goals of the health care team

Skill

The student should:
1. Know when to seek the geriatrician's help in rendering care to an individual or to a community
2. Be able to distinguish changes due to aging from those reflecting disease

PRETEST
True or false

1. Geriatric medicine emphasizes places of illness and phases of illness that are usually not emphasized in general medicine, surgery, or psychiatry.
2. Most of medicine is taught without emphasis on differences between the 75-year-old and the 40-year-old.
3. Ethical and clinical decision making for older persons is no different from that of younger patients.
4. Reducing unnecessary hospitalization and/or nursing home placement are likely methods of making health planning for the elderly cost-effective.
5. Certain illnesses, such as senile dementia, polymyalgia rheumatica, and cancer of the prostate gland are almost exclusively found in late life.
6. Illnesses common to all ages (diabetes mellitus, heart failure, etc.) have different manifestations when they occur in late life.
7. A geriatrician has special training in internal medicine (or family practice) that is followed by further training in geriatric medicine.
8. The cost of health care for an older American is three times that of a middle-aged adult.
9. Fifteen percent of the elderly are in nursing homes.

1

10. The elderly comprise 30% to 60% of patients in most acute care medical and/or surgical services in hospitals.
11. Complete heart block is usually of unknown origin.
12. The health care professions are free of ageism.

DEFINITION OF GERIATRIC MEDICINE

Geriatric medicine is that field of medicine which concerns itself with (1) the *interplay of time and disease;* (2) the *phases and settings* of illness (and health) that extend beyond, but include, the acute; and (3) the comprehensive approach to the health care problems of the elderly.

The clinical, educational, and research efforts of geriatric medicine focus on areas that have not been adequately developed within classic lines of medicine, psychiatry, and surgery.

Specific areas include:
1. Clarifying 'normal" aging changes
2. Integrating the effects of aging and disease in matters of etiology, as well as biomedical and psychosocial manifestations of clinical problems (The 70-year-old is not simply a 40-year-old, 30 years later.)
3. Attention to the long-term chronic and preventive phases of illness, not merely the acute
4. Involvement with health care settings in addition to the acute care hospital, such as the ambulatory care setting, the day hospital, the homebound, and the nursing home (There are 18,900 nursing homes with approximately 1.4 million beds; there are 1 million acute care beds in the United States.[1])

5. Extension of the knowledge, skills, and attitudes developed in the non-acute phases of illness and care settings to the acute phase and the acute care hospital setting
6. Approaches that are appropriate to the special circumstances often present in late life: (a) the team approach (interdisciplinary) and (b) age-relevant clinical and ethical decisions
7. Health planning for the unique needs of the elderly, with a focus on (a) prevention (bereavement, accidents, falls, fractures, vaccines, medication problems, etc.); (b) continuity of care; (c) excessive hospital and nursing home use; and (d) cost-effectiveness, including alternative approaches to delivery of care
8. Education of students of medicine and other health care professions, as well as graduate clinicians

The types of clinical problems encompassed within geriatric medicine in either the acute or long-term phase include (1) those that are somewhat unique to late life (senile dementia, osteoporosis, fracture of the hip, benign memory loss, polymyalgia rheumatica, chronic lymphatic leukemia, cancer of the prostate gland, etc.) and (2) those that are common to all ages but present unique issues in late life (diabetes mellitus, mental depression, stroke, heart failure, surgery, medications, etc.).

WHAT IS A GERIATRICIAN?

A geriatrician is a physician whose skills, attitudes, and knowledge are focused entirely on the elderly. The geriatrician's total field of responsibility is specified in the above definition of geriatric medicine. The usual background includes formal training in internal medicine (or family practice) followed by special training in geriatric medicine.

While assisting the community or medical center in developing an improved health care system, the geriatrician serves as teacher and clinician role model for students. The geriatrician serves as clinician in both a consulting capacity for patients, families, and/or health care professionals and a primary care capacity for the elderly (and, at times, their families) in various health care settings, such as the nursing home, acute care hospital, and ambulatory setting.

HISTORY OF GERIATRIC MEDICINE AND INTEREST IN HEALTH CARE PROBLEMS OF THE ELDERLY*

In 1889 one of the earliest articles on geriatrics in modern medical literature appeared in Great Britain and suggested a special emphasis by physicians on the healthy elderly and the latter phase of life.[2] In 1909 Nascher first used the term *geriatrics* and wrote extensively on the need for a special view of the problems of the elderly. Included in his work was the first American textbook on geriatric medicine.[3] A pathologist, he took a disease-oriented view of the latter phase of life, seeing only decline. Nevertheless, he urged his colleagues to take a particularly close and different type of look at this phase of life.

In the early 1940s Stieglitz edited a textbook of geriatric medicine that, to this day, is quite modern in its view.[4] Stieglitz was more optimistic about the latter

phase of life; he saw a good deal of positiveness in the experience of growing older and considered geriatrics an important aspect of medicine. He urged combining the basic science of gerontology and its study of natural aging with the knowledge of pathology, sociology, psychiatry, and clinical medicine with regard to the elderly. From that time through the 1950s and early 1960s, there were a number of outstanding clinicians and clinical scientists in the United States who were committed to and wrote about both clinical and research aspects of geriatrics. Their articles appeared widely, particularly in the journals of the two national societies in the field: *Journal of the American Geriatrics Society, Journal of Gerontology*, and *Gerontologist* (the latter two are publications of the Gerontological Society).

In the 1960s, J. T. Freeman taught geriatric medicine to students at several medical schools. Schools such as the University of Washington developed life cycle courses for medical students. In 1972 the first residency and fellowship training program to develop geriatricians in the United States was established by Libow at the Mount Sinai City Hospital Center* in New York; 4 years later a second program was developed at the Jewish Institute for Geriatric Care.†[5] These academic programs have trained geriatricians who have gone on to lead programs at several medical schools and have highlighted the growing strength of geriatric medicine. In 1975 the National Institute on Aging (NIA) appointed its

---

*For a discussion of the development of geriatric medicine in the United States, see Stevens, R. A.: Geriatric medicine in historical perspective: the pros and cons of geriatric medicine as a specialty, Working Paper 1, April, 1977, Tulane Studies in Health Policy. Tulane University, New Orleans, La.

*Mount Sinai City Hospital Center at Elmhurst, N.Y., is part of the Mount Sinai School of Medicine in New York.
†Jewish Institute for Geriatric Care at Long Island Jewish–Hillside Medical Center is a major clinical campus of the School of Medicine at the State University of New York at Stony Brook.

first director, Robert N. Butler, M.D., who has strongly supported the concept of geriatric medicine.

The U.S. Senate's Special Committee on Aging has long supported the need for better care of the elderly. In 1976 the committee held an open meeting before 2,000 scientists and clinicians gathered in New York at the annual meeting of the Gerontological Society. The proceedings of that meeting have been published and reveal a vigorous exchange of ideas on the issue of the need for greater emphasis on geriatrics and gerontology in U.S. medical and nursing schools.[6]

In 1970 the Administration on Aging (AOA) began to directly fund medical education projects and health care efforts for the elderly. This shift of AOA funds toward developing medical school curricula in geriatrics and gerontology was a major advance for geriatric medicine and care of the elderly. Medical student programs were established at two medical schools with AOA support.[7]

Throughout the past 25 years, many outstanding clinicians have written about the need for developing leaders in geriatric medicine in order to train students of medicine so that the elderly would have better care.[8-17]

In March 1977 the NIA convened a "first of its kind" meeting of teachers of medicine with deans and other administrators of medical schools to discuss geriatric medicine as a body of knowledge and as a component of medical school curricula. In 1977 the Veterans Administration (VA) funded fellowships in geriatric medicine at VA hospitals located at university medical centers.

Another important step in the development of geriatric medicine was the 1978 report by the Institute of Medicine on Aging and Medical Education, which strongly recommended the incorporation of geriatric medicine into medical school curricula.[18] In 1979 the National Institute on Aging, Administration on Aging, and Health Resources Administration funded new programs designed to develop curricula on aging and to train faculty members in geriatrics.

In April and May of 1979 two well-attended national meetings, one sponsored by the American Geriatrics Society and one by the American Association of Retired Persons, were convened to focus further on the teaching of geriatric medicine.

Many medical schools and teaching hospitals currently have programs in geriatric medicine. It appears likely that by the early 1980s a majority of schools will have such programs, and it should not be long before all schools accept as natural and necessary the presence of geriatric medicine and gerontology in their preclinical and clinical curricula. Similarly, all primary care residency training programs will likely include a formalized exposure to geriatric medicine.

Surveys reveal, and our teaching experiences confirm, that a majority of medical students desire formalized training with regard to the health care of the elderly.[19,20]*

DEMOGRAPHIC AND EPIDEMIOLOGICAL FACTORS RELEVANT TO HEALTH CARE OF THE ELDERLY

The rapid increase in the proportion of aged people in the advanced nations of the world has made aging the number

---

*In addition to these studies, Alvin J. Levenson, M.D., of the University of Texas Medical School at Houston surveyed students in 12 medical schools in 1977 and 1978; here, too, a majority indicated an interest in learning about geriatrics and gerontology.

one health problem in the industrialized world. The World Health Organization (WHO) has formed a new Technical Advisory Group on Health Care of the Elderly, which works closely with the directors of several national institutes on aging in various nations. The task, begun in 1978, is to study specific areas wherein health care, including preventive care, can be improved for the world's elderly.

In large part because of the efforts of medical science, more people survive to late life and less newborns come into the world. Thus, the field of medicine is doubly obligated to meet this "graying" of the population with a major commitment.

Statistics reveal an elderly population ranging from 9% to 14% or 16% in many industrialized nations.[21,22] Although the percentage is lower in the developing nations, WHO forecasts show a rapid change in the slope of the curve as the birthrate in the Third World is diminished through contraceptive techniques and as more people live to be elderly through advanced medical techniques, the availability of antibiotics, and better nutrition and child care. To highlight the development of aging populations as a major health problem, the United Nations has declared 1982 as World Aging Year.

In the United States the following factors give insight into the role of the elderly as the major consumers of health care and spenders of health care dollars:

1. Although comprising only 11% of the population, the elderly account for 29% of total personal health care expenditures ($41.3 billion out of $142.6 billion).[23]

2. Older persons have about twice as many hospital stays, and these last almost twice as long as those of younger persons.[24]

3. In the practice of internal medicine, 31% of patient visits are by patients aged 65 and older, and in the practice of family medicine the percentage is 17%.[25]

4. The leading consumers of pharmaceuticals, the elderly receive 25% of all prescriptions and a larger percentage of nonprescribed medication.[26]

5. Approximately 95% of the 1.4 million long-term beds are occupied by the elderly.[1]

6. The population 75 years of age and over is increasing at a much greater rate than that between the ages of 65 to 75. Those over 75 will constitute 45% of the elderly in the year 2000, in contrast to 30% in 1940 and 38% in 1976.[23]

7. Medication and other therapeutic and diagnostic efforts account for a considerable percentage of illnesses in the elderly (i.e., iatrogenic illness).

8. In fiscal year 1977 the cost of health care for the older individual averaged approximately $1,745 a year, which is more than three times the cost for those under 65 years of age.[27]

9. Medicare has been a remarkable insurance program and has diminished somewhat the fears and apprehensions of losing one's life savings for an illness in late life. On the other hand, Medicare has paid only for approximately two thirds of the cost of health care of the elderly and does not really provide for catastrophic or long-term illness that might necessitate either hospitalization or nursing home care for an extensive period.[27] (See Chapter 2 for a discussion of Medicare benefits.)

10. Medicaid has been an excellent financial program for the elderly at or near the poverty level, who comprise 24.5% (5.5 million) of the elderly population.[28]

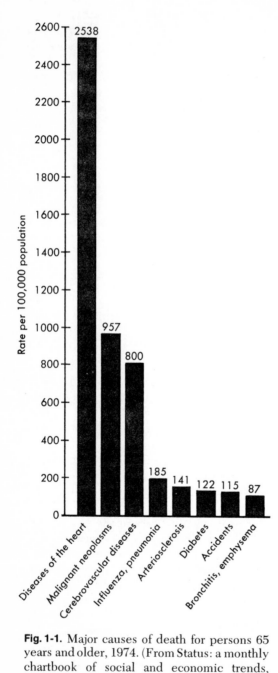

Fig. 1-1. Major causes of death for persons 65 years and older, 1974. (From Status: a monthly chartbook of social and economic trends, September 1976, U.S. Department of Commerce, Bureau of the Census.)

11. At least 10% of the elderly in the community have mental and nervous disorders but rarely receive psychiatric attention.[29]

12. Five percent of the elderly are homebound, and another 5% are in institutions. Of those in the community and not homebound, approximately 13% have difficulty with ambulation.[24]

13. Although the majority of the elderly are self-sufficient, ambulatory, and mentally alert, over 80% have reported some chronic condition.[24]

14. At the White House Conference on Aging in 1971, the elderly listed the following as major problems: income, health care, and transportation.

15. Women outlive men by approximately 8 years in late life.[30] Thus, the elderly population has a greater proportion of women; this is particularly true of the population over the age of 75. Most women over the age of 75 are widowed and many live alone.[31]

16. Black males and females do not have as great a life expectancy at birth as do white males and females. However, once the age of 65 is reached, there is no significant difference between the remaining life expectancy of whites and blacks in the United States.[30]

17. The elderly comprise approximately 33% to 60% of patients in acute care medical-surgical wards in most hospitals.[32]

18. The length of stay of the elderly in a voluntary, nonprofit hospital during an acute illness is 32% longer than that of middle-aged individuals (11.6 days compared with 8.8 days).[33]

19. In 1974 the three major causes of death for persons 65 years of age and over were diseases of the heart, malignant neoplasms, and cerebrovascular diseases (Fig. 1-1).[34]

These factors highlight the need for a special health care system for the elderly.

"NORMAL" AGING AND DISEASE

One must understand "normal" aging changes in order to properly interpret symptoms, signs, and laboratory results, as well as the etiology of disease. Some changes, such as slowing of reaction time, contribute to accidents and lowered intelligence quotient (IQ) scores. Other changes, such as increasing blood pressure, may simultaneously preserve brain intellectual function while increasing morbidity for stroke. Thus, diagnostic and therapeutic decision making necessitates knowledge of normal aging. Table 1-1 is an overview of important basic

Table 1-1. Basic changes accompanying aging and their possible extrapolation to illnesses, symptoms, signs, and problems typical of the elderly[*]

Organ or system	Basic "normal" aging change	Disease(s) or problems
Brain	Probable decrease in brain weight and/or number of cells in specific areas	Memory loss and/or senile dementia
	Alteration in sleep patterns; older persons tend to dream less and have increased periods of wakefulness	Increased complaints of insomnia
	Increased atherosclerosis of cerebral vessels	Multi-infarct dementia
	Increased activity of mono-amine oxidase enzyme	Mental depression
	Decreased reaction time	Decrease in IQ scores when speed of response is a factor; some aspects of IQ (verbal and vocabulary skills) increase in late life
Skin	Decreased response to pain sensation and temperature changes	Accidents
	Decreased response to temperature and vibration; increased pain threshold	Burns
	Decreased subcutaneous fat; loss of fat padding over bony prominences	Decubitus ulcers
	Atrophy of sweat glands	Difficulty in body temperature regulation
	Decreased ability of body to rid itself of heat by evaporation	Heat stroke

[*]With the assistance of Rein Tideiksaar, P.A.-C., Jewish Institute for Geriatric Care, New Hyde Park, N.Y., and Assistant Professor of Allied Health, Health Sciences Center, State University of New York at Stony Brook, Stony Brook, N.Y.

Continued.

Table 1-1. Basic changes accompanying aging and their possible extrapolation to illnesses, symptoms, signs, and problems typical of the elderly—cont'd

Organ or system	Basic "normal" aging change	Disease(s) or problems
Arteries	Increased peripheral resistance; diminished aortic elasticity	Abdominal pulsation, bruits, and aneurysm
	Increased systolic and diastolic blood pressure	Positive correlation between blood pressure and morbidity: unclear if this is cause and effect or simply a correlation related to a third factor; possible protective effect on brain of moderately elevated blood pressure
	Arteriosclerotic and atherosclerotic changes in blood vessels	Occlusion of arteries leading to ischemia
Gastrointestinal tract	Diminished hydrochloric acid secretion (probable)	Association with increased iron deficiency anemia as well as possible association with gastric carcinoma and/or other absorption difficulties
	Diminished large bowel motility	Diminished frequency of bowel movements
	Diminished hepatic synthesis	Diminished serum albumin
	Decreased sensitivity to thirst	Constipation; dehydration
	Decreased absorption of calcium	Malabsorption; osteoporosis
Renal	Decrease in size of urinary bladder	Incontinence and frequency
	Decrease in size of kidneys and number of glomeruli; diminished renal blood flow, glomerular filtration rate, and tubular function	Drug toxicities when kidney is a major route of excretion; greater tendency toward at least transient, if not permanent, renal insufficiency in the presence of dehydration, diuretics, hypotension, or fever
Genital tract	Enlarged prostate gland	Prostatic obstruction
	Weakening of the pelvic floor	Stress incontinence as well as cystocele and urethrocele
	Diminished vaginal and cervical secretions	Pruritus; dyspareunia
	Some, though not total, decrease in sexual function	Fear of impotence; embarrassment at sexual desires

Table 1-1. Basic changes accompanying aging and their possible extrapolation to illnesses, symptoms, signs, and problems typical of the elderly—cont'd

Organ or system	Basic "normal" aging change	Disease(s) or problems
Musculoskeletal system	Decreased synthesis and increased degradation of bone	Osteoporosis and/or fracture
	Diminished muscle size and strength	Fatigue
Eye	Decreased accommodation to light; decreased ability to distinguish between various intensities of light	Accidents
	Increased density of lens	Cataracts
	Loss of elasticity of lens	Presbyopia
	Change in aqueous kinetics	Glaucoma
Mouth and teeth	Resorption of gum and bony tissue surrounding teeth and bone of mandible	Loss of teeth and periodontal disease
	Decreased saliva flow	Malnutrition; disturbing symptom of "burning tongue" (glossopyrosis)
	Decreased number of taste buds	Weight loss
Ears	Anatomical change in inner ear as well as cochlea	Diminished hearing of high-pitched sounds (presbycusis)
Heart	Decreased cardiac muscle and catecholamine level	Diminished cardiac output (50% decrease by age 65); increased congestive heart failure
	Increased calcification of valves	Murmurs from aortic and mitral area and/or endocarditis; valve stenosis and/or insufficiency
	Calcification of the skeleton of the heart	Conduction defects; irritability of the cardiac muscle may result in alterations in rhythm
	Sclerosis of the conduction system	Most cases of complete heart block are of unknown origin
Lungs	Decreased elasticity and increased size of alveoli	Changes in lung mechanics, such as decreased vital capacity, maximal voluntary ventilation (MVV), and increased closing volume
	Decreased diffusion and surface area across the alveolar-capillary membrane	Diminished PO_2

Continued.

Table 1-1. Basic changes accompanying aging and their possible extrapolation to illnesses, symptoms, signs, and problems typical of the elderly—cont'd

Organ or system	Basic "normal" aging change	Disease(s) or problems
Lungs—cont'd	Diminished activity of cilia and decreased cough reflex	Impaired bronchoelimination and increased incidence of pneumonia
Immunological status	Decreased T cell function	Increased negativity in skin tests such as PPD; possible relationship to increased prevalence for malignancies
	Maintenance of secondary immune response (B cell antibody)	
Psychological status	Role changes	Retirement
	Losses	
	Physical	Correlation with increased death rate within 1 year of loss of spouse
	Psychological	Depression
	Social	Loss of significant others, family, and friends
Hormones	Decreased metabolic clearance rate and plasma concentration of aldosterone	Decreased sodium reabsorption
	Decreased estrogen; diminished ovarian function	Postmenopausal decrease of secondary sex characteristics
	Decreased insulin response and peripheral effectiveness	Hyperglycemia
	Increased ADH response to hyperosmolarity	Inappropriate ADH with hyponatremia
	Insensitivity of pituitary gland to TRH in older healthy men	Men less likely to develop hyperthyroidism

normal aging changes and a reasonable extrapolation to medical problems or disease.

TEAM APPROACH TO CARE OF CERTAIN ELDERLY PATIENTS: AN INTERDISCIPLINARY EFFORT

Proper health care of the frail elderly (perhaps 30% to 40% of the elderly) may require the skills of several different disciplines working together as a team.[35,36] Not all elderly patients require a team approach. Physicians often see themselves as individuals with heavy autonomous responsibilities, however, and one practitioner cannot seriously presume to deliver the multiple therapies or relieve the multiple simultaneous problems or illness faced by certain patients (and families) in the institution and/or the community.

Therapeutic and morale factor

The team is simultaneously an approach to treatment and a morale-building vehicle. The morale of the professional staff (outpatient and inpatient staff) — and of the patient and family — is a crucial consideration in dealing with chronic illness. It is easier to treat a failing heart than an older patient who has heart failure. Add to the failing heart such common accompanying problems in a 72-year-old man as (1) diminished ambulation; (2) an ill spouse; (3) limited economic resources, affecting the frequency of visits to physicians, renewal of medications, and compliance with special diets; (4) the tendency toward a low – serum potassium level when the patient is treated with diuretics; (5) diminished tolerance to fluid loss; (6) difficulty in complying with low-salt diets; and (7) the patient's concern for his adult children and relatives.

This list would be far more threatening if the illness were a stroke, amputation, fractured hip, or mental depression, or if the patient were 82 instead of 72 and had no spouse.

The physician's role in the health care team

The key difficulty is learning one's role in a team. Viewing the team as a therapeutic instrument to be used for the patient's good will help the physician define his role. Considerable commitment to a process of ideas and opinions that may at times be quite different from those held by the physician is necessary. Although he remains the leader of the team, the physician must learn to accept and value the input of his colleagues in related fields of health care. Reaching decisions about treatment prognosis, for example, often requires openness and the

ability to be challenged, as well as the ability to allow a struggle over ideas. The insights achieved, as well as the outcomes, are usually greater than those possible for an individual clinician faced with the type of problems mentioned previously. Rather than losing a crucial aspect of his professional identity, the physician will emerge with the feeling of having better achieved his mission of contributing to the diminution of suffering and to the improvement of the quality of life.

Team components

The geriatric team is multidisciplinary and varies considerably in scope, focus, and components. A team can have an institution-wide responsibility or be limited to one small unit. It's focus can extend over a community or be on one outpatient clinic or office. Whatever the scope, teams typically comprise some or all of the following; (1) physicians; (2) nurses, nurses' aides, and orderlies; (3) social workers; (4) physical and occupational therapists; (5) recreational and activities personnel; (6) speech and hearing therapists; (7) a transportation component; (8) community visiting nurses; (9) pharmacists; (10) physician assistants and geriatric nurse practitioners, and (11) other professionals to administer to the legal and religious aspects of patient care when appropriate.

Meetings of the team

Frequent meetings are crucial. These meetings should focus on patient and/or professional struggles in such areas as (1) living at home or in an institution, (2) accepting a treatment, and (3) knowledge of diagnosis and/or prognosis. Part of the meeting should involve interviews of patients and/or family members. While focusing on patient problems, however, the team meeting should produce improved staff morale and education.

AGEISM

There is prejudice against the elderly simply for what they are: old. This has been called "ageism" by Butler[37] and has been seen as analogous to racism and sexism. This prejudice is based on the fear of growing old and of dying. These fears have become especially prominent in the United States and in other industrialized cultures, where there is excessive emphasis on youth and productivity. Rather than respecting the elderly and providing them with some comforts and appropriate roles in the latter phase of life, we often tend to exclude them, not support them, ignore them, and perhaps mistreat them. This occurs in health care systems as well as in much of society. Fortunately many of the elderly are angered by this inappropriate, paternalistic treatment. Health care practitioners are no more free of this prejudice than are others in society. In fact, the physician, nurse, social worker, and other health care professionals may unknowingly employ this prejudicial mechanism more frequently than other persons, since they are so often involved with the sick and the dying elderly. An awareness of ageism is crucial to an understanding of the problem and critical to any change in attitude.

ETHICAL ISSUES

Because the latter phase of life is accompanied by a shortened life expectancy, the physician and patient (and family) are confronted with unique decisions. Furthermore, the high prevalence of dementia in late life (5% for persons over 65 and 20% for those over 80) highlights a second issue with regard to treatment of the mentally infirm.

Further compounding the ethical dilemma is the recent emphasis in the medical literature on *cost-effectiveness.* While the term is usually used in connection with efforts to halt the spiraling costs of health care, the implication is a possible set of rules as to what or who it is "worthwhile" to treat.

With ageism as a hidden prejudice, society might decide unwittingly that the triage concept should have an age-relevant component. Thus, in the extreme, we might conclude that all persons over a certain age, or residing in nursing homes, or having a certain mental state (dementia, aphasia, etc.), should not be treated for pneumonia.

One can immediately see the danger. What is necessary is enlightened debate on all such issues. The physician should continue to serve the patient as confidante, advocate, and healer. The physician should not distort his clinical and ethical decision making by misusing the cost-effective criteria and making it another form of ageism. No doubt there are situations that could lead a patient, family, and/or physician to decide on nontreatment; but each of these situations should be considered on an individual basis.

GOALS OF GERIATRIC MEDICINE

In dealing with the elderly, we must change some of our goals from those stressed in the acute care hospital setting. Although relief of acute distress (heart failure, pain, depression, etc.) is welcome at any age, smaller objective changes often have large subjective meaning to the older patient. Thus, a slight improvement in breathing, a minimal improvement in walking, less frequent urination at night, or reduced depression may have very significant meaning for the older patient. These changes have not traditionally been highlighted during medical training as being very meaningful, yet these are some of the most important problems of the elderly. The physician will do more for his patients by allowing these problems to surface and accepting and respecting these less dramatic but meaningful goals.

NEED FOR A HEALTH CARE SYSTEM

The health care system of the United States is similar to the economic system in that it is neither socialized nor nationalized. Success is left to the individual's initiatives. The elderly are at a disadvantage, because the system requires mobility, familiarity with insurance rules and terms, an adequate income, social support, and access to transportation.

More sensible would be a simply organized system to serve the needs of the elderly within the community. Most of the components of such a system already exist in many communities and merely need to be coalesced.[5,38] An integrated health care system would lead to both cost and quality effectiveness with less unnecessary hospitalization, nursing home placement, and distress. The physician should be involved in improving the health care system in his own community.

GERIATRIC MEDICINE AS A MECHANISM FOR IMPROVING HEALTH CARE FOR ALL AGE GROUPS

It is likely that studying and improving the health care of the elderly will lead to an improvement in health care for all age groups. Already we can see the lessons of Medicare being used to construct a universal health insurance program for the younger members of our society. So, too, will research into illnesses of late life and new clinical approaches be extrapolated to all age groups. For example, study of senile dementia will likely lead to invaluable insights into memory mechanisms and other brain functions.

PREVENTIVE GERIATRIC MEDICINE

Preventive medicine is not yet a major component of medical or health care training in the United States, or in most of the industrialized world. Not only do we need to consider preventing illnesses, such as influenza and pneumococcal pneumonia, from occurring, through the use of possible vaccines, but we also need to prevent the progression of already-existing illnesses (e.g., the development of a contracted limb following a stroke or the cessation of self-medication by a patient at home). Other preventive areas are support during bereavement, improved transfer of medical information, and outreach to ensure follow-up medical care.

Geriatric medicine must be mastered by all students and clinicians in order to improve health care for the elderly and those of all ages.

REFERENCES

1. National Nursing Home Survey, 1977: summary for the United States, Vital and Health Statistics Series B, No. 43, DHEW Pub. No. (P14S) 79-1794, July 1979, U.S. Department of Health, Education, and Welfare.
2. Humphrey G. M.: Old age, New York, 1889, Macmillan Publishing Co., Inc.
3. Nascher, I. L.: Geriatrics: the diseases of old age and their treatment, Philadelphia, 1914, P. Blakiston's Son and Co.
4. Stieglitz, E. J., editor: Geriatric medicine: diagnosis and management of disease in the aging and in the aged, Philadelphia, 1943, W. B. Saunders Co.

5. Libow, L. S.: A geriatric medical residency program: a four-year experience, Ann. Intern. Med. **85**:641, 1976.

6. U.S. Senate, Special Committee on Aging: Medicine and aging: an assessment of opportunities and neglect, 94th Congress, Second Session, October 13, 1976, Pub. No. 052-070-04033-5, Washington, D.C., 1977, U.S. Government Printing Office.

7. Libow, Linda G.: The development and administration of a geriatric program for freshman and sophomore medical students. In Brookbank, J.W., editor: Improving the quality of health care for the elderly, Gainesville, Fla., 1978, Publications Center for Gerontological Studies and Programs — University Presses, p. 13.

8. Wright, I. S.: Geriatrics: the challenges of the seventies; rethinking and retooling for the future, J. Am. Geriatr. Soc. **19**:737, 1971.

9. Poe, W. D.: Geriatrics: an Olympian view, N. Engl. J. Med. **290**:1020, 1974.

10. Editorial: geriatrics in medicine, Lancet **1**:663, 1974.

11. Smits, H., and Draper, P.: Care of the aged: an English lesson? Ann. Intern. Med. **80**:747, 1974.

12. Dasco, M. D.: The physician's responsibility in improvement of long-term care of the aged, N.Y. State J. Med. **75**:843, 1975.

13. Butler, R. N.: Psychiatry and the elderly: an overview, Am. J. Psychiatry **132**:893, 1975.

14. Barondess, J. A.: Old age, health policy, and social conscience (editorial), Ann. Intern. Med. **80**:769, 1974.

15. Poe, W. D.: Education in geriatrics, J. Med. Educ. **50**:1002, 1975.

16. Poe, W. D.: The scope of geriatrics (editorial), Ann. Intern. Med. **82**:842, 1975.

17. Leaf, A.: Medicine and the aged, N. Engl. J. Med. **297**:887, 1977.

18. Aging and medical education: report of a study by a committee of the institute of medicine, Contract No. 1-AG2123, Washington, D.C., September 1978, National Academy of Sciences.

19. Freeman, J. T.: A survey of education in geriatrics, Gerontologist **1**:120, 1961.

20. Libow, L. S.: The issues in geriatric medical education and postgraduate training: old problems in a new field, Geriatrics **32**:99, 1977.

21. Binstock, R. H., and Shanas, E., editors: Handbook of aging and the social sciences, New York, 1976, Van Nostrand Reinhold Co., pp. 76-77.

22. Brocklehurst, J. C., editor: Geriatric care in advanced societies, Lancaster, Engl., 1975, M T P Press Ltd., p. 1.

23. Developments in aging: 1978. 1. A report of the Special Committee on Aging, United States Senate, Washington, D.C., 1979, U.S. Government Printing Office, pp. 6, 19.

24. Brotman, H.: Every ninth American. In Developments in aging: 1978. 1. A report of the Special Committee on Aging, United States Senate, Washington, D.C., 1979, U.S. Government Printing Office, p. 20.

25. The National Ambulatory Medical Care Survey: Unpublished data, 1977, U.S. Department of Health, Education, and Welfare, National Center for Health Statistics.

26. Rabin, D. W.: Use of medicine: A review of prescribed and non-prescription medicine use, 1972 Reprint Series, DHEW Pub. No. HSM 73-3012, U.S. Department of Health, Education, and Welfare.

27. Gibson, R. M., and Fisher, C. R.: Age differences in health care spending, fiscal year 1977, Soc. Sec. Bull. **42**:3, 1979.

28. Money income and poverty status of families and persons in the United States: 1977, Current Population Reports Series P60, No. 116, U.S. Department of Commerce, Bureau of the Census, Table 16, p. 18.

29. Kayson, R.: Drugs and the elderly, 1978, Ethel Percy Andrus Gerontological Center, Los Angeles, Calif., USC Press, p. 13.

30. Statistical abstracts of the United States, 1978 ed., U.S. Department of Commerce, Bureau of the Census, Tables 98, 99.

31. Projections of the population of the United States, 1977-2050 Current Population Reports Series P25, No. 704, U.S. Department of Commerce, Bureau of the Census.

32. Somers, H. U., and Somers, A. R.: Medicine and the hospitals, Washington, D.C. 1968, The Brookings Institute, p. 57.

33. Utilization of short stay hospitals annual summary of the United States, 1977, Vital and Health Statistics Series 13, No. 41, DHEW Pub No. (PHS) 79-1792, U.S. Department of Health, Education, and Welfare, Table 12, p. 35.

34. Fact book on aging: a profile of America's older population, Washington, D.C., 1978, The National Council on the Aging, Inc.

35. Rao, D. B.: The team approach to integrated care of the elderly, Geriatrics **32**:88, 1977.

36. Sherman, F. T.: Clinical problems in geriatric

medicine—a team approach, Allied Health Behav. Sci. **2**:1-18, 1979.

37. Butler, R. N.: Why survive? Being old in America, New York, 1975, Harper & Row, Publishers, Inc., p. 11.
38. Libow, L. S., Caro, F. G., and Liota, M.: Symposium: delivery of geriatric community care, Gerontologist **14**:286, 1974.

POSTTEST
True or false

1. Geriatric medicine emphasizes places of illness and phases of illness that are usually not emphasized in general medicine, surgery, or psychiatry.
2. Most of medicine is taught without emphasis on differences between the 75-year-old and the 40-year-old.
3. Ethical and clinical decision making for older persons is no different from that of younger patients.
4. Reducing unnecessary hospitalitation and/or nursing home placement are likely methods of making health planning for the elderly cost-effective.
5. Certain illnesses, such as senile dementia, polymyalgia rheumatica, and cancer of the prostate gland are almost exclusively found in late life.
6. Illnesses common to all ages (diabetes mellitus, heart failure, etc.) have different manifestations when they occur in late life.
7. A geriatrician has special training in internal medicine (or family practice) that is followed by further training in geriatric medicine.
8. The cost of health care for an older American is three times that of a middle-aged adult.
9. Fifteen percent of the elderly are in nursing homes.
10. The elderly comprise 30% to 60% of patients in most acute care medical and/or surgical services in hospitals.
11. Complete heart block is usually of unknown origin.
12. The health care professions are free of ageism.

ANSWERS TO PRETEST AND POSTTEST

1. True. Geriatric medicine emphasizes the long-term phase (at home or in the institution) and the preventive phase.
2. True. It is a common error to simply apply non-age specific approaches to the aged.
3. False. The latter phase of life presents some very special ethical issues.
4. True. Simple "systems" of health care in each community are necessary.
5. True. Late life sets the stage for certain specific illnesses.
6. True. Late life produces symptoms and signs that may be different from those of earlier life.
7. True. A geriatrician possesses a specific body of knowledge and set of approaches that are superimposed on standard training in internal medicine (or family practice).
8. True. Older persons have multiple simultaneous illnesses, utilize multiple medications, and occupy greater numbers of hospital and nursing home beds than younger persons.
9. False. Only 5% of the elderly are in nursing homes.
10. True. The elderly are the majority of patients in acute medical-surgical units.
11. True. Arteriosclerotic heart disease is not the explanation for most cases of complete heart block.
12. False. Ageism is a society-wide prejudice.

Chapter 2

Demographic and economic aspects, including Medicare and Medicaid

LESLIE S. LIBOW, ZENA SCHECTER, and EMMANUEL MARGOLIS

EDUCATIONAL OBJECTIVES
Attitudinal

The student should:

1. Understand and develop a positive attitude toward society's efforts to meet the needs of the growing number of elderly persons in this country
2. Develop an appreciation for the inclusion of demographic and economic factors in his clinical approach to diagnosis, treatment, and prognosis
3. Increase his awareness of the physician's role as primary care provider and as advocate for the elderly patient

Cognitive

The student should:

1. Be informed about demographic and economic data relevant to the issue of health care of the elderly
2. Be familiar with the benefits and limitations of Medicare and Medicaid, know who and what is covered, and understand the personal and public components of health care costs that accompany Medicare and Medicaid
3. Be able to distinguish among the health care financing mechanisms available to the elderly (Medicare, Medicaid, private health insurance plans, Health Maintenance Organizations [HMOs], out-of-pocket contributions) and understand the impact of each on the delivery of health care services to the elderly
4. Be familiar with the institutional and community-based health care services most frequently used by the elderly and know the cost of such services to society and to the individual patient

5. Understand the effect of public policy on the health care of individuals and be aware of the difficulties in translating policies into programs that resolve specific problems

Skill

The student should:

1. Serve as advocate for the patient in accordance with his understanding of the legal and financial authority granted the physician by law
2. Render better care to the individual patient by knowing the availability of institutional and community se vice, and their financing
3. Be more involved in health care provision in the community and in the institutional setting

PRETEST

1. Which of the following statements concerning the elderly population in the United States are true:
   a. About one third of the elderly population is 75 years of age or over.
   b. Elderly people living alone or with no relations had a median income of $3,795 in 1977.
   c. Persons over the age of 65 now constitute approximately 10% to 11% of the total population.
2. Determine whether each statement refers to a Medicare and/or a Medicaid program:
   a. It is a federal health insurance program.

16

b. It is a mixed federal-state welfare program.
c. Those eligible include the categorically needy and the medically needy.
d. It covers dental services, drugs, eyeglasses, transportation, and hearing aids.
e. It provides home health-homemaker services.
3. Which of the following terms refer to long-term care facilities:
   a. Skilled nursing facility (SNF)
   b. Intermediate care facility (ICF)
   c. Domiciliary care facility
4. Which of the following statements concerning nursing homes are true?
   a. There are about 18,900 nursing homes in the United States.
   b. Medicare was the primary source of payment for 50% of nursing home costs in 1977.
   c. The average nursing home patient is 68 years of age.
   d. The patient must be seen by the attending physician at least once every 60 days in an SNF.
5. Which of the following regulatory mechanisms would involve physician participation?
   a. Utilization Review Committees
   b. Federal and state inspection teams
   c. Professional Standards Review Organizations (PSROs)
6. Which of the following statements concerning health care costs in fiscal year 1977 are true?
   a. The per capita health care expenditure for the aged was $1,745.
   b. The two largest items included in health care expenditures of the elderly were costs for hospital and nursing home care.
   c. Public funds covered 90% of the personal health care expenditures of the elderly.
   d. Government sources, including the Medicare program, paid for about 88% of the hospital care of the elderly.

OVERVIEW OF THE OLDER POPULATION
Demography

The growth of the elderly population is becoming the major health issue of developed, industrialized nations. Third world nations, too, see cause for serious concern about their aged populations in relation to demographic forecasts. Current[1] and projected[2] data forecasts for the older population in the United States make the issue quite clear (Table 2-1 and Fig. 2-1).

There was a sevenfold increase in the aged population from 1900 to 1970, while the general population increased only 2.5 times.[2] By the year 2030, the elderly will represent 18.3% of the general population (the figure is approximately 11% at present). The fastest growing segment of the elderly population is composed of those over 75 years of age, who now make up about one third of the elderly population.

We need to accelerate and strengthen our efforts in dealing with this commanding data. Improved planning is needed in areas of health manpower, training in geriatric medicine, health services, and preventive measures.

Physical and mental health

The elderly population resides primarily in their own homes; only about 5% are in nursing homes. Of those at home, 7% need assistance in getting out-of-doors and another 5% are confined to their homes.[3] More than 80% of the elderly have one or more chronic illnesses,

Table 2-1. America's older population: current and projected data*

	1900	1940	1965	1975	2000†	2030†
Population of persons 65 years of age and over						
Number (in millions)	3.1	9.0	18.5	22.4	31.8	55.0
Percent of total population	4.1	6.8	10.0	10.5	12.2	18.3
Population of persons 75 years of age and over						
Number (in millions)	0.9	2.7	6.6	8.5	14.3	23.2
Percent of total population	1.2	2.0	3.0	4.0	5.5	7.7
Population of persons 75 years of age and over as a percent of the elderly population (65 years of age and over)‡	29	29	36	38	45	42

*Modified from Health in the United States, 1976-1977, DHEW Pub. No. (HRA) 77-1232 (PHS) 78-1232, 1978, U.S. Department of Health, Education, and Welfare, National Center for Health Statistics.
†The population is projected to reach 260 million people by the year 2000 and 300 million by the year 2030.
‡The population of persons 75 years of age and over is the fastest growing segment of the aged.

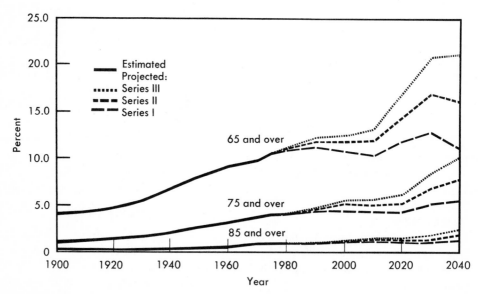

Fig. 2-1. Percent of the total population in the older ages: 1900 to 2040. (From Projection of the population of the United States, 1977-2050, Current Population Reports Series P25, No. 704, U.S. Department of Commerce, Bureau of the Census.)

such as hypertension, diabetes, arthritis, arteriosclerosis, cardiac disease, or visual or hearing loss.[4] Dental care in particular is underutilized; less than 28% of the elderly see a dentist during the course of a year.[5]

Health care for the elderly is somewhat splintered. Most elderly people have access to medical care, but not to an organized system of care. Such a system would provide for integration of various services, including physicians' services, community nursing services, transportation, pharmaceutical services, house visits, dental and podiatric care, and psychiatric and social services.

Health manpower needs for the elderly have not been planned for. Recently, however, the U.S. House of Representatives held special sessions attempting to clarify these manpower needs and their accompanying costs.[6]

Financial status

The average income of the elderly population is obviously significantly less than that of the younger population. It is difficult to maintain financial security in late life, since fixed incomes cannot keep up with the inflation rate. Close to 25% of the elderly are at or near the poverty level.[8]

In 1977 families headed by a person 65 years of age or over had a median income of $9,110, as compared with $17,203 for younger families.[8] Elderly people living alone or with no relatives have exceptionally low incomes: the median was $3,829 for men and $3,762 for women in 1977.[9] At retirement, the income drops by about 50%. Although it is probably true that the economic needs of the elderly are less than those of the young, it is not true that their needs are reduced by one half at retirement.[9]

Living arrangements

The majority of elderly people continue to live in a family setting (Table 2-2 and Fig. 2-2), with the married-couple

Table 2-2. Living arrangements of men and women 65 years of age and over: 1975 (percent)*

	65-74 years	Over 75 years
Male		
Family	85	74.5
Alone	12.1	18.2
Institutionalized	2.9	7.4
Female		
Family	64.6	49.4
Alone	32.9	40.6
Institutionalized	2.5	10.0

*From Current Population Reports, Special Studies, Series P23, No. 59, May 1976, U.S. Department of Commerce, Bureau of the Census, p. 48.

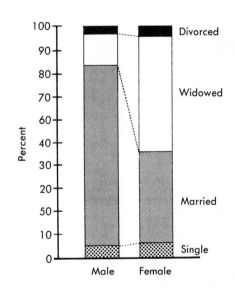

Fig. 2-2. Marital status of persons aged 65 and over, 1975. (From Status: a monthly chartbook of social and economic trends, September 1976, U.S. Department of Commerce, Bureau of the Census.)

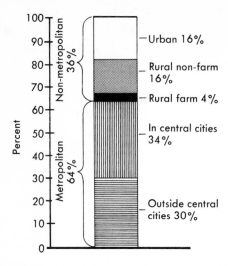

Fig. 2-3. Residential status of persons aged 65 and over, 1970. (From Status: a monthly chartbook of social and economic trends, September 1976, U.S. Department of Commerce, Bureau of the Census.)

setting being the most prevalent. Since older women outlive older men, the woman lives alone in about one third of all situations.[10] This latter fact significantly affects health planning and the necessity for institutionalization. The absence of a spouse greatly increases the likelihood of institutionalization following illness.

Two thirds of the elderly population live in metropolitan areas and make up a large portion of the population in most central-city areas and small towns (Fig. 2-3). Florida plus six other states contain almost half of the entire U.S. elderly population.[10]

Transportation

Since the use of automobiles declines with age, and since public transportation is often nonexistent in suburban and rural settings and difficult to use in urban

settings, the elderly are adversely affected.

Even in the central city, where public transportation exists, the linkage of adequate and inexpensive transportation to health care remains a serious and important problem. At the White House Conference of 1971, the elderly listed transportation as a key problem.

DEVELOPMENT OF NATIONAL PROGRAMS AIMED AT IMPROVING HEALTH CARE FOR THE ELDERLY

As the elderly "population explosion" came into view in the era of 1940 through 1960, it became clear that national plans were necessary. Medicare and Medicaid, and the Older Americans Act establishing the Administration on Aging (AOA) were developed during the 1960s. Programs to assist the elderly included funds to develop new efforts in health care and social services, nutrition projects, senior citizens' centers, housing, volunteer programs, and manpower training for older workers.[11]

The National Institute of Aging (NIA) was established in the 1970s with a mandate to develop research and educational efforts in aging and in health care for the elderly. The NIA and AOA have been committed to the development of geriatric medicine.

Each community needs a simple and integrated system. Such a system must combine the economic benefits of Medicare and Medicaid with the service skills of the various key disciplines in the community and its institutions. The physician's involvement is essential for an integrated system to work. The physician needs this system in order to render appropriate care to elderly patients with multiple problems, frailty, isolation, and/or poverty.

NURSING HOMES

Nursing home is a general term that encompasses more official terminology, such as skilled nursing facility (SNF), intermediate care facility (ICF) or health-related facility, and domiciliary care facility. In this text the term *nursing home* is used to mean all three categories of long-term care facilities described below.

1. *Skilled nursing facility:* The SNF is for patients needing the highest level of nursing, medical, and rehabilitation services. Federal regulations require SNFs to provide rehabilitation, dietetic, pharmaceutical, laboratory, and radiological services, as well as patient activities and social services. Reimbursement and regulations are generally from Medicare and Medicaid, although private-paying patients exist at SNFs in small numbers.

2. *Intermediate care facility or health-related facility:* These institutions are licensed under state law to provide health-related care and services on a regular basis to individuals who are less ill than those requiring SNF care. The patients in an ICF require more health care attention, however, than simply room and board. Reimbursement and regulations are via Medicaid, and there are a modest number of private-paying patients.

3. *Domiciliary care facility:* These facilities (homes for the aged; old-age homes) provide room and board and, in some cases, recreational and/or social services. There is no reimbursement to the institution via Medicare or Medicaid. Usually these facilities are regulated by the state's department of social services.

In the United States there are more nursing home beds (over 1,400,000) than general hospital beds (approximately 1 million). There are about 18,900 nursing homes, of which about 7,000 are SNFs.

Four to five percent of the elderly population reside in nursing homes, and the average age of nursing home patients is 82 years. However, approximately 20% to 30% of all elderly people will spend some time in a nursing home.

Two thirds of nursing homes are privately owned for profit (proprietary). The remaining one third are voluntary, public, and/or governmental. This is the reverse of the hospital situation in the United States, where the voluntary, not-for-profit sector is dominant. Thus, the nursing home industry is largely in the private arena. The not-for-profit nursing homes have generally been innovative in services.

Mental impairment (generally senile dementia of the Alzheimer type [SDAT] and multi-infarct dementia [MID]) is present in about 50% of nursing home patients, and ambulation difficulties in about 40% to 50%. Many have difficulty with speech (aphasia), hearing, and/or vision. About 30% are incontinent.[12,13] Most patients have four to eight major medical problems and are taking three to six medications, yet their major reasons for admission to the nursing home are difficulties with ambulation and/or mentation.

Regulations affecting health care in the nursing home

The following are federal regulations pertaining to nursing homes:[*]

1. Health care policies must be developed by an advisory group made up of one or more physicians as well as reg-

---

[*]Federal regulations pertaining to SNFs can be found in Title 42 of the Code of Federal Regulations, Part 405 (Sect. 42, CFR 405); federal regulations pertaining to ICFs can be found in Title 42 of the Code of Federal Regulations, Part 442 (Sect. 42, CFR 442).

istered nurses. Each patient must be under the care of a physician.

2. Admission to an SNF is only on the recommendation of a physician. A patient care plan must be evolved. Patients are to be seen at least once every 60 days. Any patient in need of special rehabilitative care must be seen by his physician at least once every 30 days.

3. Medical records are to be kept.

4. There must be an independent review of patient care and of each patient's need for institutionalization. (These committees are made up of physicians and others and are generally called Utilization Review Committees or Professional Standards Review Organizations [PSROs].)

5. Federal regulations are generally enforced by state inspection teams (usually including a physician, a hospital administrator, a nurse, a sanitation expert, a nutritionist, and an engineer) who simultaneously enforce state standards. The inspections focus on medical matters, such as medical records, progress notes, and orders being signed, and on nonmedical matters, such as fire safety.

The inspection procedures are aimed at maintaining a minimum standard of appropriate care. The inspection system, however, is not very capable of evaluating the quality of care rendered.

Title XVIII of the Social Security Act of 1965 was an outstanding advance in federal efforts to improve the financing of health care of older Americans. Only the original Social Security Act of the 1930s was of similar impact. Although they did much to reduce the financial burden and provide access to health care for most of the older population, however, these landmark federal acts did not provide regulations for a change in the system of health care delivery for the elderly.

The physician's role concerning health care in the nursing home

The physician has, until recently, been a too-distant participant in the development of the quality of care in the nursing home. How will the quality of health care reach its proper level without physician input? The physician, working in collaboration with his colleagues in the other health care disciplines, can remarkably improve the health care, morale, and humanity within the nursing home.

The contribution of physicians to enlightened, institution-wide programs in nursing homes has been most evident in the not-for-profit sector. (In the private sector, physician involvement has been largely in primary patient care.) In both the private and the voluntary sectors, however, there is a need for greater physician involvement in the development of health services. This involvement could be through roles such as medical director or member of the medical board or committee(s) of the institution.

MEDICARE: HEALTH INSURANCE FOR THE ELDERLY

Part A of Medicare provides hospital and nursing home *insurance*, financed through the Social Security system and applicable to all those eligible for Social Security benefits. Part B of Medicare is a federally subsidized program providing reimbursement for physician services and for a variety of outpatient services. Older persons voluntarily buy this insurance (Part B) by paying a premium that supplements the federal subsidy. The money is handled by insurance companies, so-called "third parties."

A summary of Medicare benefits is given in Table 2-3. There are no income requirements for eligibility, as there are with Medicaid. When it was started in

Table 2-3. Summary of Medicare Benefits*

Covered	Not covered
Medicare, Part A	
Semiprivate room	Physicians' services
Meals and special diets	Personal conveniences, such as television,
Regular nursing services	radio, or telephone in the room
Intensive care unit costs	Private-duty nurse
Drugs used in the hospital	Private room unless medically indicated
Laboratory services in the hospital	The first 3 pints of blood in a benefit
X-ray services (diagnostic and therapeutic)	period
Medical supplies, such as casts, surgical dressings, and splints	
Use of a wheelchair	
Operating and recovery room costs	
Rehabilitation, physical, occupational, and speech therapy	
At home	
Up to 100 visits	More than 100 visits
Part-time skilled health care (if medically necessary after illness) or or injury provided by home health care agencies	Home care services (home health aid, homemaker-housekeeper) to help in domestic needs
Medicare, Part B	
Medical and surgical services, including inpatient hospital or SNF emergency room or outpatient clinic	Routine physical examinations and tests that are part of such examinations
Diagnostic tests and procedures that are part of the above treatment	Routine foot care
X-ray services (diagnostic and therapeutic)	Eye or hearing examinations for fitting of eyeglasses or hearing aids
Nursing services in the physician's office	Immunizations (unless required because of an injury or immediate risk of infection)
Drugs and biologicals that can be self-administered	
Medical supplies	Cosmetic surgery (except if resulting from accidents or to improve a malfunctioning part of the body)
Speech and physical therapy	
Therapeutic foot care by a podiatrist.	
At home	
Up to 100 visits	More than 100 visits
Part-time skilled nursing care	Full-time nursing care
Physical or speech therapy	Drugs and biologicals
If one of the above services is needed, Medicare will also pay for:	Meals delivered to the home
Occupational therapy	Housekeeping-homemaker services furnished primarily to assist in meeting personal, family, and domestic needs
Part-time services of homemaker	
Home health aides	
Medical social services	
Medical supplies and equipment provided by the home health care agency	

*Data from Social Security Administration, U.S. Department of Health, Education, and Welfare: DHEW Pub. No. (SSA) 77-10050, January 1977; and from Medicaid-Medicare: Pub. No. (HCFA) 77-24091, March, 1977.

1965, Medicare covered only the aged who were eligible for Social Security benefits. A 1972 amendment extended coverage to:

1. Disabled individuals of any age entitled to Social Security disability benefits for the previous 24 consecutive months, such as persons requiring hemodialysis or renal transplantation
2. Persons entitled to railroad retirement benefits because of disability
3. Persons over the age of 65 who are not entitled to Social Security benefits, including migrant agricultural workers, home domestics, and federal and state employees
4. Persons under the age of 65 who are not entitled to Social Security benefits but who voluntarily enroll under a special provision requiring the payment of a monthly premium

Part A

Part A of Medicare pays much of the costs of acute care hospital expenses, some of the costs of SNF care, and some of the costs of home health care. Hospital coverage includes up to 90 days per spell of illness; SNF coverage includes up to 100 days per spell of illness following discharge from a hospital or SNF.

Spell of illness

A *spell of illness* is arbitrarily defined as an illness requiring institutionalization in a hospital or SNF. It begins on the first day on which the patient is institutionalized and ends following 60 days during which the person is not a patient in a hospital or SNF.

Lifetime reserve

All Medicare beneficiaries have a 60-day *lifetime reserve*. Each day may be used only once and is not renewable.

Psychiatric services

Psychiatric care in the hospital is available for 90 days during the elderly person's lifetime.

SNF and home health care

To obtain SNF coverage, a patient must spend at least 3 consecutive days in an acute care hospital and enter the SNF within 14 days of discharge from the hospital. A physician must certify that skilled nursing and/or rehabilitation services are necessary on a daily basis. A Utilization Review Committee or a PSRO must, on review, approve the patient's stay.

Home health care services are available only if they are requested within 14 days of discharge from an acute care hospital (at which the patient stayed for 3 consecutive days) or from an SNF. (Home health care under Part B of Medicare does not require prior hospitalization or SNF stay.) A physician's certification is also necessary.

Problems faced by the patient and physician because of the limitations of Part A Regulations

Patients at home who need skilled nursing and/or rehabilitation services (e.g., for treatment of stroke) cannot come directly into the SNF unless they pay privately. Furthermore, some patients need more time at the SNF than the period allowed by Medicare. This period may be much less than 100 days, since the patient's status is under regular review by the Utilization Review Committee or PSRO. The status is also reviewed by Medicare, and the criteria do not always capture the patient's level of dysfunction. This "hospital before SNF" sequence was presumably established to prevent SNFs from acting like hospitals. However, certain SNFs are actually geriatric hospitals with fine rehabilitation services and could well serve selected patients directly admitted from their own homes.

Part B

Part B of Medicare is voluntary and is insurance to cover much of physicans' services, hospital outpatient services, physical therapy services, diagnostic x-ray and laboratory services, radiation therapy, surgical dressings etc. (Table 2-3).

Home health care coverage under Part B is limited to 100 visits per year but does not require an antecedent hospitalization (as with Part A, a physician's certification of need is required). These 100 visits may be added to the 100 visits under Part A and total 200 visits per year for patients who have been institutionalized. Even this quantity may be insufficient for the very ill homebound, since total visits include all those made by the nurse, physical therapist, speech pathologist, occupational therapist, home health aide, and physician.

Psychiatric outpatient coverage is limited to $250 per year. This is obviously inadequate at today's fees.

Health care services excluded from coverage

Medication prescriptions, eyeglasses, "routine annual examinations," vaccinations (pneumococcal, influenza, or tetanus), cosmetic surgery, orthopedic shoes, dentures, dental services, and hearing aids are not covered. Much criticism has occurred over some of these exclusions. The matter appears to be a financial issue.

Payment mechanisms

Under Part A of Medicare, as mentioned earlier, hospitals and SNFs receive payment via "intermediaries," who handle the federal dollars of Medicare.

Under Part B of Medicare, the physician may charge the patient directly and have the patient apply for reimbursement, which is 80% of the "allowable" charge, rather than 80% of the physician's fee. The physician may decide to accept payment directly from Medicare (80% of Medicare's allowable charge); this is called "accepting assignment." *Example:* The patient is charged $30 for a visit; he pays the physician directly and is reimbursed by Medicare, under Part B, for 80% of the allowable charge. Medicare's allowable charge for this visit is $20; thus, the patient is reimbursed for $16 ($20 × 80%) of the $30 fee. Therefore, this $30 visit actually costs the patient $14.

This incomplete coverage under both Part A and Part B of Medicare requires the elderly to pay a significant portion (close to 30% to 40%) of their annual health bill. The annual amount paid by the elderly was about $300 per person before Medicare and was $613 in 1977, 12 years after Medicare was started.[14] Thus, the cost of health care continues to burden the elderly.

Additional patient financial responsibilities

Costs under Medicare include deductibles, copayments, and premiums (Part B), as can be seen in the following:

A. Deductibles*:
   1. When admitted to a hospital, the patient pays the first $160 and for the first 3 pints of blood.
   2. In an SNF or under home health care, the patient pays for the first 3 pints of blood.

---

*Figures given are from 1979; these change yearly to keep up with increasing costs.

3. The patient pays the first $60 of charges for physicians' services.
B. Copayments*:
   1. In the hospital the patient pays $40 per day for the sixty-first through the ninetieth day and $80 per day for each lifetime reserve day. Thus, the cost for a 92-day hospitalization would be $1,520 (30 × $40 = $1,200; 2 × $80 = $160; $1,200 + $160 + $160 = $1,520).
   2. In the nursing home the patient pays $20 per day for the twenty-first through the one-hundredth day. Thus, for a 100-day stay the cost to the patient would be $1,600 (80 × $20 = $1,600).
   3. After the initial deductible of $60, the patient pays 20% of allowable charges for physicians' services. *Example:* One hundred twenty visits at $25 allowed per visit would cost the patient $648 (120 × $25 = $3,000 − $60 = $2,940 × 0.2 = $588 + $60 = $648).
   4. For a *catastrophic* illness lasting 190 days, the patient might pay $3,768 ($1,520 for a 90-day hospitalization + $1,600 for a 100-day stay in an SNF, + $648 for 120 visits by a physician at $25 allowed per visit).
C. Premiums (Part B): In 1979 the cost was $8.70 per month.

The cost of health care annually for older Americans is about $1,700 per year (based on 1978-1979 figures), as compared with approximately $660 per year for middle-aged Americans.[14] As stated earlier, about 30% to 40% of this total cost ($500 to $700) is not covered by Medicare and is paid by the elderly person.

The physician's role, responsibilities, and burdens

In both the hospital and the SNF, it is necessary for the physician to certify and constantly recertify the patient's need for institutional care. Reviewing this need further are committees of the institution and/or community made up of physicians and others. These reviews are mandated by Medicare and Medicaid and are aimed, it appears, primarily at cost containment through a focus on the necessity of hospitalization or an SNF stay. These committee (Utilization Review Committee and PSRO) decisions may lead to crises for the patient and medical staff, since alternative placement situations are often lacking. A system emphasizing quality of care and less surveillance and paperwork is necessary.

The physician is challenged to balance his role on behalf of the patient and on behalf of carrying out governmental regulations.

Home health care services

The physician recertifies the need for home health care every 2 months.

MEDICAID*

Medicaid, established under Title XIX of the Social Security Act of 1965 (Public Law 89-87), is aimed at those persons receiving public assistance and those who are not eligible for public assistance but whose finances are such that they cannot afford their necessary major medical expenses: the so-called "medically indigent."

This combined federal-state-local program is not uniformly practiced over the

*Material adapted from:
1. Title XIX: Grants to states for Medical Assistance Programs, Pub. No. (HCFA) 79-24001, revised January 1979, Health Care Financing Administration, Medicaid Bureau.
2. Beten, C. L.: Medicaid and you: a scriptographic booklet, Pub. No. 1656A-1-79, Greenfield, Mass.
3. Medicaid-Medicare, Pub. No. (HCFA) 77-24901, March 1977, Health Care Financing Administration.

*Figures given are from 1979; these change yearly to keep up with increasing costs.

country; there are variations in eligibility requirements and services from state to state. Financing is in the range of 50% federal, 25% state, and 25% local comunity.

The elderly are a major group utilizing the benefits of Medicaid.

Eligibility*

The *categorically needy* are automatically covered and include all persons receiving cash benefits under the Supplemental Security Income (SSI) program because of age, blindness, or disability. States may exclude some of these SSI cash assistance recipients from automatic Medicaid eligibility if they are eligible only because the standards for the federal program are more liberal than those previously utilized by the state.

The *medically needy*, established at the state's discretion, are persons who fit into one of the categories of those covered by the cash welfare program (aged, blind, or disabled individuals) and who have enough income to pay for their basic living expenses but not enough for their medical care. They are not recipients of welfare.

Services required by federal regulation

The following services are required by federal regulation under a state's Medicaid program:

1. Inpatient hospital care
2. Outpatient hospital care and rural health clinic services
3. Other laboratory and x-ray services
4. SNF and home health care services for individuals 21 years of age and over

---

*Aspects of Medicaid eligibility specifically applicable to the young have not been included.

5. Early and periodic screening, diagnosis, and treatment for individuals under 21 years of age (a bias against the elderly)
6. Family planning services
7. Physician services

Optional services

In addition, states may provide the following services:

1. Private-duty nursing services
2. Clinic services
3. Dental services
4. Physical therapy, occupational therapy, and treatment of speech, hearing, and language disorders
5. Prescribed drugs, dentures, prosthetic devices, and eyeglasses
6. Other diagnostic, screening, and rehabilitation services
7. Inpatient hospital services, SNF services, and ICF services for persons 65 years of age and over in institutions for tuberculosis or mental disease
8. ICF services, including services for the mentally retarded in institutions other than tuberculosis hospitals or mental institutions, for persons determined to be in need of such care as specified in the Social Security Act
9. Inpatient psychiatric services for those under 21
10. Any other type of medical or remedial care recognized under state law and specified by the Secretary of the Department of Health, Education, and Welfare (HEW)

Medicaid services, state by state, are shown in Fig. 2-4, which lists a number of the optional services that can be covered under state Medicaid programs.

*Basic required Medicaid services: Medicaid recipients receiving federally supported financial assistance must receive at least th[e] skilled nursing facility services and home health services for individuals 21 and older; early [...] participation is also available to states electing to expand their Medicaid programs by cover[...] offer the services required for financial assistance recipients or may substitute a combination[...]

Services provided only under the Medicare buy-in or the screening and treatment program for individuals under 21 are not shown on this chart.

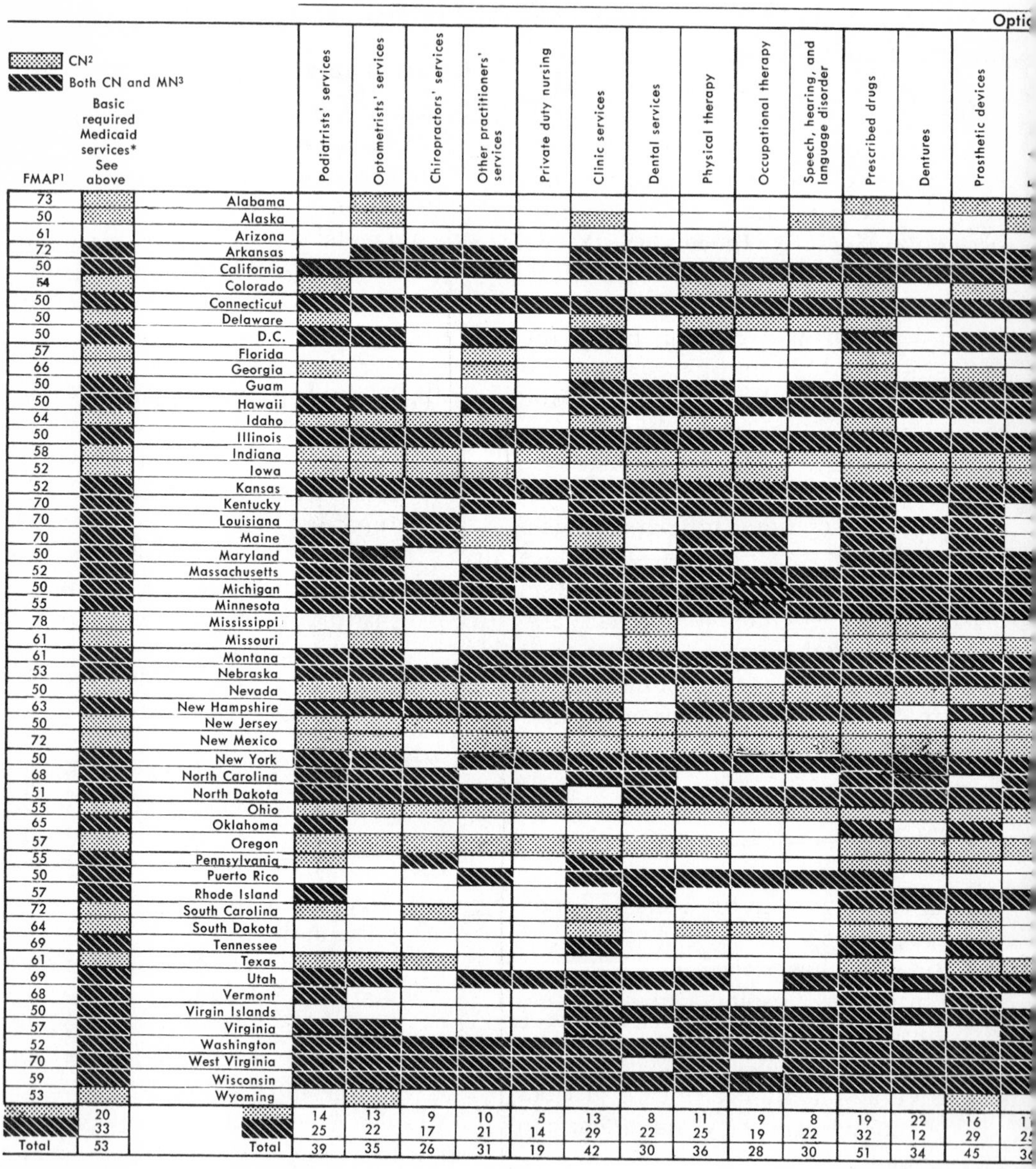

Optic[...]

Legend:
- CN[2]
- Both CN and MN[3]
- Basic required Medicaid services* See above

FMAP[1]	State	Podiatrists' services	Optometrists' services	Chiropractors' services	Other practitioners' services	Private duty nursing	Clinic services	Dental services	Physical therapy	Occupational therapy	Speech, hearing, and language disorder	Prescribed drugs	Dentures	Prosthetic devices
73	Alabama													
50	Alaska													
61	Arizona													
72	Arkansas													
50	California													
54	Colorado													
50	Connecticut													
50	Delaware													
50	D.C.													
57	Florida													
66	Georgia													
50	Guam													
50	Hawaii													
64	Idaho													
50	Illinois													
58	Indiana													
52	Iowa													
52	Kansas													
70	Kentucky													
70	Louisiana													
70	Maine													
50	Maryland													
52	Massachusetts													
50	Michigan													
55	Minnesota													
78	Mississippi													
61	Missouri													
61	Montana													
53	Nebraska													
50	Nevada													
63	New Hampshire													
50	New Jersey													
72	New Mexico													
50	New York													
68	North Carolina													
51	North Dakota													
55	Ohio													
65	Oklahoma													
57	Oregon													
55	Pennsylvania													
50	Puerto Rico													
57	Rhode Island													
72	South Carolina													
64	South Dakota													
69	Tennessee													
61	Texas													
69	Utah													
68	Vermont													
50	Virgin Islands													
57	Virginia													
52	Washington													
70	West Virginia													
59	Wisconsin													
53	Wyoming													
CN = 20		14	13	9	10	5	13	8	11	9	8	19	22	16	1[...]
Both CN and MN = 33		25	22	17	21	14	29	22	25	19	22	32	12	29	2[...]
Total 53	Total	39	35	26	31	19	42	30	36	28	30	51	34	45	3[...]

[1]FMAP-federal Medicaid assistance percentage: Rate of federal financial participation in a state's medical vendor payment expenditures on behalf of individu[...]
[2]Categorically needy: People receiving federally supported financial assistance.
[3]Medically needy: People who are eligible for medical but not for financial assistance.

Fig. 2-4. Medicaid services, state by state, 1979. (Modified from the U.S. Department

rvices: inpatient hospital services; outpatient hospital services; rural health clinic services; other laboratory and x-ray services; riodic screening, diagnosis, and treatment for individuals under 21; family planning; and physician services. Federal financial ditional services and/or by including people eligible for medical but not for financial assistance. For the latter group states may ven services.

finitions and limitations on eligibility and services vary from state to state. Details are available m local welfare offices and state Medicaid agencies.

rvices in state Medicaid programs

Diagnostic services	Screening services	Preventive services	Rehabilitative services	Services for age 65 or older in TB institutions A. Inpatient hospital services	B. SNF services	C. ICF services	Services for age 65 or older in mental inst. A. Inpatient hospital services	B. SNF services	C. ICF services	ICF services	ICF for mentally retarded	Inpatient psychiatric service for under age 22	Christian Science nurses	Christian Science sanitoria	SNF for under age 21	Emergency hospital services	Personal care services	Total additional services
																		12
																		10
																		22
																		29
																		14
																		24
																		9
																		19
																		9
																		13
																		9
																		20
																		13
																		29
																		24
																		19
																		26
																		17
																		14
																		22
																		16
																		28
																		22
																		31
																		9
																		15
																		26
																		26
																		20
																		24
																		27
																		17
																		29
																		19
																		24
																		23
																		10
																		23
																		14
																		13
																		10
																		12
																		13
																		14
																		10
																		18
																		10
																		9
																		16
																		28
																		20
																		32
																		5
	3	4	9	8	2	2	13	9	12	23	22	10	1	6	18	17	2	
18	12	16	19	19	10	9	28	17	17	27	26	23	5	12	24	28	9	
23	15	20	28	27	12	11	41	26	29	50	48	33	6	18	42	45	11	

nd families eligible under Title XIX of the Social Security act. Percentages, effective from October 1, 1977, through September 30, 1979, are rounded.

ealth, Education, and Welfare, Health Care Financing Administration.)

Relationship between Medicaid and Medicare

Most of the elderly who are eligible for Medicaid additionally have Medicare coverage. State Medicaid programs may elect to pay the premiums, deductibles, and copayments for their Medicare-eligible clients. In addition, many state Medicaid programs provide services for the elderly and disabled that are not provided by Medicare (e.g., SNF coverage beyond the 100 days, posthospital coverage provided by Medicare; eyeglasses; prescription drugs; and hearing aids.

Home health care

In some states these services are covered extensively under Medicaid.

COSTS OF GERIATRIC CARE
National health care expenditures

Health care expenditures for all ages represented about 9.15% of the gross national product (GNP) in 1978 (Fig. 2-5). Health care expenditures are increasing at a more rapid rate than is the GNP. Those under 19 years of age, representing one third of the population, accounted for 13% of the total health dollar,

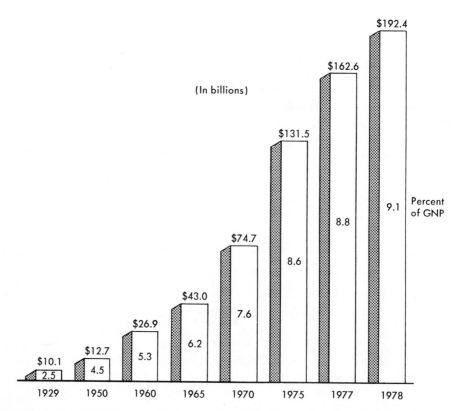

(In billions)

Percent of GNP

Fig. 2-5. National health expenditures and percent of gross national product: selected calendar years, 1929 to 1978. (Modified from Gibson, R. M.: National health expenditures, 1978, Health Care Financing Rev. 1[1]:1, 1979.)

while those over 65 years of age, representing about one tenth of the population, accounted for about 26% of the total health dollar (Fig. 2-6).[14]

Personal health care expenditures

As seen in Fig. 2-7, the $41.3 billion accounted for by the aged amounted to $1,745 per elderly person in 1977. Hospitals ($769), nursing homes ($446), and physicians' services ($302) accounted for 87% of the $1,745.

About two thirds of this total came from government financing (Medicare, Medicaid, and other public programs), and the remaining one third from private payments made by the elderly.

Hospital costs[14]

Hospital costs accounted for approximately 45% of the total health care costs of the elderly ($18 billion or $769 per person) in 1977 (Fig. 2-7). About 88% of the hospital bill was paid by government sources, with 74% coming from Medicare.

Nursing home costs.[14]

Nursing home costs accounted for approximately 25% of the total health care costs of the aged ($10.5 billion or $446 per person) in 1977 (Fig. 2-7). Contrary to the situation with the hospital bill, Medicare paid very little (3.3%) of this bill. Medicaid paid about 50% of the bill, and

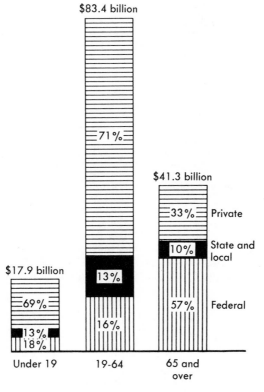

Fig. 2-6. Percentage distribution of expenditures for personal health care by source of funds and age group, fiscal year 1977. (From Gibson, R. M., and Fisher, C. R.: Age differences in health care spending, fiscal year 1977, Soc. Sec. Bull. **42**[1]:3, 1979.)

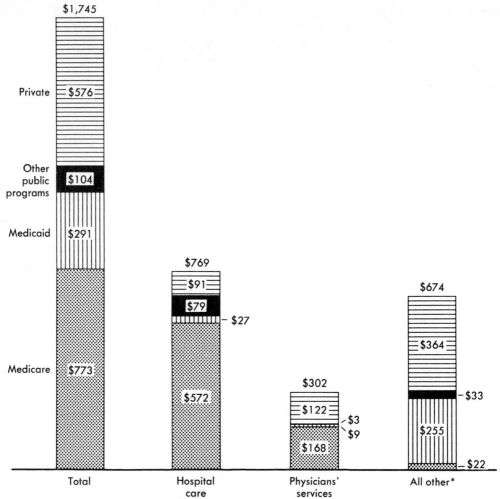

Fig. 2-7. Per capita health care expenditures for the aged, by source of funds and type of care, fiscal year 1977. (From Gibson, R. M., and Fisher, C. R.: Age differences in health care spending, fiscal year 1977, Soc. Sec. Bull. **42**[1]:3, 1979.)

the remaining 46.7% came from patients' private funds. Nursing home costs varied in 1977 from $25 to $100 per day, depending on geography, quality, and type of facility and services.

Physician costs[14]

The third leading cost of health care in 1977 was that of physicians' services

($7.1 billion or $302 per person). Fifty-six percent of this was covered by Medicare, but this figure is reduced to 41% if one considers the cost of coinsurance and the deductible (Fig. 2-7).

Other costs[14]

Eighty-seven percent ($35.8 billion) of the $41.3 billion was related to hospital, nursing home, and physician costs in 1977. The remaining "other costs" included the costs of eyeglasses, podiatric services, physical therapy, orthopedic appliances, medications, etc. The costs of dental care, eyeglasses, and medications were paid largely with patients' private funds. For example, of the $2.9 billion spent on drugs during 1977 ($120 per person), only about 10% came from public funds; the remainder came from personal funds.

CONCLUSION

Medicare and Medicaid have been giant steps forward in the provision of medical care for older Americans.

Medicare does not cover the full cost of health care for older persons, however, and is not linked to requirements for improved "systems" of health care delivery.

Medicaid quite appropriately provides more extensive coverage for health care needs of the indigent or near indigent elderly than Medicare provides for those at any income level. However, the linkage of Medicaid to the necessity of proving indigency status appears to detract from the excellent coverage provided.

Knowledge of the interplay of economic, social, and health care factors should help the student and clinician, both, to be more effective in primary care delivery and in leadership roles in the community.

REFERENCES

1. Health in the United States, 1976-1977, DHEW Pub. No. (HRA) 77-1232 (PHS) 78-1232, 1978, U.S. Department of Health, Education, and Welfare, National Center for Health Statistics.
2. Projection of the population of the United States, 1977-2050, Current Population Reports Series P25, No. 704, U.S. Department of Commerce, Bureau of the Census.
3. Current estimates from the Health Interview Survey: United States, 1977, DHEW Series 10, Report 126, U.S. Department of Health, Education, and Welfare, National Center for Health Statistics, Table 14, p. 24.
4. Health Interview Survey: chronic conditions and limitations of activity and mobility, United States, July 1965 – June 1967, U.S. Department of Health, Education, and Welfare, National Center for Health Statistics, Table 1, p. 19.
5. America's health care system, a comprehensive portrait, Chicago, 1978, Center for Health Administration Studies, University of Chicago. Special report.
6. Libow, L. S.: Future of health care and the elderly (geriatric medicine), Comm. Pub. No. 95-151, p. 8. Joint hearing before the Subcommittee on Health and Long-Term Care and the Subcommittee on Human Services of the Select Committee on Aging, House of Representatives, Ninety-fifth Congress, Second Session, May 17, 1978.
7. Money, income and poverty status of families and persons in the United States: 1977, Current Population Reports Series P60, No. 116, 1979, U.S. Department of Commerce, Bureau of the Census, Table 16, p. 18
8. Older Americans, DHEW Pub. No. (OHDS) 79-20006, 1978, U.S. Department of Health, Education, and Welfare.
9. Money income in 1977 of families and persons in the United States, Current Population Reports Series P60, No. 118, U.S. Department of Commerce, Bureau of the Census, Table 21, p. 83; Table 20, p. 70.
10. Fact book on aging: a profile of America's older population, Washington, D.C., 1978, The National Council on the Aging, Inc.
11. 1971 White House Conference on Aging: Towards a national policy on aging, Federal Report V, No. 1, DHEW Pub. No. (OHD) 74-20911, U.S. Department of Health, Education, and Welfare.
12. Kovar, M. G.: Elderly people: the population 65 and over in Health in the United States, 1976-1977; DHEW Pub. No. (HRA) 77-1232 (PHS) 78-1232, U.S. Department of Health, Education, and Welfare, National Center for Health Statistics.
13. The National Nursing Home Survey, 1977 – summary for the United States, Vital and Health Statistics Series B, No. 43, DHEW Pub. No. (P14S) 79-1794, U.S. Department of Health, Education, and Welfare.
14. Gibson, R. M., and Fisher, C. R.: Age differences in health care spending, fiscal year 1977, Soc. Sec. Bull. **42**(1):3, 1979.

PROBLEM-SOLVING EXERCISES*
Case one

Mr. R. is 68 years old and entitled to Social Security benefits. He has never applied for benefits, because he earns $20,000 per year and he will not need Social Security until he retires. On May 1, he is ill and admitted to a hospital. After leaving the hospital, he decides to apply for Part A Medicare benefits.

Questions

1. Will Mr. R. obtain retroactive payment for his hospitalization?
2. If yes, under what conditions?

Case two

Miss Y. is admitted to the hospital on January 1. She is released on February 1; she is readmitted on March 15 and remains until April 20.

Questions

1. Is she still under the same spell of illness for Medicare purposes?
2. How much does she have to pay to the hospital?

Case three

Mrs. Z. is admitted to a hospital on February 1. After 2 weeks she is transferred to an SNF; she remains there 61 days; then, because of a sudden change in her condition, she again enters the hospital.

Question

1. Is Mrs. Z. under the same illness?

Case four

Mr. W. is hospitalized for 90 days and needs to stay in the hospital for a more prolonged, undefined period of time. The first 90 days of hospitalization are covered somewhat by Medicare.

Questions

1. Can he find a way to stay in the hospital without out-of-pocket payment to the hospital?
2. Once lifetime reserve days are used, can they be used again for a future spell of illness?
3. Would you advise him to use his reserve days at this time?

Case five

Mr. J. is admitted to an SNF, where he remains for 97 days.

Question

1. Given that the copayment is $20 per day, how much will he have to pay?

Case six

Mrs. S. is discharged from an SNF, and her physician certifies that home health care services are necessary for the continued treatment of the illness for which she was institutionalized.

Question

1. What is the maximum number of home health care visits she is entitled to in a calendar year if she has both Part A and Part B of Medicare?

ANSWERS TO PROBLEM-SOLVING EXERCISES
Case one

1. Yes.
2. If he applies before May 1 of the following year. If a person applies for benefits after the month of attainment of age 65, protection can be retroactive for 12 months preceding the month the person filed the application.

Case two

1. Yes. Less than 60 days have elapsed between the time of her release and the time of her readmission.
2. $440. The total of 31 days + 36 days = 67 days. Thus, the 7 days beyond the basic 60

*Thanks are due to the Institute of Law and Rights of Older Adults, New York, N.Y., for allowing us to use some of their teaching cases.

cost the patient $40 per day ($7 \times $40 = $280 + $160 deductible = $440).

Case three

1. Yes. Although she has been out of the hospital for more than 60 days, the stay in the SNF extends her spell of illness.

Case four

1. Yes. He can use his lifetime reserve days for his continued hospital stay. He has to pay $80 per day for each reserve day he uses.
2. No.
3. Yes; as a general rule, the lifetime reserve days should be used at the first opportunity.

Case five

1. $1,540 ($77 \times $20 [because there is no payment for the first 20 days] = $1,540).

Case six

1. 200 visits. Home health care services are reimbursable under both Part A and Part B of Medicare, provided that Mrs. S. meets the necessary requirements. She could receive up to 100 visits for the condition related to the prior SNF stay under Part A and an additional 100 visits for the same condition or a condition arising after the inpatient stay, under Part B.

POSTTEST

1. Which of the following statements concerning the elderly population in the United States are true:
   a. About one third of the elderly population is 75 years of age or over.
   b. Elderly people living alone or with no relations had a median income of $3,795 in 1977.
   c. Persons over the age of 65 now constitute approximately 10% to 11% of the total population.
2. Determine whether each statement refers to a Medicare and/or a Medicaid program:
   a. It is a federal health insurance program.
   b. It is mixed federal-state welfare program.
   c. Those eligible include the categorically needy and the medically needy.
   d. It covers dental services, drugs, eyeglasses, transportation, and hearing aids.
   e. It provides home health-homemaker-services.
3. Which of the following terms refer to long-term care facilities:
   a. Skilled nursing facility (SNF)
   b. Intermediate care facility (ICF)
   c. Domiciliary care facility
4. Which of the following statements concerning nursing homes are true?
   a. There are about 18,900 nursing homes in the United States.
   b. Medicare was the primary source of payment for 50% of nursing home costs in 1977.
   c. The average nursing home patient is 68 years of age.
   d. The patient must be seen by the attending physician at least once every 60 days in an SNF.
5. Which of the following regulatory mechanisms would involve physician participation?
   a. Utilization Review Committees
   b. Federal and state inspection teams
   c. Professional Standards Review Organizations (PSROs)
6. Which of the following statements concerning health care costs in fiscal year 1977 are true?
   a. The per capita health care expenditure for the aged was $1,745.
   b. The two largest items included in health care expenditures of the elderly were costs for hospital and nursing home care.
   c. Public funds covered 90% of the per-

sonal health care expenditures of the elderly.

d. Government sources, including the Medicare program, paid for about 88% of the hospital care of the elderly.

ANSWERS TO PRETEST AND POSTTEST

1. All of these.
2. a, Medicare; b, Medicaid; c, Medicaid; d, Medicaid; e, Medicaid and Medicare. Program e is under Medicare only if the person receives part-time skilled nursing care, physical therapy, or speech therapy.
3. All of these. Facility a provides skilled nursing care and rehabilitation services; facility b provides health-related care and services; facility c is a nonmedical residential institution.
4. a and d. Statement b is false because Medicaid was the primary source of payment for 50% of nursing home costs in 1977. Statement c is false because the average patient is 82 years of age.
5. a. All of these. a—The physician reviews the medical necessity of the initial admission and continued institutionalization. b—The physician is a member of the inspection team, along with the hospital administrator, a nurse, a sanitation expert, a nutritionist, and an engineer. c—Physicians in local areas conduct "peer reviews" of the specific ways that services are provided.
6. a, b, and d. Statement c is false because public funds covered only 60% to 70% of expenditures for health care of the elderly. Pertaining to statement d, the 12% not covered by public funds amounted to $2.1 million and reflects direct payment by the elderly for services not covered by public funds, such as Medicare deductibles and copayments, and private health insurance premiums.

Chapter 3

Interviewing and history taking

LESLIE S. LIBOW and FREDRICK T. SHERMAN

EDUCATIONAL OBJECTIVES
Attitudinal

The student should:

1. Know how normal aging affects the elderly (not all elderly people are senile or incontinent, and not all of them live in nursing homes)
2. Be aware of the increased time needed to deal with the history and physical examination of the elderly individual
3. Be aware of the potential frustration in obtaining this history and physical examination because of sensory deficits, aphasia, or dementia
4. Recognize his reluctance to discuss certain sensitive subjects (death, sex, diagnoses) with the elderly patient
5. Be aware of how the age difference between the student and the older patient may affect the interview
6. Understand the implications of confirming the elderly patient's history in the presence of a relative or friend
7. Recognize his feelings toward the elderly individual who cries during the interview
8. Recognize his feelings about physical contact with elderly people
9. Recognize his feelings about discussing major losses (friends, spouse, children, job, income, etc.) with the elderly individual

Cognitive

The student should:

1. Be aware of the following challenges in history taking with the elderly:
   a. The fact that symptoms are often underreported
   b. The fact that certain symptoms may have different implications
   c. The possible need for alternative sources of history
   d. The possible need for different interview

techniques to overcome sensory deficits (hearing or vision), to deal with family dynamics, and to structure the time and duration of the interview
   e. The fact that attitudes toward proposed surgical or invasive procedures may differ from those found in younger persons

Skill

The student should:

1. Know how to diagnose and initiate treatment for the many problems of communication encountered with the elderly (hearing loss, aphasia, dementia, etc.)
2. Be able to use the techniques of life review and reminiscence in interviewing the elderly patient
3. Be able to introduce into the interview sensitive areas, such as forced retirement, sexual function, and "heroic" measures to prolong life in the elderly
4. Know how to seek out alternative sources of history and determine their reliability (e.g., past medical records or interviews of others)
5. Know how to get complete information about such subjects as nutritional history, medication history, social history, and psychiatric history
6. Know when to involve family members and how to effectively interview them

PRETEST*

1. Which of the following is (are) characteristic of interviewing and history taking with the elderly?
   a. More time is required to complete an initial evaluation than with the middle-aged patient.

*Some questions may have more than one correct answer.

b. A family member should always be present during the initial interview.

c. The oral history may have to be complemented by other sources of information.

d. It is often necessary to obtain a sexual history, but not necessarily during the first interview.

e. The appropriate time and setting are important factors in determining the outcome of a mental status examination.

2. Which of the following attitudes or biases on the part of the interviewer can present potential problems in interviewing the elderly patient?

a. Biases about normal aging

b. Biases about sexual activity in old age

c. Ideas based on previous experiences with grandparents

d. The idea that nursing homes are to be avoided

3. In comparing history taking with elderly patients and history-taking with young or middle-aged patients, one would expect which of the following to be true?

a. Symptoms specific for illness in the young or middle-aged may have different significance in the elderly.

b. Multiple chief complaints are more frequently expressed by elderly patients.

c. The elderly patient tends to underreport illness more than the young or middle-aged patient.

d. Signs of depression arising from loss of job, home, or spouse are less frequently encountered with elderly patients.

4. When interviewing an elderly patient with functional deficits in communication, particularly in the acute care hospital or nursing home, the interviewer may need to:

a. Optimize the setting so the patient can lip-read, and face the patient directly, allowing for proper light on the interviewer's face.

b. Ask the patient to insert his dentures

c. Check to see whether the patient has cerumen in his ear canals and remove it

d. Ask the patient to insert his hearing aid before starting the interview.

5. What information would you wish to obtain at a minimum, from an elderly patient in order to complete the:
   • Nutritional history?
   • Medication history?
   • Social history?
   • Psychiatric history?

6. Sources of additional history include:

a. The relative's description of the patient's symptoms and dysfunction

b. The transfer summary on the previously hospitalized patient just admitted to a skilled nursing facility and vice versa

c. Reports of pathological specimens

d. All other medical records, including those from prior physicians and institutions

e. The "bag" of medications brought from the patient's home

7. A sexual history in the elderly:

a. Should be pursued because sexual dysfunction can result from multiple medical, surgical, and psychological problems encountered in late life

b. Should always be done during the first interview

c. Need not be explored in older women

d. May be valuable in understanding the patient's life-style

8. The family history of the elderly patient may be helpful in suggesting a diagnosis of:

a. Glaucoma

b. Idiopathic hypertrophic subaortic stenosis

c. Diabetes mellitus

d. Coronary artery disease

e. Cancer

Obtaining a thorough history from the older patient is often a challenge to the skills of the clinician.[1] While the student or physician should have no difficulty interviewing the majority of elderly patients who are ambulatory, mentally clear, and without visual or auditory deficits, certain issues arise that require a special approach. Interviewing and history taking with an elderly patient who has multiple sensory deficits and memory impairment will be rewarding if proper techniques are used. The methods described in this chapter will assist the student or physician in interviewing and history taking with the variety of elderly patients that he may encounter.

SPECIAL ASPECTS OF HISTORY TAKING WITH THE ELDERLY

Certain aspects of history taking with the elderly require a different approach by the interviewer.

Reporting of illness

The elderly often tend to underreport illness. They may think that breathlessness, hearing loss, incontinence, difficulty in walking, and a variety of aches and pains are all part of normal aging. The interviewer must treat each of these symptoms or signs as potentially reversible illnesses and not equate pathological events with normal aging. A presenting symptom, such as constipation or weakness, may appear insignificant and therefore go unreported when, in fact, colonic carcinoma or polymyalgia rheumatica can be diagnosed and treated. Clinical judgment, not a battery of tests, is called for.

Interpreting symptoms and signs

The chief complaints may be multiple, overlapping, and nonspecific, fitting no well-defined illness pattern. For example, a fractured hip, resulting from a syn-copal episode from a dysrhythmia, may manifest itself not by local pain and tenderness over the hip, but by the inability to ambulate, referred knee pain, and/or mental confusion. A specific symptom of illness in the young or middle-aged may have different significance in the elderly. In addition, multiple minor complaints must be sorted out and scrutinized. Remember that seemingly minor symptoms may be the tip of the iceberg.

Alternative sources of history

History taking has its limitations as a data-gathering process with all ages and must be supplemented by a physical examination and laboratory tests. With the elderly patient, the history is obviously more extensive, sometimes incomplete because of memory loss, and sometimes delayed because of memory loss, mental illness, or lack of physicians' records. Other sources of history, such as the spouse, adult children, or a home health aide who may be providing services for the patient, must be sought.[2] Particularly important are medical records from physicians, hospitals, and nursing homes.

Interview techniques

Multiple sensory deficits, inattention, fatigue of the patient and/or interviewer from a lengthy interview, desire to reminisce, and the inability to recall exact symptomatology force the interviewer to use other kinds of interview techniques with the elderly patient. Making sure that the interviewer's face is well lighted and that the patient is wearing his dentures, eyeglasses, and a working hearing aid is important.

Ageism

Ageism, described in Chapter 1 as prejudice against an individual merely because of his age, may influence both the interviewer and the elderly patient.[3] The interviewer should deal with his own biases as well as with those of the patient when dealing with certain aspects of the interview. The following relate to' possible biases:

1. Normal age-related changes, though often in the direction of decline, are occasionally in the direction of improvement or superiority when compared with younger adults. For example, it takes an older person longer to do complex movements (such as completing a standardized history form or removing clothes for the physical examination), to react, and to make decisions. The older person's verbal intelligence quotient (IQ) score, creativity, and problem-solving ability, however, do not decline. In fact, verbal intelligence of the healthy elderly has been shown to be superior to that of young college students.

The interviewer may have to alter the tempo of the interview or divide the interview into two parts and be prepared to give his elderly patient more time to respond to questions and perform such tasks as undressing or transferring from chair to bed or examining table.

2. Personality patterns persist through old age. The "grouchy," self-centered elderly man may have been this way for his entire adult life. The interviewer should not attribute these personality "changes" to old age when, in fact, the patient may have always been a difficult person with whom to deal. Elderly people are just as heterogeneous in their personalities as are younger individuals, and stereotypes are not helpful. The interviewer should not generalize an occasional negative experience from one elderly patient to the next.

3. The sexual history is frequently en-

tirely omitted, even when indicated, such as after transurethral or suprapubic prostatectomy or in the diabetic patient. This omission may be due to the following:

   a. The interviewer may have general discomfort about discussing sexuality with a patient of any age.

   b. The interviewer may have the attitude that sexuality is not expressed in old age.

   c. Because of the taboo on discussion of sexuality in old age, the patient may be afraid to admit to having sexual feelings.

4. The reality of personal, family, and job losses and, ultimately, of death increases with age. Discussion of these realities, which are often denied by young and middle-aged individuals, may be easier for elderly people, who expect such losses and may better accept the news of serious illness. The interviewer must explore his own fears of loss.

5. Because of age and sex differences between the interviewer and the patient, the interviewer must examine his feelings of ageism, which may emerge during the medical interview.

The medical interviewer (student or physician) is usually younger than the patient, and the elderly patient may make the younger interviewer feel uncomfortable by referring to the latter's age and inexperience. The interviewer should be prepared to deal with statements such as "You're a nice young doctor," "Are you a doctor?" or "You're too young to remember that." Feelings and biases that the student or physician may have toward older members of his own family may influence his reactions to the patient.

Since two thirds of the older population are women while more than one half of medical students are men, the interview often takes place with an older woman alone with a younger male physician. Previous relationships, such as between mother and child or grandmother and grandchild, may have subtle influences.

INTERVIEW TECHNIQUES
Timing and duration

Since a thorough initial interview with an elderly patient may be lengthy, it is best to schedule at least two interview sessions. The patient himself may limit the length of these sessions because of fatigue, inattention, or anger. Thus, one should not expect to use the initial meeting as a "total evaluation session," as in the young or middle-aged patient. Unless the patient has had an unusually healthy life history, there will probably be considerable medical, surgical, social, and medication histories to be obtained.

The elderly patient (or family member, when indicated) should be asked to bring in as many medical records and previous and current medications as possible. This request can be made by phone or mail, preferably before the initial meeting. In the case of a patient with mental deterioration, past records are vital. A useful option is to send a "geriatric oriented" questionnaire to the patient and/or relative, to be filled out prior to the patient's coming in for the initial evaluation or clinic interview.

The time of the interview, although not always within the control of the patient or the interviewer, should preferably take place in the midmorning or afternoon to avoid any changes in mental status that may occur because of oversedation from nighttime hypnotics. In some cases additional interviews may need to be performed at different times of the day to get an overall picture of the patient's mental

function. Afternoon confusion ("sundowning") may occur in mildly demented patients who are living at home or in an institution from a decrease in auditory and visual stimuli that occurs as evening comes.

Determining who should be present

Who should be present during the interview of the elderly patient? For the patient accompanied by a family member or friend, the clinician must decide whether the interview should be conducted in private or whether the family member(s) or friend should be allowed to participate. This decision requires the clinician to be sensitive to issues of privacy, family dynamics, and the mental status of the elderly patient.[4]

The elderly patient should be interviewed by himself unless the patient's mental status is so poor that a relative is needed to give the history. Interviewing the family and patient together, however, may make it difficult or impossible for the elderly patient to mention personal or private problems. The family members may talk about their elderly relative as if the relative were a nonfunctional, invisible third party. An interview with the family and patient may show how family members inappropriately relate to their older relative because the relative has been labeled "senile," "demented," or just "old." Such interviews often demonstrate fascinating family dynamics and social interplay.

Objectivity is mandatory if the interviewer is to properly assess mental status, since it will affect almost all future therapeutic decisions. Since there is a large spectrum of mental ability among patients with dementia (mild to severe), determining the mental status in front of a relative may embarrass the patient who remains sensitive to his memory loss. Therefore, initial history taking with the apparently demented patient, as well as with the mentally clear patient, should be done with only the patient and the interviewer present.

In the case of the mentally deteriorated person, a brief initial interview alone with the patient to assess mental status can be followed by an interview at which the family member(s) or friend is included.

Having a relative or friend present when he is not needed implies both to this third party and to the patient that the patient is incapable of telling the entire history. Privacy is also violated. Asking the relative or friend to "Excuse us while I talk to Mrs. Smith" (the patient) shows that you respect the patient's privacy and also allows you to hear the patient's medical history without being biased by another individual.

While it is best to interview the patient alone initially, the clinician may choose to ask the elderly individual his preference; and often the patient will state that he wants his spouse or child, etc., present: "I have no secrets." Unfortunately, asking "Do you want him [the family member or friend] present?" places considerable pressure on the elderly individual to demonstrate his trust in the accompanying person. Thus, it is best not to ask this question and merely ask the relative or friend to leave, as you would a person accompanying a young or middle-aged patient.

The most inappropriate route to take would be to ask the patient to leave and remain in the waiting room while the relative or friend is interviewed; this approach could limit any potential for a positive physician-patient relationship.

The majority of families remain involved with their elderly relatives. Because the family is concerned with supporting their older relative in the community, it is often necessary to meet with the family and the patient together. The patient and family should be asked about their feelings regarding such a meeting, since some patients may not want to discuss their need for support with family members.

Privacy is important in any interview and should not be neglected in interviewing the elderly. A lack of privacy inhibits not only the sensitive interviewer, but also the sensitive patient. The problems of trying to keep discussions of the patient's health confidential arise most often in ambulatory care clinic settings and emergency rooms. They also can arise at the bedside in nursing homes and acute care hospitals.

Overcoming auditory, visual, and/or language difficulties

If the patient has functional deficits in vision and hearing, the following steps should be taken:

First, the patient's own glasses, contact lenses, functioning hearing aid, and/or dentures should be in place before the interview begins to ensure optimum conditions for conversation. The interviewer may have to assist the patient in inserting dentures and either turn on or insert the hearing aid; therefore, the interviewer must have a working understanding of each. (See Chapters 9 and 14.)

Second, if functional deficits in hearing are present, the interviewer should initially determine whether the patient has cerumen in his ear canals. If removing cerumen does not improve hearing, the interviewer should:

1. Enable the elderly patient to lipread by moving closer, directly facing the patient, and putting proper lighting on the interviewer's face

2. Speak slowly, allowing more time between words (Shouting into the better ear is usually self-defeating, because it makes lipreading impossible.)
3. Eliminate extraneous noises, such as the television, radio, or page system, which may be present in emergency rooms, hospital clinics, or nursing homes

The aphasic elderly patient offers other challenges to the interviewer. Asking questions that require a "yes" or "no" answer may give valuable information. Open-ended questions will often elicit replies that have little value and cause much frustration for both the interviewer and the aphasic patient (See Chapter 8 for methods of interviewing the aphasic patient.)

Reminiscence and life review: getting to know the patient as a person

The medical student or physician who focuses only on "diseased organs" may completely miss the human being behind the illness. In addition to missing the rich life history of the elderly person, he will fail to learn how the patient handled major life crises. Allowing a period of reminiscence early in the interview may also help establish rapport; it assures the patient that the interviewer is interested not only in his health but also in his life story (life review).[3]

For example, the entire tone of the interview will probably change once the interviewer learns that his 80-year-old patient is the parent of several children, some of whom have grown to have their own children. The interviewer may also learn that the patient immigrated to the United States after having faced some difficult situation in another country and that he sustains himself economically and has managed to "survive" for 70 to 80

years.* The fascinating "roots" of the patient will unfold.

The late-life social experience pertinent to the medical history includes the following:

1. Loss of a spouse, siblings, children, friends, neighbors, job, pets, and/or one's home
2. Change of a physician because the previous physician died, retired, or moved or the patient moved to a new residence
3. Retirement
4. Widow(er)-hood and remarriage or couple relationship without marriage
5. Economic difficulties brought about by inflation and a fixed income

The interviewer should obtain a general description of a "typical" day or week in the patient's life, since there is a positive correlation between an elderly person's typical day being varied and goal directed and that person's survival into late life. If there has been a significant recent change in health status, then the typical day before the change as well as the typical day after the change should be understood. The typical day activities to be discussed include social contacts, family visits, reading, television viewing, eating (frequency and diet), work, hobbies, and goal setting. If this information is obtained gently and with interest, the patient will develop trust and confidence in the interviewer.

Touching

The elderly patient may cry while discussing major losses. Attempts by the interviewer to comfort the patient should be delayed while the patient cries. Tis-

---

*The work history, the challenges surmounted, the gains and losses withstood—all enhance the interviewer's understanding of the elderly person being evaluated and treated.

sues may be offered. Verbal intervention is appropriate when the initial release seems to be ending. At times, the interviewer may feel it would be comforting to the elderly patient to hold the patient's hand. The younger interviewer (male or female) is much more likely to hold the hand of an older female patient than that of an older male patient. In the case of the younger interviewer (male or female) and older male patient, anxieties about the inappropriateness of such a gesture may impede the interviewer from comforting the elderly man. Touching the elderly patient, even if only to shake hands or a light touch on the shoulder, may be important in establishing a meaningful relationship.

Determining the reliability of the history

There is generally no question about the reliability of the history in young and middle-aged patients. First, the patient is usually mentally clear. If he is not, he is usually accompanied by a spouse who knows the brief, complete history. In the younger patient, the history is usually not lengthy but consists of a chief complaint and elaboration of this complaint. There are fewer illnesses, operations, hospitalizations, and medications to be forgotten.[5] The elderly patient, however, is different. Not only is the history lengthy, making it difficult to recall dates, treatments, and operations, but diagnoses and conversations between patient and physician that took place three or four decades ago may have been forgotten. Most histories obtained from the elderly, however, are generally reliable.

If the patient's memory, orientation, logic, or emotional state appears to be affecting the reliability of the history, it may be necessary to perform a mental sta-

tus evaluation early in the interview. The evaluation should be done tactfully, without denigrating the patient or making him feel defensive. For example, one could say, "I'd like to ask you a few questions that will help me evaluate your thinking. Some of the questions will be simple and some difficult." The mental status examination could also begin without an introductory statement if the interviewer does not want to influence the patient's response to the questions. Not introducing the mental status examination, however, may make the elderly patient defensive, apprehensive, or hostile. A negative attitude on the part of the interviewer can be communicated to the elderly patient by rapid-fire questioning that includes, "What time is it?" "What place are you in?" and "What is your full name?" The mentally clear, anxious elderly patient may become hostile when such simple mental status questions are asked. Care should be taken not to offend the patient. Often the patient will say, "Do you think I am stupid or crazy?" when he realizes that the interviewer is testing his memory and/or mental function. The reasons for the mental status examination may have to be explained. In the majority of interviews with elderly patients, the initial casual conversation will help determine whether further mental status evaluation is needed.[6] FROMAJE an easily remembered mental status evaluation technique, is described in Chapter 5.

In some situations it will be readily apparent that the patient's mental status is compromised. In a minority, however, the initial conversation will appear normal, though significant deficits exist. An assessment of mental status should take place whenever the interviewer believes that the patient is not responding normally to the conversation. Performing a mental status test early will often save time in further interviews.

The elderly patient may also react to the medical history by rejecting the interviewer, telling him, "Go away and don't bother me," or asking, "Why are all these questions important?" Or he might interject humor into the conversation. These reactions may be a sign of the patient's fatigue, anxiety, or preoccupation with other concerns, in which case a future time should be arranged for completing the interview. On the other hand, rejecting the interviewer may be the patient's way of extricating himself from a situation wherein he may be forced to make it known that he has a failing memory or other mental inadequacy. Therefore, the interviewer, recognizing that the rejection may be a sign of early or undetected organic brain disease, should ask the patient why he wants to conclude the interview. A mental status examination should follow at an appropriate time.

Using alternative sources of history
Relatives, friends, and agencies

If the patient is mentally unclear because of an acute or chronic brain syndrome, stroke, or psychotic behavior, it will be especially important to interview others who know him.[7] Friends and relatives, and particularly individuals who have lived with the elderly patient in the recent past, may provide valuable functional history.

Past medical records must be obtained through phone calls and letters to physicians, hospitals, pharmacies, and social agencies. This additional history should be obtained with the patient's permission if he is mentally clear. Often a relative can expedite the transfer of medical documents, such as x-ray studies and copies of old charts, by actually obtaining and transporting them to the clinician. Medical transfer summaries from hospitals or nursing homes, however, may be inaccurate in their diagnoses and treatment plans. The clinician should get recent transfer summaries, scrutinize them closely, and confirm the information with other sources.

Written interview

If hearing poses a problem in communication that cannot be overcome by the methods described, a written interview may be performed. A thorough geriatric history questionnaire can be completed by the patient prior to the time of the interview and make an interview possible where previously none would have occurred.

Dealing with the chief complaint

All too often the focus of an encounter with an elderly patient is on what appears to be the "major problem." This is an incorrect extrapolation from the approach applied to younger patients. Multiple chronic medical illnesses are common among the elderly. Many of these illnesses are known to the clinician, but others may be unknown to him or to the patient. The chief complaint can be a manifestation of an already known problem or of a newly discovered one. Often multiple chief complaints are present. The patient may believe that a problem is a result of normal aging and therefore not bring it to the attention of the clinician.

The patient's main problem may be loss of function, such as ambulation, continence, or memory; or it may involve a specific medical complaint, such as constipation, dizziness, or chest pain. In addition to the main problem(s), there are often three to six other problems present, often of a chronic nature. As stated, not all of these problems may be known to the clinician. A relative or friend may disagree with the patient as to the reason for coming to the clinician. This is not to say that the third party's list of problems is more accurate than that of the patient. Often both sets of problems are important.

The medical student or physician usually looks for such major illnesses as coronary artery disease, hypertension, stroke, depression, malignancy, arthritis, and diabetes. To be sure, all or some of these are frequently present in the history of the elderly. There are many problems, however that beset the elderly that may be overlooked by the interviewer because they are not considered significant or major "diseases." Among these problems may be urinary stress incontinence; nocturia; diminished sexual activity; decreased hearing; malfitting dentures; inability to rise from a chair; dizziness; falls; anxieties; loss of home, wife, job, or children; and the need for outside support systems. Dealing with these symptoms and ameliorating some of the distress are important to the patient. Modest objective changes may be accompanied by remarkable subjective improvement.

APPLYING THE CLASSIC MEDICAL HISTORY FORMAT TO THE ELDERLY

At the initial evaluation, after establishing the usually extensive list of past and present problems, the interviewer must obtain proper details about each. The initial evaluation should be followed by the classic format of history taking (which has been modified for the elderly), including (1) review of systems; (2) medical and surgical history, including allergies; (3) family history; (4) social history; (5) nutritional history; (6) medica-

tion history; (7) sexual history; and (8) psychiatric history.

Review of systems

This section will not attempt to repeat the classic questions addressed to the "average" patient that are well described elsewhere.[8,9] Rather, it focuses on questions of particular importance in interviewing the older patient.

Head

Headaches, particularly new symptoms and any related to visual difficulties, may signal temporal arteritis, a disease almost exclusively found in the elderly.

Eyes

Loss of near vision (presbyopia) is normal with age. Loss of peripheral fields may relate to glaucoma or stroke (homonymous hemianopia), whereas loss of central vision may relate to macular degeneration. Pain over the eyes could reflect glaucoma or temporal arteritis. Glare from lights at night may result from cataract formation.

Ears

Hearing loss is not universal in late life, although loss of the high-frequency range is common.

Mouth

Questions about dentures not fitting correctly and about changes in taste perception are useful.

Throat

Voice changes may relate to a tumor on the vocal cords, to thyroid dysfunction, or occasionally to sex hormone abnormalities. Dysphagia may result from neurological or muscular causes or from local obstruction.

Endocrine glands

Following diabetes mellitus, the most common type of endocrine disorders of the elderly involve the thyroid gland. These disorders occur at least as often in the elderly as in the middle-aged. The clinician should focus on changes of behavior. The typical clinical picture of hyperthyroidism may be absent. In the elderly hyperthyroid patient, a multinodular goiter is usually present. Hyperthyroidism may present with a cardiovascular or nervous system picture. Hypothyroidism may be suggested by the patient's chronic constipation, confusion, and lethargy. These conditions, however, may be unrelated to a thyroid disorder. A previous thyroidectomy 20 to 40 years earlier or treatment with radioactive iodine should alert the interviewer to the possibility of hypothyroidism.

If a patient has had diabetes or is taking hypoglycemic agents, he should be asked about hypoglycemia (fainting, dizziness, chest pains) and hyperglycemia (frequency of urination, fungus infections in the mouth or crural areas of the vagina). If a patient is losing weight and maintaining a satisfactory appetite, the interviewer should be alert to the diagnosis of diabetes mellitus as well as neoplasm, hyperthyroidism, and chronic infectious diseases.

Cardiovascular system

There may be a history of mental confusion related to unknown cardiac dysfunction. Similarly, swollen ankles (bilaterally) or difficulty in sleeping or eating may be related to heart failure. Myocardial infarction may occur with no chest pain or with atypical symptoms. Occasionally, patients with rheumatic fever in childhood, and subsequent valvular disease, will remain asymptomatic until very old.

Heart failure may also occur as a result of long-standing hypertension or the patient's use of salt-retaining medications, such as steroids or nonsteroidal anti-inflammatory drugs. Dietary indiscretion is a common precipitant of heart failure. Moreover, one third of acute heart failure cases in the elderly occur soon after some type of emotional turmoil (within 3 days). Thus, questions must be addressed to any anxiety-producing situations in the recent past.

Asymptomatic hypertension is common in the elderly. Hypotension occurs frequently and is associated with a change in position (supine to standing), especially in stroke patients, and with medications (diuretics, antihypertensives, antidepressants, antipsychotics).

Gastrointestinal system

Epigastric and retrosternal distress is a common problem that results in a difficult differential diagnosis. Benign peptic ulcer and peptic esophagitis are much more common as causes of symptoms than are carcinoma of the stomach and esophagus. Pancreatic, biliary, and cardiac problems may cause nocturnal discomfort. The etiology of acute abdominal distress may be obscure in late life. Generalized malaise and confusion may be the dominant complaint, rather than pain or fever.

It is common for older persons, particularly those less physically active, to have one bowel movement every 2 to 3 days. As a chronic history, this usually does not warrant any diagnostic tests or intervention. A bowel movement every 3 days is probably normal for an elderly individual; and unless it causes discomfort, no therapy is indicated. Any recent change in bowel habits, however, is significant. Excessive hardness of the stool may indicate dehydration, dietary, or therapeutic factors, such as diuretics, low-fiber content, or aluminum-containing antacids for peptic ulcer. Fecal impaction in relatively immobile elderly people may cause intestinal obstruction, with pain, constipation, or vomiting. Occasionally, diarrhea may result from fecal impaction (paradoxical diarrhea). In rare cases fecal impaction may cause fever in an elderly patient.

Fecal incontinence may be related to cerebral dysfunction or to local large bowel abnormalities, such as fecal impaction or carcinoma of the rectum.

Urinary tract

Common symptoms of benign prostatic hypertrophy include nocturia, dysuria, and urgency, as well as difficulty in starting or stopping urination. Incontinence in men and women is a serious and socially embarrassing symptom. Incontinence may be due to cerebral dysfunction; to local bladder, prostate, or pelvic dysfunction; or to local neurogenic causes, such as an autonomic neuropathy from diabetes mellitus. Previous surgical intervention may result in incontinence or urinary retention. In elderly women, stress incontinence precipitated by coughing, is common. Senile vaginitis with pruritis may be associated with urinary incontinence and vaginal bleeding. Carcinoma of the prostate gland may be manifested by urinary obstructive-like symptoms, even without actual anatomical obstruction, probably through some hormonal mechanism. Bladder stones or a tumor may be manifested by many of the above-mentioned symptoms, including retention. Asymptomatic bacteriuria is common in the elderly. Symptomatic urinary tract infections may present as dysuria, frequency, suprapublic discomfort, fever, or confusion.

Musculoskeletal system

Proximal muscle weakness resulting from a myopathy is found in patients who experience difficulty when carrying packages, in shaving, or in standing up from the sitting position. Hyperthyroidism, polymyalgia rheumatica, and corticosteroids (exogenous or endogenous) may be etiological factors.

Rheumatoid arthritis may occur for the first time in late life, and early-morning joint stiffness is a cardinal symptom. Similarly, gout and pseudogout are not uncommon in the elderly. The incidence of fracture increases in late life. If multiple simultaneous fractures occur, or if a sequence of fractures occurs, one should seek out possible causes of osteoporosis and/or osteomalacia, such as malabsorption, multiple myeloma, and hyperparathyroidism.

Neurological system

Dizziness and/or falling (e.g., drop attacks) may be related to movement of the head to either side or to extension of the neck, resulting in vertebrobasilar insufficiency. If a fall has occurred, it is necessary to determine if there was a loss of consciousness (resulting from postural hypotension, cardiac dysrhythmia, or a seizure, for example) or if consciousness was maintained (vertebrobasilar or carotid artery ischemia). The possibility of the patient's tripping over an obstruction in the environment must also be considered. Transient interference with speech, muscle strength, or sensation may reflect transient cerebral ischemia.

Medical and surgical history

With increasing age, there is a greater likelihood that the patient will have experienced more medical and surgical events. Some of these will have been acute and one-time episodes; others will have been chronic. In view of these multiple problems, it is often surprising how well the patient looks and functions. This is a basic point of geriatric medicine. A unique combination of genetics, environment, fortune, and, perhaps, willpower have produced the older person who is being interviewed; actually, this person is a "survivor." The interviewer should not, therefore, confuse the forest for the trees and become overly involved with only one of the patient's problems unless that problem is clearly causing the patient considerable disability or distress. *Remember:* Do not treat the diagnosis; treat the patient, always emphasizing function and how therapeutic intervention will reverse disability.

A patient may not accurately recall a medical event that occurred 30 years ago. Hospital records or physician office records are unlikely to be available. The clinician may have to settle for sound medical guesswork. For example, a thorough search for abdominal, neck, and breast suture lines will confirm operations that have been forgotten or denied. Often past history may not be too significant, and more recent years will have brought new ailments of greater importance.

Such words as "heart attack" and "stroke" may be used interchangeably by the patient. The interviewer must simultaneously interpret what the patient is saying and translate his own medical jargon to the patient so that the two understand each other. It is often difficult for the elderly patient to differentiate between dizziness, light-headedness, and vertigo, each of which may result in a fall. Attempts by relatives or friends to interpret the patient's symptoms may be

inaccurate. The assessment of such third parties is much more reliable in relation to the elderly person's functional deficits ("He stopped walking and went to bed," "She can't remember to keep her checkbook up to date," or "He lost his way"). Asking the relative about the quality of the patient's chest pain, for example, is likely to yield less valuable information.

The history of modern medicine may unfold before the interviewer as he obtains a history. Allowing time for the patient to do a brief life review, punctuated by highlights of his health, will often bring to the interviewer's attention historical events in medicine. The interviewer may learn, for example, that a patient:

1. Was one of the first patients treated with insulin
2. Had an appendectomy or other abdominal surgery when the only anesthesia was ether
3. Was an immigrant placed in the Ellis Island Hospital in New York for isolation and "treatment" of typhoid and typhus
4. Regarded the hospital as "the place to die"
5. Had all the family children delivered at home by the family doctor
6. Was the first patient to have a carotid endarterectomy for a transient ischemic attack

Family history

The family history is quite important, since survival patterns and longevity as well as diagnoses will often be related to parental and sibling history. For example, senile dementia appears to occur more often in patients whose parents and/or siblings have a history of the disease. One often learns that the parent and/or sibling of the demented patient developed a dementia like illness at about the same age as the patient. Idiopathic hypertrophic subaortic stenosis (IHSS), an unusual cause of the common aortic systolic murmur heard in the elderly, may be suggested by the history of an adult child diagnosed as having IHSS. The clinician will then order an echocardiogram to confirm the diagnosis in the elderly patient. Definite familial trends are also found for coronary artery disease, diabetes mellitus, manic-depressive psychosis, neoplasms, and glaucoma.

The family history will also tell the interviewer about the elderly patient's experiences with past diseases. For example, the patient's reaction to the suggestion that surgery is necessary for colonic cancer may be influenced by a relative's experience with the same disease and operation. If the surgery failed and the relative died, the older patient may not want to consent. If the interviewer knows the patient's family history, he may understand the refusal and not regard the patient as unreasonable. Similarly, the attitudes and experiences of siblings or children with chronic diseases, such as hypertension or diabetes, will influence the attitude and decision-making process of the elderly patient.

Social history

Physical separation of an elderly patient from his adult children is common in industrial societies. This physical separation is usually *not* accompanied by emotional abandonment. The family, or at least one member of the family, usually remains quite involved with the older patient whether the patient resides in the community or in a nursing home.

Knowledge of the patient's attitudes toward the family and vice versa ("Never got along with my daughter," "Was al-

ways independent," "My son-in-law doesn't want me to live in his house," or "We always had a good relationship") is important, as is the ability of the family to assist their elderly relative. If all of the adult children work full time, little daytime support can be given to a partly dependent older parent. Traveling time and distance to the older person's home, apartment, or nursing home and the health of the adult children ("My son had a stroke and can't visit me") may also influence how often visits are made and what services are provided. An interview with the family at a later date complements the interview with the patient and allows the interviewer to actually assess the health of the various family members, their attitudes toward the patient, and their ability to assist in taking care of the patient. Other important aspects of the social history include the patients reaction to retirement, death of a spouse, and/or loss of money and status, as well as to living arrangements, future plans, and/or the need for community services. There are many who develop increased religious feelings as life draws to its inevitable end; others, in contrast, disavow their religion for the first time.

Alcoholism is quite prevalent in late life. The elderly, more than those in other age groups, tend to deny their alcoholism. This probably reflects their generation's reaction to what they may perceive as antisocial behavior. The alert interviewer should detect the symptoms.

The clinician may, through the patient's spontaneous comments, learn how the patient feels about heroic medical measures in the case of life-threatening illness. Because this is an emotional issue, the clinician should probably not explore such measures at the initial interview unless the subject is introduced by the patient. As the patient-physician relationship develops, however, the patient's views may be explored. Discussions of the "living will" will be relevant for the elderly patient who wants to control or limit any efforts to prolong his life in the case of an acute, life-threatening illness. A "penultimate will" can be written by the mentally clear elderly individual who wants to name his guardian and thus control his economic, residential, and medical situation should he develop a chronic, irreversible dementia or aphasia that is not life threatening.[10]

Nutritional history

Clinical nutritional problems are not common in the elderly, except for obesity and protein-calorie malnutrition, which can easily be diagnosed. Protein-calorie malnutrition often occurs during a major illness in the hospital and in the demented individual who refuses food. Deficiencies in various vitamins and minerals in the elderly, such as vitamins A and C, riboflavin, iron, and calcium, have been detected. Except for iron, the implications of these deficiencies and other prolonged subclinical nutritional deficiencies in the elderly are unclear.

The interviewer should question the patient about practical matters related to nutrition, including:

1. How much and what he eats
2. How well he can chew
3. What diets were prescribed by previous physicians and what unusual fad diets he has been following
4. How much money he spends on food
5. Whether food stores are easily accessible
6. Whether fear of crime or of falling keeps the elderly person homebound
7. Whether proper kitchen facilities are available and if he can cook
8. How many hot meals he eats each week, which may provide a general indication of his nutritional status (Hot meals are offered to the elderly at many senior citizens', day care, and nutrition centers. Hot meals under such programs as Meals on Wheels can also be delivered to the homebound elderly.

A dietary history will reveal any diets that physicans have prescribed in the distant past and that are no longer suitable, as well as any long-term fad diets. The diabetic or low-sodium diet can often be altered with satisfactory patient compliance. Long-term fad diets, however, are difficult to manipulate, and vitamin supplements may be helpful in these cases. The possibility of alcoholism, the patient's level of activity, and his intake of dietary fiber should be investigated. Vitamins in over-the-counter preparations can cause complications in the elderly patient. For example, the folic acid found in many nonprescription preparations can induce a hematological response in patients with pernicious anemia, while the neurological manifestations continue to progress. A history of weight loss should not be attributed to diet alone without other causes searched for.

Medication history

Older people are the leading consumers of medications and account for 25% of all prescriptions in the United States. Multiple simultaneous medications are the rule, with a fortunate few taking no medications. An elderly patient who is ill and ambulatory may be taking 2 to 4 medications at the same time; a nursing home patient may be taking 3 to 6 medications; an acutely ill, hospitalized elderly patient may be taking 6 to 12 medications. In some instances, the number of medications is excessive. Often, there are multiple physicians and clinics prescribing for the same patient, so that he will come in with a "bag full." The clinician should examine and, with the aid of the *Physicians' Desk Reference,** identify all of the medications being taken. Prior physicians and pharmacies may also have to be contacted. Many symptoms and illnesses result from side effects of medications, including chemical effects, allergic effects, and drug interactions. Drug-related side effects are usually reversible on withdrawal of the medication. Symptoms may also develop because a patient does not take a drug in the prescribed frequency or amount. Nonprescription medications are frequently taken for pain, colds, sleep, and rheumatism. The interviewer should ask whether such medications are being taken.

Habituation and addiction to such medications as barbiturates (for sleep) and benzodiazepines (for sleep and anxiety) are not infrequent. The clinician should not discontinue a nighttime barbiturate taken for 20 years because he knows of a "paradoxical reaction by the elderly" to barbiturates. This reaction is occasionally found in an older person but not in a patient who has slept well for 20 years because of nighttime secobarbital or similar medication.

Sexual history

A sexual history is not essential in every clinical situation. In many cases, however, a sexual history will be valuable in understanding the patient's symptomatology and life-style.[11] To get this information, the interviewer must be

*Published by Medical Economics Co., a Litton division.

gentle, confident, and skillful. There may be many psychological difficulties for the younger interviewer in dealing with the older patient's sexuality.

The younger interviewer will quite often presume that there is little sexual activity and few sexual thoughts or impulses on the part of the older patient. Sexual activity continues, however, for a considerable percentage of older men, although often less frequently and with less extensive periods of intercourse. Older women living alone may be frustrated because they lack a sexual partner. At the same time, older persons are more likely to have sexual dysfunction because of the accumulation of illnesses, drugs, operations, and psychological and physical trauma that occur in late life.

Obtaining a sexual history requires a setting of privacy and confidentiality, an appearance of calm and confidence on the part of the interviewer, and a readiness to deal with relevant questions.

Questions by the interviewer should address such issues as:

1. Level of satisfaction
2. Sexual experience in comparison with earlier life
3. Sexual desire in comparison with earlier life
4. Frequency of masturbation
5. Effects of operations (prostatectomy, hysterectomy, abdominal perineal resection, lumbar sympathectomy, abdominal aortic aneurysmectomy), medications (diethylstilbestrol, methyldopa, diazepam, tricyclic antidepressants), and/or diseases (aortic-iliac occlusive disease, depression)
6. Effects of disability from a stroke or myocardial infarction on sexual function (The history should include a discussion of any self-im-

posed limitations because of a medical illness. For example, sexual function need not be curtailed because of compensated congestive heart failure or for arthritis unless these conditions are severe and disabling.)

Case histories

The following brief cases illustrate the kinds of situations that may be encountered:

Case 1. A 70-year-old retired accountant, in generally good physical and mental health, was scheduled for a transurethral prostatectomy as treatment for his bothersome benign prostatic hypertrophy. Prior to surgery, he made several long-distance calls to a physician in whom he had considerable confidence to ask extensive questions about the effect of this operative procedure on sexual function. He had not been told anything by his local physicians and had been too embarrassed to bring up the subject. Pertinent issues that should have been discussed include sterility from retrograde ejaculation and the infrequent occurrence (about 5%) of impotence with a transurethral prostatectomy.

Case 2. An 80-year-old man was seen in geriatric medical consultation because his wife had complained of his increasing "rage" behavior. She said (and he concurred) that when they argued over minor matters, he would at times come close to violence; once he threatened to strike her. This pattern had existed for about 2 to 3 years and was in sharp contrast to the relative calm that had existed between them for the previous 50 years of their relationship. The patient revealed that he had lost his potency about 3 years before and felt quite disturbed by this loss. The patient attributed his anger to his feeling of sexual inadequacy. His wife said that throughout their marriage he had been more aggressive and more interested in sexual activity than she had. A diagnostic evaluation to determine any possible occult neurological explanation for the rage reactions was negative.

Case 3. A 73-year-old woman had developed intractable itching of the perineum over the previous 4 years. The itching and scratching had led to an atrophic condition of the perineum. A medical and gynecological evaluation revealed no explanation. The patient's husband had died 5 years before and her brother-in-law, to whom she had been quite close, had died 4½ before. She had been actively masturbating for the previous 4 to 5 years.

Psychiatric history

Since almost all aspects of the elderly patient's functional ability will be affected by emotional illness, the psychiatric history is crucial. Mental illness is at least as frequent in the elderly as in the young and middle-aged. Some illnesses unique to late life are senile dementia of the Alzheimer type (SDAT) and nonprogressive benign memory loss. Depression is common and easily overlooked. Insomnia, constipation, or somatic complaints, all signs and symptoms of depression in middle age, may be present in the elderly patient with depression. The interviewer should ask directly about the patient's feelings of sadness, depression, and hopelessness; episodes of crying; recent losses of family, home, or pets; and, when privacy is assured, about suicidal thoughts.[12] A history of antidepressant or electroconvulsive therapy, institutionalization, or visitation to a psychiatrist or community mental health center should be specifically elicited.

Anxiety states are frequent among the elderly. Paranoid ideation and manic depressive behavior are seen occasionally. Acute or chronic dementia (organic brain syndrome) occurs in approximately 3% to 5% of the elderly living in the community and in 50% of those living in nursing homes. Perhaps 10% of these dementias are false dementias, or pseudodementias ("pseudosenility"), that are treatable and, at times, reversible. Specific techniques are described in Chapter 4.

SUMMARY

In summary, the interviewer must have a solid grasp of the techniques of conducting medical and psychiatric interviews and know how to adapt these techniques to the older person.[13]

The interviewer should recognize that ageism and sexism may bias his interview with the elderly patient. Special interview techniques, such as the life review, must be employed; and alternative sources of history may have to be used to confirm illnesses that have not been reported or that have presented with altered symptoms. The student or physician must be aware of the time and duration of the interview, the presence of family members and friends, and the problems of interviewing an elderly patient with multiple sensory deficits. The classic history-taking format must include questions directed at specific aspects relevant to the elderly, including nutrition, medication, and social history.

History taking and interviewing with the elderly can be a rewarding and fascinating experience if proper techniques are used.

REFERENCES

1. Steel, K.: Evaluation of the geriatric patient. In Reichel, W., editor: Clinical aspects of aging, Baltimore, 1978, The Williams & Wilkins Co., p. 3.
2. Hodkinson, H. M.: An outline of geriatrics, New York, 1975, Academic Press, Inc., p. ii.
3. Butler, R. N., and Lewis, M. I.: Aging and mental health, St. Louis, 1973, The C. V. Mosby Co., pp. 141–143.
4. Anderson, W. F.: Practical management of the elderly. (ed. 3), Oxford, Eng., 1976, Blackwell Scientific Publications Ltd., pp. 81–82.
5. Agate, J.: The practice of geriatrics (ed. 2), Springfield, Ill., 1970, Charles C Thomas, Publisher, pp. 53–55.
6. Comfort, A.: Non-threatening mental testing of the elderly, J. Am. Geriatr. Soc. **26:**261, 1978.
7. Caird, F. I., and Judge, T. G.: The assessment of the elderly patient, London, 1975, Pitman Medical Publishing Co. Ltd., p. 15.
8. De Gown, E. L., and De Gown, R. L.: Bedside diagnostic examination (ed. 3), New York, 1976, Macmillan Publishing Co., Inc.
9. Bates, B.: A guide to physical examination, Philadelphia, 1974, J. B. Lippincott Co.
10. Libow, L. S., and Zicklin, R.: The penultimate will: its potential as an instrument to protect the mentally deteriorated elderly, Gerontologist **13**(4):440, 1973.
11. Butler, R. N., and Lewis, M. I.: Sex after sixty, New York, 1976, Harper & Row, Publishers, Inc.
12. Williamson, J.: Depression. In Anderson, W. F., and Judge, T. G., editors: Geriatric medicine, New York, 1974, Academic Press, Inc., p. 74.
13. MacKinnon, R. A., and Michels, R.: The psychiatric interview in medical practice, Philadelphia, 1971, W. B. Saunders Co.

PROBLEM-SOLVING EXERCISES

1. Explore with your colleagues the types of satisfactions and problems you have had when interviewing elderly patients. What do you like or dislike about such interviews?
2. You, an elderly patient, and her adult daughter are seated in the room of an acute care hospital after the patient has been admitted for abdominal pain. How would you handle this triangle in the initial interview?
3. You have spent 15 minutes interviewing an 82-year-old woman with idiopathic Parkinson's disease and an extensive medical history who has come to the outpatient clinic of your medical school hospital. The resident who is supervising you says that the clinic is backed up and that you should hurry. What are your reactions to this situation and what would you do?
4. With the help of a colleague who wears your glasses and has cotton in his ears to simulate a conductive hearing loss, as with

impacted cerumen, demonstrate the proper techniques used to assure communication with an elderly patient whose vision and hearing are impaired. Discuss the techniques and methods used to overcome your colleague's visual and hearing deficits.

5. Without an introductory statement as to what you plan to do, perform a FROMAJE mental status examination (see Chapter 5) on an elderly individual who is mentally clear. Then, perform the examination on another patient with an introductory statement. Discuss the patient's reaction to each approach.

6. Attempt the life review technique with an elderly patient. Explore your feelings and reactions to this type of emotionally charged information.

7. Explore your preconceptions about the sexual life of a 75-year-old woman with hypertension and diabetes who has recently undergone an amputation of her left leg below the knee and comes under your care during her rehabilitation. Consider two situations: (a) she lives in an apartment, and (b) she lives in a nursing home. How would you introduce the topic of sexual function or dysfunction with this patient?

8. How would you deal with an elderly patient who, in the middle of the mental status evaluation interjects: "Why are you asking me all these stupid questions? Go away and ask somebody else!"

9. Obtain a nutritional history from Mr. S., and 80-year-old man who is retired, lives alone in a two-room apartment in New York City, and has a net annual income of $3,800.

ANSWERS TO PROBLEM-SOLVING EXERCISES

1. Potential satisfactions include learning about the patient's life history by allowing him to reminisce, learning about some of the advances in medicine through patients who actually lived through them, and feeling respect and admiration toward the older survivor of life's course. Potential problems include the length of the interview, the need to talk to the family to clarify the history, difficulty in overcoming the sensory deficits of the patient, and the need to seek alternate sources of history.

2. Possibilities include the following. Consider the dynamics of each.
   - Asking the daughter to leave the room while you talk with her mother
   - Asking the mother whether she minds if the daughter stays with you while you interview both of them
   - Talking to the daughter in the waiting room while the mother stays in her room

3. Reactions include:
   - Speeding up the interview and examination in an attempt to cover all aspects of the usual clinical history and physical examination
   - Asking the patient to return for another visit
   - Discussing with the resident your ideas that doing an adequate history and physical examination with some elderly patients takes longer and that fewer patients should be scheduled on days when the number of elderly patients is large
   - Staying late at the clinic to finish all the patients assigned to you

4. You should use the following techniques:
   - Face the patient with light falling on your face.
   - Speak clearly and somewhat slower than usual.
   - Do not yell into the patient's ear.
   - Exclude all background noise such as radios and paging systems.

5. A mental status evaluation need not be done on every elderly patient. When it is indicated, you should be cautious about how you introduce the examination. Launching into an intense, rapid-fire series of questions requiring factual recall may cause the elderly patient to become anxious and resent you. On the other hand, introducing the fact that you will be examining the mental status of the patient ("how

you think") may also make the elderly patient uncomfortable and anxious.

6. Your reactions to the life review may include:
    - Interest in the patient's fascinating life history
    - Uneasiness about numerous losses
    - Uneasiness about the necessity of discussing death
    - Uneasiness about desires to physically comfort the elderly individual
    - Uneasiness about the length of the life review

7. You should discuss sexual function and dysfunction with this patient because of the problems that she may be having from her amputation, her diabetes mellitus, and any visual loss from the diabetes. This discussion should take place regardless of her living arrangements. Sexuality can be discussed at the first interview or at any subsequent interview, depending on the nature of the chief complaint and how comfortable you feel about the subject.

8. The reaction of anger toward you can result from the elderly patient's real anger at the length of the interview, the questions being asked, uneasiness about loss of control, or anxiety because he cannot answer all of the questions you are asking him. On the other hand, anger may be a means by which the patient with mild or moderate organic mental syndrome can hold you at a distance rather than have you become aware of his decline in cognitive function.

9. You should ask the following questions while taking an initial history:
    - How well can the patient chew?
    - How many hot meals does he eat per day?
    - What about his past and present diet? Have there been any fad diets?
    - How far is the grocery store from his home?
    - Can he cook?
    - Has he had a recent weight loss?
    - What is his intake of alcohol? Of vitamins?
    - Is he taking any medications that could conceivably interact with vitamins?

- Has he had any loss or change in appetite?

POSTTEST*

1. Which of the following is (are) characteristic of interviewing and history taking with the elderly?
    a. More time is required to complete an initial evaluation than with the middle-aged patient.
    b. A family member should always be present during the initial interview.
    c. The oral history may have to be complemented by other sources of information.
    d. It is often necessary to obtain a sexual history, but not necessarily during the first interview.
    e. The appropriate time and setting are important factors in determining the outcome of a mental status examination.

2. Which of the following attitudes or biases on the part of the interviewer can present potential problems in interviewing the elderly patient?
    a. Biases about normal aging
    b. Biases about sexual activity in old age
    c. Ideas based on previous experiences with grandparents
    d. The idea that nursing homes are to be avoided

3. In comparing history taking with elderly patients and history-taking with young or middle-aged patients, one would expect which of the following to be true?
    a. Symptoms specific for illness in the young or middle-aged may have different significance in the elderly.
    b. Multiple chief complaints are more frequently expressed by elderly patients.
    c. The elderly patient tends to underreport

---

*Some questions may have more than one correct answer.

illness more than the young or middle-aged patient.

d. Signs of depression arising from loss of job, home, or spouse are less frequently encountered with elderly patients.

4. When interviewing an elderly patient with functional deficits in communication, particularly in the acute care hospital or nursing home, the interviewer may need to:
   a. Optimize the setting so the patient can lip-read, and face the patient directly, allowing for proper light on the interviewer's face.
   b. Ask the patient to insert his dentures
   c. Check to see whether the patient has cerumen in his ear canals and remove it
   d. Ask the patient to insert his hearing aid before starting the interview.

5. What information would you wish to obtain at a minimum, from an elderly patient in order to complete the:
   • Nutritional history?
   • Medication history?
   • Social history?
   • Psychiatric history?

6. Sources of additional history include:
   a. The relative's description of the patient's symptoms and dysfunction
   b. The transfer summary on the previously hospitalized patient just admitted to a skilled nursing facility and vice versa
   c. Reports of pathological specimens
   d. All other medical records, including those from prior physicians and institutions
   e. The "bag" of medications brought from the patient's home

7. A sexual history in the elderly:
   a. Should be pursued because sexual dysfunction can result from multiple medical, surgical, and psychological problems encountered in late life
   b. Should always be done during the first interview
   c. Need not be explored in older women

d. May be valuable in understanding the patient's life-style

8. The family history of the elderly patient may be helpful in suggesting a diagnosis of:
   a. Glaucoma
   b. Idiopathic hypertrophic subaortic stenosis
   c. Diabetes mellitus
   d. Coronary artery disease
   e. Cancer

ANSWERS TO PRETEST AND POSTTEST

1. a, c, d, and e. The presence of a family member at the initial interview is sometimes desirable. Interviewing a family member may be necessary. Whether done in the presence of the patient depends on clinical judgment. Even if the patient has impaired mental function, however, it is still important to interview the patient alone initially to get an unbiased assessment of the patient's mental status and functional ability. Obtaining a sexual history may be necessary because of the increased, yet often unreported, prevalence of sexual dysfunction in the elderly associated with physical illness, medications, past prostatic or gynecological operations, or psychological problems.

2. All of these. Since the majority of elderly patients are women, the interviewer will more often be dealing with an elderly woman. Biases about how normal aging affects function, sexuality in late life, and the interviewer's previous experience with older women (mother, grandmother, teacher, etc.) may subtly affect the interviewer's approach. Nursing homes are a necessity for many older persons who require a variety of services and supportive care beyond that available in the community.

3. a, b, and c. Altered presentation of illness, multiple chief complaints, and underreporting of illness are basic concerns in geriatric history taking. Losses, which are more frequent in the elderly, play a major role in causing depression.

4. All of these. All are measures that will maximize communication.

5. Nutrition history:
   • How well can the patient chew?
   • How many hot meals does he eat per day?
   • What about his past and present diets? Have there been any fad diets?

- How far is the grocery store from his home?
- Can he cook?
- Has he had a recent weight loss?
- What is his intake of alcohol? Of vitamins?

Medication history
- What are the patient's medications (prescription and nonprescription)? What has he taken in the past? Ask the patient and/or relative to bring all medications to the interview.
- Have there been any problems with compliance?

    Can the patient tell the difference between similar-looking medications?

    Does he know his medication regimen?

    Do any of the medications cause side effects that have caused him to discontinue them?

    Does he have his medication regimen in writing?

Social history:
- Where does the patient live?
- What family or friends support him and in what ways?
- What community services (senior citizens' center, Meals on Wheels, visiting nurse service, etc.) is he using?
- What are his feelings about retirement, death of a spouse, and other losses?

Psychiatric history:
- Is there any past history of depression? Of suicidal thoughts? Does the patient take any antidepressant medications? Has he had electroconvulsive therapy? Any medications for sleep?
- Has he, or is he using, any outpatient community mental health center?
- Has he used any antianxiety medications in the past?

6. All of these. A relative's description of the patient's functional abilities (his ability to walk, care for himself, manage his finances, etc.) is usually more accurate than his description of the patient's specific symptoms (chest pain, urinary symptoms, etc.). Transfer summaries on hospitalized patients admitted to skilled nursing facilities are often inaccurate. Reports of pathological specimens, when available, are reliable sources of additional history.

7. a and d. The sexual history should be obtained when the patient-doctor relationship seems appropriate. This may be during the first interview. Regardless of the timing, the sexual history should be obtained from the elderly patient if there is any likelihood that it will enhance the diagnostic and therapeutic situation.

8. All of these.

Chapter 4

Geriatric psychiatry

FRED B. CHARATAN, FREDRICK T. SHERMAN, and LESLIE S. LIBOW

EDUCATIONAL OBJECTIVES
Attitudinal

The student should:

1. Deal with the biases that he may have about how normal aging affects the mind, including the ideas that:
   a. A person's intellect declines with age
   b. A person's intelligence quotient (IQ) and verbal ability decline with age
   c. Normal aging leads to senility
2. Confront the myth that all mental illness in late life leads to or is equivalent to senility°
3. Develop a positive outlook toward the diagnosis and treatment of mental disorders in late-life
4. Develop a positive outlook toward the diagnosis and treatment of acute and chronic organic brain syndromes in the elderly

Cognitive

The student should:

1. Understand the psychology of normal aging
2. Know the epidemiology and classification of the mental disorders of old age, including depression, dementia, paranoid states, psychoneurosis, and transient situational disorders
3. Understand the concept of reversible organic mental states (pseudosenilities) in the elderly and their differential diagnoses
4. Know the various treatments available in geriatric psychiatry, including the use of psychopharmacological agents (different doses), electroconvulsive therapy (ECT), reality orientation therapy (pros and cons), psychotherapy, and community health care centers

5. Know how to:
   a. Diagnose and treat the emotionally ill elderly, including the acutely confused psychotic and nonpsychotic elderly patient
   b. Weigh the factors for and against institutionalization of the mentally impaired elderly
   c. Manage interrelating medical and psychiatric illness
6. Understand the rationale for the use of the team approach

Skill

The student should:

1. Be able to take a psychogeriatric history
2. Be able to conduct a psychiatric interview and elicit the main symptoms and signs of the common mental disorders of old age
3. Know the differential diagnoses of dementia and confusion in the elderly
4. Be able to perform a mental status examination using the FROMAJE or other technique (see Chapter 5)
5. Be able to explain to the patient and/or family what dementia is and the various problems arising from it (financial decisions, institutionalization, selling of home or apartment, etc.)

PRETEST°

1. Objective evidence of aging is found in all the items below *except:*
   a. Slowing of responses
   b. Lower IQ

°Senility is a nonmedical term that refers to an overall decline in mental function, usually an organic brain syndrome

°Some questions may have more than one correct answer.

c. Nonprogressive memory impairment
d. Reduction in sexual activity
2. The prevalence of chronic organic brain syndrome in the population above age 80 is:
   a. 5%
   b. 12%
   c. 22%
   d. 30%
   e. 45%
3. List the three major diagnostic groupings of the *psychoses* of old age.
4. The neurohistology of senile dementia of the Alzheimer type (SDAT) characteristically shows:
   a. Wallerian degeneration
   b. Inclusion bodies
   c. Giant cells
   d. Large numbers of senile plaques
   e. Basophil granules
5. In multi-infarct dementia, can the degree of mental impairment during life be correlated with the volume of infarcted brain observed at autopsy?
6. A causal relationship to so-called secondary dementia can be found in all of the following conditions *except:*
   a. Hypothyroidism
   b. Neurosyphilis
   c. Vitamin B_{12} deficiency
   d. Head injury
   e. Paranoia
7. Senile paranoid states respond exceptionally well to:
   a. Benzodiazepines
   b. Phenothiazines
   c. Antidepressants
   d. Anticonvulsants
   e. Amphetamines
8. List any five losses that occur in old age that may lead to depression.
9. The most important question in the psychiatric evaluation of elderly depressed patients is:
   a. Paranoid feelings

b. Homicidal impulses
c. Thought disorder
d. Suicidal feelings
e. Hallucinations
10. An early feature of parkinsonism associated with the use of the major tranquilizers is:
    a. Tardive dyskinesia
    b. Emotional incontinence
    c. Sleep reversal
    d. Cogwheel rigidity
    e. Akathisia

Age is best defined as change associated with the passage of time.[1] Some of the changes in the aging body are obvious; equally important are the psychological changes that gradually develop as youth evolves into middle age and, eventually, old age. Butler has argued effectively that aging is an intrinsic part of the human developmental cycle.[2] The psychological profile of the older person, then, displays both strengths and weaknesses, declines and gains. Understanding the intellectual, emotional, and behavioral characteristics of the aging person will help one become more effective in providing health care to this group.

PSYCHOLOGY OF NORMAL AGING

If one asks an older person, "When did you first become aware of being old?" the person may reply as follows:
1. "When I had difficulty walking or fell" (There is a breakdown of the locomotor apparatus.)
2. "When I became nervous" (There are increasing tendencies to fret or worry, with a greater susceptibility to depression.)
3. "When my hearing and vision got worse" (There is gradually increas-

ing hearing loss (presbycusis) and reduced visual acuity with impaired night vision.)

4. "When my skin became wrinkled and my hair turned gray" (There is graying and loss of hair, and wrinkling of the skin together with the appearance of "age spots" or pigmented areas on the hands and face. Increasing depositions of subcutaneous fat lead to thickening of the figure. The integument also loses its elasticity, so that the nubility of youth is replaced by the loose skin folds of age. These changes are particularly serious narcissistic wounds for women.)

5. "When I started to feel tired and got out less" (There is a reduction in stamina, and recuperation after effort takes longer.)

6. "When I started to need daytime naps" (Aging is associated with lighter nighttime sleep [reduced amounts of rapid eye movement—REM—and stage 4 sleep], frequent wakening, and decreased total sleep.[3] Complaints of insomnia by elderly people must be evaluated in the light of this altered sleep pattern.)

7. "When I started to forget minor details" (A mild, nonprogressive memory impairment, mainly affecting recent memory, is seen in the elderly. In some cases this is sufficient to interfere with the person's ability to function socially; for example, the person cannot recall the name of a familiar acquaintance or forgets to keep an appointment.)

8. "When I started to lose my sexual desires" (Sexual activity declines with age; about 50% of persons 60 to 71 years of age have regular and frequent intercourse, whereas only about 15% to 25% of persons over the age of 75 remain sexually active.[4,5])

Being old is also a function of the perception of other people. For example, some youths regard anyone over the age of 30 as being "old." Nevertheless, every aging person reaches a point in his development when he is recognized as having joined the community of elders. Society, government, and tradition have, unfortunately, made 65 or 70 the age when this acknowledgment frequently occurs.

Chronological, biological, and psychological age, however, do not necessarily coincide. Some elderly people retain a remarkable youthfulness of spirit, just as there are young people whose thoughts, feelings, and behavior bear the stamp of premature age. Longevity in elderly men has been correlated positively with the organization and complexity of the day's activities.[6] Creativity and achievement are often preserved into advanced old age, as exemplified by Michelangelo, who completed the dome of St. Peter's at the age of 75; by Grandma Moses, who began painting at the age of 75 and completed her most famous painting, "Christmas Eve," at the age of 100; and by the writer P. G. Wodehouse, a tribute to the persistence of so-called verbal intelligence, who died at the age of 95, writing to the end.

INTELLECTUAL CHANGES OF NORMAL AGING
Slowness

A decline in the speed of response is a well-recognized characteristic of the elderly. This decline is probably not due to slowing in the conduction time of nerve impulses, since the conduction rate in old single nerve fibers is only 15% less

than that in young ones.[1] Sensory deprivation resulting from sensorineural deafness and/or visual impairment may contribute to slowness.

Memory impairment

Elderly people frequently suffer from a
mild, nonprogressive memory impairment. This condition is in contrast to the
severe, progressive, global impairment of
memory that is observed, for example, in
patients with senile dementia of the Alzheimer type (SDAT) or multi-infarct
dementia (MID). (Such patients make up
a minority of the elderly population.) The
healthy elderly know that when they forget something, it will "come back," without special effort on their part, at a later
time.

Memory for recent events is more affected than remote memory. There are
two explanations for the older person's
difficulty with registration, retention, and
recall of current experience. One explanation is that age-related neuronal loss
reduces the number of functioning cir-
cuits available for new memory storage.
The second explanation is that the older
person may have less interest in current
events. His interest is invested in his vast
store of old memories. This interest and
emotion are often related during remi-
niscing, a favorite activity of the elderly.

Changes in creativity and originality

Lehman[7] has studied the effects of aging on many fields of achievement:
chemistry, practical inventions, chess,
medical discoveries, philosophy, music,
art, and literature. In general, for persons
in all fields, originality and creativity
tend to "peak" (with few exceptions)
between the ages of 30 and 40. Work in
metaphysics, politics, literature, history,
and philosophy improves slightly with
age. On the other hand, mathematical

and chemical discoveries usually origi-
nate before the person is 30. Projective
psychological testing in elderly people
demonstrates their thinking to be more
"concrete," routine, and stereotyped.
Yet, creativity in late life is common.

Prolonged learning time

Learning depends to a large degree on
efficient memorization. Learning in the
elderly is slower than in the young. Difficulty in reproducing recently acquired
material is common to all aging mammals
and can be demonstrated in elderly rats
running mazes in the psychological testing laboratory.

Intelligence tests reveal little or no
decline in vocabulary or information
scores in the elderly, but they do show a
relative decline in performance (digit
symbol, picture arrangement, etc.). When
tests are speeded up, the elderly do poorly in comparison with the young.

Work performance

Decline in psychomotor skills with
aging suggests that older persons should
not be placed in work situations requiring continuous rapid action. Loss of
speed, however, tends to be compensated for by greater accuracy and attention
to detail. Elderly workers are no less
productive, reliable, or accident prone
than younger workers.[8]

EMOTIONAL CHANGES OF AGING

It has been said that people age as they
have lived. Nevertheless, there are some
emotional changes associated with growing old.

Changes in motivation

Bromley[9] points out unequivocally that
"motivation in general (drive) appears to
decrease in old age, probably because of

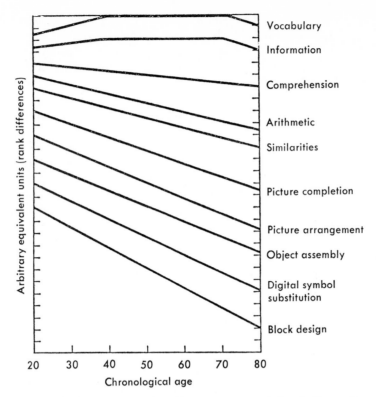

Fig. 4-1. Simplified illustration of age differences in Wechsler-Bellevue functions expressed in equivalent units (From Bromley, D. B.: The psychology of human aging, ed. 2, Harmondsworth, Eng., 1974, Penguin Books Ltd, p. 196. © D. B. Bromley, 1966, 1974. Reprinted by permission of Penguin Books Ltd.

decreased energy and poorer arousal mechanisms; some kinds of motivation, including sexuality, fall off fairly steadily." He qualifies this statement by pointing out that "age changes in motivation, however, are very much a matter of continuity and development, depending upon temperamental qualities and experiences in life." Some elderly people need strong incentives, support, and encouragement to embark on new ventures.

Engagement versus disengagement

In late life, motivations toward withdrawal, avoidance, and substitution predominate. This is quite commonly be-

cause the older person's psychological resources cannot sustain the demands being made on them. These tendencies toward withdrawal into a more limited, private, and family-centered life-style have been called disengagement.[10] Some gerontologists argue that disengagement is not only correlated with successful aging, but is essential for aging; others point out that the majority of aging people maintain fairly steady amounts of activity and do not withdraw from society.

Hence, the amount of engagement or disengagement may be influenced more by past life-styles and socioeconomic forces than by any intrinsic or inevitable process. Comfort[11] maintains that society has negative expectations of the elderly, who are expected to be invisible, non-contributory, and sexually inactive. Such expectations might well lead to disengagement of older persons who, in a more favorable climate, could still make significant contributions to society.

Elderly people are more aware of their bodies as functions decline and disorders accumulate within. Functions such as defecation, urination, eating, and sleep, become more gratifying and meaningful than in youth. Hypochondriasis is very common in even the mentally well-preserved elderly.[12] Its importance lies in the tendency of elderly people to "shop around" from physician to physician in an endless search for relief from such feelings; this practice adds enormously to the cost of health care as investigations are duplicated and admissions to hospitals multiply. Hypochondrias may be the initial manifestation of depression. Furthermore, it is known that elderly people who are hypochondriacal are more liable to become severely depressed and to attempt suicide.[13] Finally, the hypochondriacal elderly, especially where the feeling is covert, may, in an effort at rejuvenation, become involved with the promises of eternal youth, through such means as queen bee jelly, megavitamin therapy (e.g., vitamin E), and injections of embryonic salts.

NOSOLOGY OF MENTAL DISORDERS IN OLD AGE

Geriatric psychiatry began at the end of the nineteenth century. At that time senile dementia, arteriosclerotic dementia (now called multi-infarct dementia [MID]), and the presenile dementias were differentiated from each other and from other organic psychoses, such as neurosyphilis. Some benign psychoses were recognized as occurring in old age, but their natural history and significance were doubtful. Most psychiatrists at that time believed that even affective and paranoid psychoses were early manifestations of senile dementia. It was believed that whatever the psychosis occurring in old age, the final common pathway was inexorable dementia and death.[14]

Kay and associates,[15] however, showed that the outcome of mental illness with predominantly depressive or paranoid features in elderly subjects was comparatively favorable, that it did not progress to dementia, that it did not necessarily shorten life expectancy (as does chronic dementia) and that it had a favorable outcome when properly treated.

According to Roth,[16] "In earlier life, organic psychosis are comparatively rare; in old age they are commonplace, and their manifestations so protean that they can never be omitted from consideration when arriving at a diagnosis. Moreover, if organic disorders are common, organic damage of a less obvious and more limited kind is ubiquitous in advanced age."

Butler[17] has warned against the use of the term *senility:* "Senility is not, properly speaking, a medical diagnosis, but is instead a wastebasket term for a range of symptoms that include (minimally) some memory impairment or forgetfulness, difficulty in attention and concentration, decline in intellectual grasp and ability, and decreased emotional responsiveness to others." Senility can be a term of dismissal for what others are unwilling to understand about the elderly individual. Accurate diagnosis is, therefore, just as important in geriatric psychiatry as in any other branch of medicine.

The following is a simple and practical

classification of mental disorders in old age:

I. Organic brain syndromes
   A. Acute (all potentially reversible)
   B. Chronic
      1. Senile dementia of the Alzheimer type (primary dementia)
      2. Multi-infarct dementia (vascular dementia)
      3. Secondary dementias (some potentially reversible)
II. Paranoid states
III. Affective disorders
   A. Depression
   B. Mania
IV. Psychoneuroses
V. Personality disorders
VI. Transient situational disorders (anxiety and/or depression, for example, caused by changes in life situations, such as losses of relatives and/or change of place of residence)

Acute organic brain syndrome
Clinical features

Acute organic brain syndrome, a common condition, is the response of the aged brain to physical or psychosocial stress. The brain of the elderly person may respond with confusion under stress. Other terms used for this condition are acute confusional state, acute delirium, and acute brain failure. The acute organic brain syndrome is caused by a potentially reversible impairment of neuronal function: anoxic, toxic, nutritional, metabolic, or traumatic. Many of the causes are extracerebral.

A pathognomonic feature is the presence of lucid intervals wherein the patient may temporarily be mentally clear, followed by a worsening of symptoms. The lucid interval soon disappears, and the patient displays clouded consciousness, accompanied by one or more of the following: disorientation, impaired attention and concentration, impairment of memory, an intellectual defect, poor judgment, and/or a labile mood.

The patient's conversation may be rambling and irrelevant, with occasional hallucinations or delusions. He may become aggressive and uncooperative, especially if attempts are made to restrain him. Refusal of food and fluid are not uncommon, and insomnia may be severe. The neurological examination is usually negative, except for the abnormal mental status.

Underlying causes

There are a number of possible causes of acute organic brain syndrome, both cerebral and extracerebral; and it is important to methodically look for the cause of an acute confusional state in an elderly patient, since it may be reversible. Depression or acute emotional stress, usually following the death of a spouse, may appear similar to organic brain syndrome and must be differentiated from it.

Potentially reversible causes of acute and/or chronic organic brain syndromes (pseudosenility) have been outlined as follows[18]:

I. Medication-induced disorders
   A. Errors in self-administration
   B. Drug interactions, such as alpha-methyldopa and haloperidol, or ethyl alcohol and chlorpropramide
   C. Use of L-dopa, indomethacin, steroid compounds, cimetidine, and rifampin, as well as many other drugs that can cause confusion
   D. Use of chlorpropramide and, to a much lesser extent, tolbutamide, which can lead to hyponatremia from inappropriate ADH secretion
   E. Use of all drugs that act on the central nervous system (CNS), including major and minor tranquilizers, hypnotics, and tricyclic antidepressants

II. Metabolic imbalance
 A. Hypercalcemia secondary to multiple myeloma, primary hyperparathyroidism, ectopic parathyroid hormone (PTH) secretion from carcinoma of the lung, thiazide diuretics, or inappropriate doses of vitamin D
 B. Hypocalcemia secondary to malabsorption syndrome or hypoparathyroidism after thyroidectomy
 C. Hypoglycemia associated with oral hypoglycemic agents or overzealous attempts to control blood glucose with insulin
 D. Hyperglycemia associated with ketoacidosis, lactic acidosis, or hyperosmolar states
 E. Hypothyroidism secondary to previous thyroidectomy or idiopathic causes
 F. Hyperthyroidism presenting as apathy, depression, or a confusional state
 G. Hypernatremia secondary to dehydration in ill patients being fed by tube
 H. Hyponatremia due to inappropriate ADH effects secondary to medication, pneumonia, or primary brain disorders, such as a stroke
 I. Azotemia secondary to obstructive uropathy or overzealous diuresis (e.g., with furosemide)
 J. Miscellaneous: hepatic failure, renal failure, alcohol withdrawal syndrome, hypothermia

III. Cardiovascular disorders
 A. Acute myocardial infarction (acute myocardial infarction will present mainly as confusion in 13% of elderly patients)
 B. Decreased cardiac output secondary to congestive heart failure (CHF), dysrhythmia, or pulmonary embolism

IV. CNS disorders: vascular
 A. Transient ischemic attacks (TIAs)
 B. Cerebrovascular accidents (CVAs)
 C. Subdural hematoma (20% of all intracranial masses in the elderly)
 D. Tumors

 1. Metastasis from lung, breast, and others
 2. Primary

V. Respiratory disorders
 A. Pneumonia from fever, hypoxia, or associated CNS infection
 B. Chronic lung disease with hypoxia or hypercapnia
 C. Pulmonary emboli

VI. Miscellaneous disorders
 A. Normal-pressure hydrocephalus characterized by incontinence, ataxia, and progressive dementia
 B. Agitation and confusion due to fecal impaction
 C. Postoperative dementia secondary to hypotension or an as-yet-to-be-explained mechanism
 D. Posttraumatic disorder, such as after a fall or a fractured hip
 E. Any febrile condition, such as urinary tract infection or pneumonia
 F. Relocation or transfer confusion occurring as the result of a move from one setting to another, as from a hospital to a nursing home
 G. Nutritional deficiencies: vitamin B_{12}, folic acid deficiencies, etc.
 H. Nonmetastatic CNS effects of neoplasm (e.g. mental depression or multifocal demylinating lesion).

Prognosis

About 50% of all cases of acute organic brain syndrome will clear after several weeks or months when it is properly diagnosed and the patient treated. Of the remainder of patients with this disorder, half will die within a year and the other half will develop a clinical picture similar to SDAT.[19]

Chronic organic brain syndrome: the dementias
Clinical features

Chronic organic brain syndrome comprises a group of conditions wherein there is a decline, usually irreversible and permanent, in mental function because of cerebral disease. There is a decline in intellect and personality, in memory, in orientation, in the capacity for conceptual thought, and, often, in affect. Early signs may be impaired judgment, such as wandering; inability to handle money or marketing; or self-exposure in the case of elderly men. Progressive forgetfulness, disorientation, and confusion appear, followed by difficulty in grasping new situations, with regression to a childish level of behavior and conversation.

The majority of these patients suffer from SDAT, a disease of unknown etiology. It is generally believed that the neuropathology of SDAT is identical with that found in presenile Alzheimer's disease.[20] Both are characterized by nerve cell fallout, especially in the neocortex, and by the widespread emergence of neurofibrillary tangles, senile plaques, and granulovacuolar degeneration. The prevalence rate of chronic organic brain syndrome rises steeply to as much as 22% of the elderly population over the age of 80 (Fig. 4-2).

In both sexes life expectancy of patients suffering from SDAT is shortened to around 2 years from the time the disease is definitely established.[21] The customary terminal illness, pneumonia, may be overdiagnosed.[22] Other possible causes of death include so-called benign neglect, incorrect diagnoses and treatments, malnutrition, dehydration, and, finally,

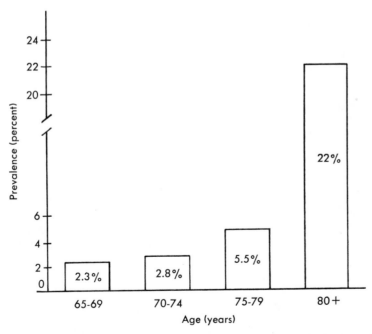

Fig. 4-2. Prevalence of chronic organic brain syndrome in the elderly. (Based on data from Kay, D., and others: Mental illness and hospital usage in the elderly: a random sample followed up, Comprehens. Psychiatry **2**:26, 1970.)

some unknown systemic disease that produced both the dementia and the increased death rate.[22]

Diagnosis

The diagnosis of chronic organic brain syndrome is made on the basis of the history, physical examination, and laboratory tests. Reversible causes should always be looked for.

History. Mental deterioration (severe memory impairment, loss of self-motivation, tendency to wander, and inability to carry out the activities of daily living (ADL) without continuous supervision) is progressive over a period of months or years. Often there is a worsening of symptoms at night ("sundown syndrome"). Habit deterioration as well as urinary and/or fecal incontinence are not uncommon.

Physical examination. A complete mental status examination using the FROMAJE technique (see Chapter 5) or another test of mental status should be performed.[18,23,24] The patient should have a thorough physical examination, with the clinician particularly looking for those diseases that can lead to reversible chronic dementia, such as hypothyroidism; hyperthyroidism; vitamin B_{12} or folic acid deficiency; chronic infectious diseases, such as pulmonary tuberculosis or bacterial endocarditis; or heart failure.

The neurological examination does not usually show signs of focal deficit in SDAT. In MID and dementia from cerebral masses, however, there can be both focal findings and a poor mental status. Primitive reflexes (snout, suck, grasp, and palmar-mental) should also be performed. These reflexes, while present in some normal elderly people, are found more frequently in patients with chronic organic brain syndrome.[25] It should be remembered that there are certain age-related changes in the neurological examination, including (1) loss of the ankle jerk in about 5% to 10% of the elderly population; (2) loss of the superficial abdominal reflexes in 20% of elderly men and approximately 50% of elderly women;[26] and loss of vibratory sense, especially over the medial malleolus. Being aware of these potential alterations in the physical examination will prevent confusion with focal findings.

Laboratory tests. Certain laboratory tests should be done in all patients with chronic (or acute) cognitive decline in order to explore any possibility of a reversible cause. These screening tests include:

A. Routine
  1. Complete blood count (CBC)
  2. Erythrocyte sedimentation rate
  3. Serum sodium, potassium, and chloride concentrations, blood urea nitrogen (BUN)
  4. Serum calcium and phosphorus concentrations
  5. Liver function tests, including SGOT, SGPT, total bilirubin, and alkaline phosphatase
  6. Serum B_{12} and folate concentrations
  7. Serological test for syphilis (VDRL)
  8. Serum T_4 and T_3 resin uptake or TBG level
  9. Chest x-ray study
  10. Electrocardiogram (ECG)
B. Recommended but not routine: computerized axial tomography (CAT) scan of the head (Although the diagnosis of SDAT cannot be made by CAT scan, one can observe the 4% to 8% of focal brain lesions presenting as dementia.)
C. Elective
  1. Skull x-rays (Because of the increased incidence of a calcified pineal gland with aging, a midline shift is likely to be seen if an intracranial mass is present. Skull x-ray studies, however, can

usually be omitted if a computerized axial tomography is to be performed.)

2. Spinal tap (It may be difficult to assess whether nuchal rigidity in an elderly individual is from local cervical spine disease, muscle rigidity, or inflammation of the meninges. An examination of the cerebrospinal fluid is indicated if physical examination cannot clarify the cause.)

3. Brain scans (Radioisotopic scanning has become less popular in the evaluation of mental decline and has been replaced by the CAT scan.)

4. Electroencephalogram (The electroencephalogram [EEG] is likely to be abnormal in the elderly patient with SDAT and usually demonstrates diffuse slowing. The severity of the slowing on the EEG, however, does not correlate with the degree of cerebral atrophy as measured by the CAT scan.)

5. Radionuclide cisternography (This test is used when normal-pressure hydrocephalus [NPH] is suspected. Clinically, NPH should be suspected if the patient develops the following symptoms: ataxic gait, dementia, and urinary and/or fecal incontinence. The CAT scan will show large ventricles without cortical atrophy.)

6. Pneumoencephalography (This test is seldom used in the elderly because of its high morbidity and because the information gleaned from the CAT scan is more helpful.)

Multi-infarct dementia

Less common than SDAT is MID. As its name (multi-infarct dementia) implies, MID is caused by multiple small strokes or infarcts that occur over time.[27] The condition has a stepwise course, occurs at a younger age, is more common in men, is associated with hypertension, and frequently is accompanied by neurological signs. See Table 4-1 for a differentiation of MID from SDAT.

Thrombosis, embolism, and, less commonly, hemorrhage cause cerebral infarction, resulting in areas of softening. Roth[16] and his colleagues in England have been able to demonstrate a correlation between the degree of dementia measured during life and the volume of infarction observed and calculated at autopsy. They believe that the cutoff point is about 50 cc of infarcted brain.

Underlying causes

It has been found that only about 10% to 15% of all cases of chronic organic brain syndrome are due to potentially reversible causes, such as myxedema, vitamin B_{12} or folate deficiency, brain

Table 4-1. Differentiation of MID from SDAT

MID	SDAT
Men more commonly affected	Women more commonly affected
Younger: 60 years and over	Older: 80 years and over
Stuttering or episodic course	Insidious, progressive course
Hypertension common	Usually normotensive
Focal neurological signs common	Focal neurological signs rare
Signs of arteriosclerotic heart disease, peripheral vascular disease, and/or embolization elsewhere common	May or may not be signs of arteriosclerotic heart disease or peripheral vascular disease

tumor, and neurosyphilis.[18,28] It should be noted that even though an underlying cause is diagnosed and treated, the dementia may persist. The mental status of a chronically confused patient with myxedema, for example, may not improve with thyroid replacement, because the patient also has SDAT. The list of potentially reversible causes of acute and chronic organic brain syndromes is essentially the same (see pp. 65 and 66).

Paranoid states: clinical features in late life

An elderly person in a senile paranoid state believes himself to be the object of hostile attention by others, often neighbors or members of his own family. He may have ideas of reference or frank paranoid delusions (e.g., that he is being spied on by Communists or unknown persecutors). The most common types of delusion are that the patient's family is trying to steal his money or possessions, and that the food is poisoned. Paranoid ideas may generate grandiosity. For example, if the patient believes he is the target of persecution, he may be convinced that he is a superior or important person, such as an inventor, a national leader, or a deity.

There are several predisposing conditions in the evolution of the paranoid state in elderly individuals. These include:

1. *A suspicious, sensitive, socially isolated premorbid personality:* Typically, an elderly widow or spinster who has lived alone for many years becomes increasingly eccentric.

2. *Deafness:* Deafness may predispose an elderly person to paranoid feelings on the basis of misinterpretation of what others say.

3. *Feelings of being distinctive or different:* Such feelings may result from membership in a minority group or from the presence of a birthmark or deformity; or they may have some other basis.

4. *Alcoholism:* Accusations of infidelity and misconduct directed at the spouse are common when the alcoholic's potency is reduced. This is seen more commonly in elderly male alcoholics. Prolonged use of alcohol may result in alcoholic paranoia or alcoholic hallucinosis.

5. *Amnesia:* Paranoid delusions can readily occur on the basis of loss of memory. The patient forgets where he placed some personal item; and when he cannot find it again, he assumes it must have been stolen.

Clinical experience shows that paranoid states in late life do not ordinarily lead to personality deterioration; nor do they shorten life expectancy like SDAT does. Twenty percent of all patients with paranoid states develop an organic brain syndrome that may not be caused by the paranoid state.[14] Finally, paranoid states have one striking feature in common: they respond well to the major tranquilizers.

It has been suggested that most of the paranoid states in the elderly may be forms of schizophrenia developing in late life (paraphrenia). The illness takes a benign course, perhaps because of reduced genetic susceptibility; also, the fact that the personality is more rigid in late life may protect the individual against the kind of schizophrenic deterioration seen when the disease affects young adolescents.

Depression in old age

Many people think of old age as intrinsically depressing because of the felt decline of energies; the constant reminders of narcissistic wounding (the loss of hair and teeth, the development of wrinkles, and other body changes); and other threatened, fantasied, or actual losses. Depression is probably the most common mental disorder affecting the elderly and may be underdiagnosed. Depression may be manifested by hypochondriasis, fatigue, loss of interest, withdrawal from society, and even alcoholism. Since older persons rarely attend mental health clinics or consult psychiatrists, the primary care physician's responsibility for diagnosing and treating depression among his elderly patients is an important one.[29]

Prevalence

While it is generally agreed that depression is probably twice as common in elderly women as in elderly men living in the community, completed suicide is three to four times as common in elderly white men (**Fig. 4-3**).

Reasons suggested for the high prevalence of depression in elderly women are (1) women live longer, so many of them live out their final years as lonely widows, often economically and socially deprived; and (2) the concentration of monoamine oxidase (MAO), an enzyme that destroys neurotransmitters in the

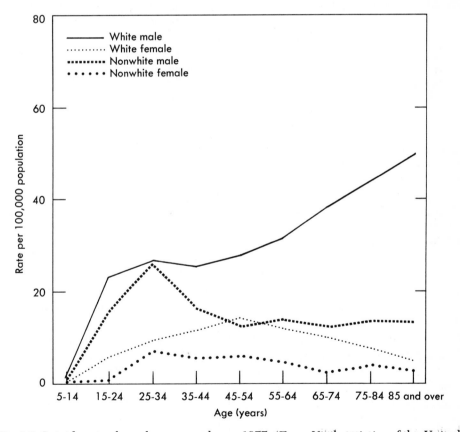

Fig. 4-3. Suicide rates by color, sex, and age: 1977. (From Vital statistics of the United States, vol. 2, Mortality, Mortality Statistic Branch, Division of Vital Statistics, National Center for Health Statistics [published and unpublished data].)

brain, rises with age—and the rise is greater in the female brain. This might render the elderly woman more vulnerable to depression. Tyrosine hydroxylase, the rate-limiting enzyme in norepinephrine synthesis, is also decreased in the aged brain.

The following losses make up what has been called "the season of loss," in other words, old age:

1. Physical vigor and stamina
2. Mental energies and capacities (alertness, memory)
3. Senses (sight, hearing, taste, smell)
4. Sources of affection (spouse, family, friends, contemporaries)
5. Peer group (employment)
6. Status (especially after retirement)
7. Income
8. Location (after retirement; the "empty nest syndrome")
9. Nutrition (malnutrition in extreme poverty)
10. Body parts (hair, teeth, sometimes limbs—from peripheral vascular disease)

Most depressions in old age appear to be reactive. A family history of depression is uncommon. Earlier attacks of depression (occurring before the age of 50) are also unusual. The central clinical feature is the dysphoric or depressed mood or affect, which includes prominent feelings of sadness associated with feelings of hopelessness or worthlessness. Other psychic symptoms include a general withdrawal of interest and an inhibition of activity better known as psychomotor retardation. There may be guilt and self-reproachful ideas. The patient's powers of attention and concentration are reduced, so that he is likely to reject questioning and display a negative attitude toward the examiner. He feels hopeless about his future and on inquiry may ad-

mit to suicidal preoccupations. It is essential to question the patient closely about suicide, including any thoughts of suicide he has considered and whether he has begun to plan any actions for carrying them out.

The biological signs of depression include severe and intractable insomnia, decreased appetite, and weight loss. Sexual interest and activity, once present, disappear. Depressed patients may suffer from extreme fatigue and spend much of their time lying on a bed or couch. They may also display anxiety or agitation as well as a depressed mood. Constipation is another symptom of depression and may eventually lead to fecal impaction. Since many elderly persons consider themselves constipated, this symptom may not be of any help. Likewise, total sleep time decreases with normal aging, thereby making insomnia a less reliable symptom of depression in old age.

Hypochondriasis

With aging, the individual may become more preoccupied with the interior of the body, and this preoccupation may lead to severe hypochondriasis in some depressed patients. One may observe the following mechanisms:

1. Withdrawal of psychic interest from other persons and objects and a centering of this interest on one's own body and its functioning
2. A shift of anxiety from a specific psychic area to the less threatening concern with bodily pain and discomfort
3. Physical symptoms used as a means of self-punishment for unacceptable hostile or vengeful feelings toward persons emotionally close to the patient

4. Physical symptoms used to show aggression against, and induce guilty feelings in, those caring for the patient (doctors, nurses, aides, etc.)
5. Physical symptoms used to excuse the patient from all social responsibilities because he is "sick" (secondary gain)

Diagnosis

History. It is necessary to inquire closely about the occurrence of important events, particularly losses, in the life of the patient and the relationship they bear to the onset of the depression. Losses, however, may not always be present. One should be alert to attacks of depression or elation earlier in the patient's life, although as already noted, this is not common in the depressions of late life.

Physical assessment

The primary care physician will undoubtedly diagnose and treat the majority of depressions of late life. Several important medical illnesses that closely imitate depression must be differentiated by history, physical examination, and laboratory tests. These include:

1. *Hypothyroidism:* The patient's slowness; vague bodily complaints, such as fatigue, weakness, and coldness; sluggish cerebration; and depressed mood can lead to a misdiagnosis.
2. *Apathetic hyperthyroidism:* Depression may be the most prominent symptom.
3. *Neurological disease:* Depression may be an early accompaniment of a minor stroke or cerebral neoplasm, or even be part of an insidiously developing dementia. In its early stages parkinsonism may be confused with dementia. In parkinsonism, the stooping gait, bradyki-

nesia, masked face, and lack of overt emotional response during the interview may sometimes suggest depression.

4. *Hidden neoplastic disease:* Such disease may give rise to depression as an early symptom. Traps lying in wait for the unwary are cancer of the pancreas and bronchial carcinoma.
5. *Malnutrition, with or without iron-deficiency anemia:* Malnutrition may result in depression as a prominent complaint. It is often difficult to know which came first. Did the patient become depressed gradually, lose his appetite, and become secondarily malnourished and anemic? Or did malnutrition from poverty, social isolation, and self-neglect result in the depressed mood? In many instances, one can only say that a vicious circle developed.

Mental status evaluation. The interviewer should observe the patient's overt behavior for evidence of retardation of motor activity; self-neglect; and facial expression betraying sadness, anxiety, or suspiciousness.

The patient's talk may reveal repetitiveness, depressive retardation, and poverty of ideation. The patient should be encouraged to describe his mood, and one should not hesitate to question him closely to assess the depth of the depressive feeling, its variation during the day, and what the patient believes to be its cause.

Because depression and dementia may have similar symptoms and even exist in the same patient, the interviewer should be alert for evidence of disorientation, amnesia, and decline of intellectual abilities, as well as for any other evidence of organic impairment, such as mild degrees of dysphasia, perseveration, or loss of abstracting ability. A formal effort should be made to assess the patient's performance in orientation, memory, reasoning, and judgment through use of the FROMAJE mental status technique described in Chapter 5. The most important element in the mental content in depression is the question of suicidal thoughts or intentions, which should especially be inquired about with the elderly individual. Paranoid feelings, guilt, and self-reproach should also be noted. It is often helpful to record, either on paper or audiotape, a representative sample of the patient's mental content.

Case history: depression complicated by acute organic brain syndrome

Mrs. B. T., a 78-year-old widow, was admitted to an acute care hospital after an accidental fall resulting in a fracture of the left femoral neck. This was treated by the insertion of an Austin-Moore prosthesis. She was then transferred to a skilled nursing facility for rehabilitation.

She also suffered from adult-onset diabetes mellitus, controlled by an oral hypoglycemic agent and diet, and congestive heart failure (CHF), controlled by digoxin and furosemide. She had been in a psychiatric hospital for the treatment of recurrent depression 4 months before her fall.

On admission she was noted to be depressed and have psychomotor retardation.

She showed considerable aversion during the interview. Her memory seemed impaired through inattention and loss of interest. Although she attended the rehabilitation program, progress was slow because of her poor motivation.

About 1 week after admission, her mental state deteriorated. She became febrile and dehydrated, and developed leukocytosis. A latent infection was suspected. She was coughing, and a chest x-ray study showed some infiltration. *Klebsiella* was suspected from the Gram stain of her sputum and was subsequently isolated on culture. A clear-catch midstream urine culture revealed 10^5 *Escherichia coli*. It was believed that the positive urine culture was merely asymptomatic bacteriuria. The patient was treated with a cephalosporin antibiotic and normal saline solution intravenously. The mental condition was diagnosed as acute organic brain syndrome due to *K. pneumoniae*.

Two weeks later, the patient had recovered insight and admitted that she had had ideas that everyone was against her and that the staff were trying to poison her. She could not account for why she had developed these ideas, but said that she had had "a change of mind" and no longer held these beliefs.

The final psychiatric diagnosis was recurrent depression complicated by acute organic brain syndrome due to pneumonia.

Mrs. T.'s depression improved when she was given a combination of a tricyclic anti-

Table 4-2. Prognostic factors in depression[*]

Favorable factors	Unfavorable factors
Age less than 70	Serious physical illness
Positive family history	Signs of organic brain syndrome
Recovery from earlier attack before age 50	Age over 70
Extroverted personality	Depression lasting 2 years or more
Even temperament without psychopathic/ dysthymic trends	
Previous favorable response to tricyclic antidepressants or ECT	

[*]Modified from Post, F.: The clinical psychiatry of late life, Oxford, Eng., 1965, Pergamon Press, Ltd.

depressant and a phenothiazine. With improvement in her motivation, her physical therapy progressed. She soon returned to her apartment and was followed in the geriatric outpatient department.

Prognosis

Generally in the elderly, depressive states show a far better prognosis than organic brain syndromes. Clinical presentation, however, is a poor guide to prognosis. There are no symptoms that predict outcome accurately. Recurrence is not uncommon. Table 4-2 may be helpful in attempting to assess the prognosis.

ANXIETY STATES

Anxiety is the well-known feeling of tension, together with psychophysiological manifestations, such as a rapid heart rate, muscle tension, and sweating. Anxiety is the response to some internal problem of which the subject may not be fully aware. In old age, anxiety rarely occurs in pure form; it is much more likely to be associated with depression and hypochondriasis. One of the commonest causes of anxiety in old age is the gradually increasing problem of dependency. To be dependent on others, no matter how willing or generous they may be, evokes feelings of frustration, impotence, and anger. Other causes include conflicts with children in association with the reversal of roles.

Obsessional symptoms in the form of recurring thoughts associated with tension and distress are common with anxiety states in the elderly. Worrying preoccupations and hypochondriacal concerns accompanied by a depressed and anxious mood are often seen. Successful treatment may be through psychotherapy or the use of antianxiety drugs.

CLINICAL PRINCIPLES IN WORKING WITH PSYCHOGERIATRIC PATIENTS*

Interviewing an elderly person calls for a comfortable setting with as few distractions as possible, whether visual or auditory. The interview should never be so long as to fatigue the older person. Considerable patience and a willingness to pace oneself at the slower rate of the elderly are needed for successful interviewing. The time of day is quite relevant, as many elderly people are at their best, not shortly after rising, but after they have had a few hours to be up and about.

The high prevalence of deafness has already been discussed. The interviewer should assure himself that the patient can actually hear what is being said. Furthermore, the interviewer should keep his face in a good light so that the patient may lip-read if he has that capacity. Informality, touch, and reassurance are interviewing techniques especially helpful in improving rapport, and, hence, the flow of important material from the elderly.

THERAPEUTIC MANAGEMENT IN GERIATRIC PSYCHIATRY

The treatment of elderly patients with psychiatric disorders should be individualized and comprehensive, and should include the following aspects: milieu as therapy, psychotherapy, psychotropic medication, somatic therapy, and counseling with the patient's family.

Milieu as therapy

Milieu refers to the physical and human environment in which the patient lives. It is obvious that the physical environment must be closely matched to the

---

*This section should be read in conjunction with Chapter 3.

patient's needs and abilities. Thus, a patient who is wheelchair-bound is going to need a setting with doors wide enough to permit the passage of his chair and a bed with an adjustable height to permit him to transfer from bed to chair and vice versa. The human environment must also be compatible with the patient's personality, background, cultural attributes, level of taste and education, and personal preferences.

Within a long-term care facility, for example, it may not be therapeutic to locate well-integrated patients next to patients who are severely regressed because of advanced organic brain syndrome. The well-integrated patients would be distressed when forced to witness deteriorated habits, incontinence, and mental confusion. Patients should live with others who are at the same functional and behavioral level. In this way, the level of stimulation of group activities can be suited to the patients' remaining mental capacities. Patients with severe memory impairment, for example, could not participate in tasks requiring this ability, but might still be able to take part in and enjoy old-time musical sing-alongs.

Over 50% of geriatric patients in long-term care institutions have psychiatric disorders, with many suffering varying degrees of chronic organic brain syndrome. The technique of reality orientation is used to help these patients remember the day of the week, the date, and the schedule of activities they are expected to follow.[30] Part of this "imprinting" involves repetition.

It is also important for men and women to mix freely. Just as in psychiatric facilities for younger persons, mixing of the sexes tends to promote more pride in appearance and grooming. Short periods of therapeutic leave are often recommended for patients and offer a valuable stimulus. Patients should be encouraged to attend important family events, such as weddings, graduations, and confirmations.

Psychotherapy

It is not true that the elderly are inaccessible to psychotherapy. There are many opportunities for psychotherapy (explorative, supportive, or group) in both community and institutional settings, such as when a patient must be informed of the death of a family member or when a patient needs help in working through the anxiety of an impending operation. Discussion about the following topics can be helpful: dealing with and accepting disability and dependency, venting feelings of resentment toward family members or feelings of neglect or abandonment, and correcting unwarranted feelings of mistrust and suspicion.

Although amnesia, long-standing patterns of defense, and blunting of emotional responses may pose problems in psychotherapy with the elderly, both long-term inpatients and community-residing elderly people appreciate and often benefit from help in working through the common crises and conflicts of this stage of human development.

Group psychotherapy for the elderly is a valuable approach.[31] It is important that the group share some homogeneity regarding problems, needs, and mental capacities, and that meetings should take place regularly at a specific time and place. Whether based in the community or in an institution, these groups tend to be open-ended because of the recurring loss of members through death or discharge. Group psychotherapy provides a means for patients with common problems such as strokes, amputations, and depression, to find mutual support through the sharing of their feelings.

Psychotropic medication

Problems of absorption, side effects, incompatibilities, metabolism, and excretion of drugs commonly used in treatment are discussed in Chapter 6. Poor compliance by the elderly is also discussed.

Psychotropic medications in geriatric psychiatry may be classified as follows: major tranquilizers; minor tranquilizers; antidepressants; and miscellaneous (vasodilators, anticoagulants, ergot alkaloids, and hormones).

Major tranquilizers

Major tranquilizers include the phenothiazines, thioxanthenes, and butyrophenones. They are indicated to control target symptoms of acute or chronic organic brain syndromes or paranoid states. These target symptoms are hallucinations, delusions, agitation, hostility, lability of affect, restlessness, paranoid outbursts, and self-punitive behavior.

As a routine, treatment should be started with the lowest possible doses, with the medication given by mouth when the patient can swallow. The motto in geriatric psychopharmacology is, "Start low, go slow." In an emergency it may be advisable to give the drug by intramuscular injection. The drugs listed in Table 4-3, with the exception of thioridazine (Mellaril), are available in injectable form. It is important to titrate the dose carefully, guided by the level of behavioral disturbance and medication side effects.

Side effects, which should be carefully monitored, fall into two groups: anticholinergic and extrapyramidal (Table 4-4). Although the anticholinergic side effects

Table 4-3. Psychotropic drugs and oral dose equivalents (in milligrams)

Chlorpromazine (Thorazine)	Thioridazine (Mellaril)	Thiothixene (Navane)	Haloperidol (Haldol)
25	25	1 to 2	0.5
50	50	1 to 3	1
100	100	5	2

Table 4-4. Side effects of major tranquilizers

Anticholinergic	Extrapyramidal
Dry mouth	Akathisia (motor restlessness)
Palpitations, tachycardia, dysrhythmias	Dystonia (nuchal, truncal)
Postural hypotension	Tremor
Constipation	Rigidity
Urinary retention	Excessive salivation
Nausea, vomiting	Festinant gait and risk of fall
Dizziness, faintness	Tardive dyskinesia
Blurred vision	
Acute confusion (central anticholinergic effect)	

are usually peripheral, there exists the possibility of a central anticholinergic effect occurring in a small number of patients, giving rise to a confusional state.

Less common side effects include cholestatic jaundice; leukopenia; occasional agranulocytosis; rashes, pruritus, and urticaria; and altered glucose metabolism.

Patients with behavioral disturbances caused by chronic organic brain syndromes can be maintained on low dosages of the major tranquilizers for long periods of time, provided that they are carefully monitored. Vital signs and blood pressure should be monitored regularly. Patients should be periodically reevaluated for the need for maintenance therapy.

Minor tranquilizers

Minor tranquilizers include the benzodiazepines and meprobamate. The half-lives of some of the benzodiazepines (e.g., diazepam) is prolonged in the elderly; therefore, the dosage should be modified.

Antidepressants

There are two types of antidepressants: monoamine oxidase (MAO) inhibitors and tricyclic antidepressants. Ordinarily, only the tricyclic antidepressants are used in treating depression in the elderly. The MAO inhibitors can cause hypertensive crises when foods rich in tyramine, such as cheese, wines, and organ meats, are ingested.

Tricyclic antidepressants may be subdivided into sedating and nonsedating types. Sedating types include amitriptyline (Elavil) and doxepin (Sinequan). Nonsedating types include imipramine (Tofranil) and protriptyline (Vivactil).

The side effects of the tricyclic antidepressants are similar to those of the major tranquilizers. In particular, the effects on the heart are anticholinergic, adrenolytic, and quinidinelike. It is better to prescribe tricyclic antidepressants in divided doses during the day rather than as a single nighttime dose. A high blood level of an antidepressant at nighttime might predispose the patient to orthostatic hypotension or dysrhythmia and a subsequent fall. Beginning with low doses of the order of 10 mg tid, the dosage is raised in increments every few days until 50 mg tid is reached. An exception is protriptyline, where the dose is 5 mg tid or qid. Doxepin has been shown to have weaker anticholinergic side effects and less cardiotoxicity than the other compounds.[32]

Miscellaneous drugs

With patients suffering from dementia of the multi-infarct type, there has been an emphasis on the use of vasodilators, such as nitrites, nicotinic acid, papaverine, and cyclandelate. While these drugs may in some cases improve cerebral blood flow (CBF), there is at this time no convincing evidence that their use has improved mental function in patients suffering from MID. There is no substantial evidence that conjugate ergot alkaloids (e.g., Hydergine or vasodilators) have caused clinically significant, long-term improvement in patients with SDAT.[33,34]

A promising approach to the prevention of cerebrovascular disease is the use of anticoagulants, such as dicumarol, or antiplatelet agglutinators, such as aspirin. While valuable in preventing transient ischemic attacks (TIAs) that have not yet been followed by cerebrovascular accidents (CVAs) leading to neurological impairment, these drugs have never been shown to reduce or reverse mental impairment resulting from cerebrovascular disease.

Somatic therapy

The most important somatic therapy in the treatment of depression in the elderly is electroconvulsive therapy (ECT). According to the American Psychiatric Association's task force report on ECT,[35] it is "an effective treatment in cases of severe depression where the risk of suicide is high and/or where the patient is not taking adequate food or fluids and/or where the use of drug or other therapy entails high risks and/or will take an unacceptably long period to manifest a therapeutic response."

The only major contraindications to ECT are recent myocardial infarction and space-occupying intracranial lesions. The technique has been generally standardized. After the patient has been medically cleared and premedicated with 0.5 mg atropine 15 minutes previously, he is anesthetized with an intravenous injection of an ultra short–acting barbiturate, such as methohexital (Brevital). Succinylcholine chloride (Anectine) is then injected intravenously in a dose of from 10 to 30 mg to modify the muscle contractions during the convulsion and avoid fractures or dislocations. A suitable electrical stimulus sufficient to induce a grand mal convulsion is then administered by means of saline-moistened pad electrodes applied to the temporal regions of the scalp. During the apneic phase induced by the muscle relaxant, the patient must be ventilated until he begins to breathe spontaneously. An anesthetist always attends to monitor respiration and cardiac status.

Treatments are given twice weekly for a total of 8 to 12 treatments, depending on the clinical response. Some degree of retrograde amnesia and slight confusion may be seen as immediate aftereffects of ECT. These usually disappear over a few weeks or months following the completion of the course of treatment and may be minimized by the use of a unipolar electrode.

Counseling the patient's family

The spouse, siblings, and children of the geriatric patient often seek guidance on a number of topics, including:

1. *The prognosis of the mental condition:* When the patient is suffering from chronic organic brain syndrome, the family will wish to know the outcome, the expectation of life, and will often bring up for discussion alleged treatments and cures they may have read about. It should be emphasized that although the patient appears severely impaired mentally to the medical and nursing staff, the family tends to see the patient through the eyes of the past and will often deny or ignore the most obvious disorder. It is important to be candid with the family, to let them know what to expect, and to remain supportive.

2. *Deaths in the patient's family:* Relatives may want to conceal the fact that a death has taken place. The physician should point out to the family that it is usually inappropriate to withhold such news from the patient, thereby depriving him of the important human experience of mourning.

3. *Questions concerning the patient's property:* In the case of a patient incompetent to handle his Social Security payments or other property he owns, the family may wish to apply for a conservatorship and may seek advice on how to do this. The physician may be asked to testify about the patient's competency by affidavit or in court.

4. *Retaining the patient's residence when he enters an institution:* It is often difficult to decide whether to retain the patient's residence, especially when his mental and physical states are in question. Giving up the home significantly reduces the patient's chance of returning to the community. It is necessary to discuss the prospects for mental improvement in such cases with the family and help them arrive at a decision. Sometimes a compromise can be reached, with the family agreeing to pay the rent for a limited period, perhaps 3 months. This will allow for the prospect of some mental and physical recovery without an excessive outlay of funds.

Finally, whether the patient lives in an institution or in the community, it should never be forgotten that his family represents his major support system. The elderly, contrary to popular belief, are not abandoned by their families.

REFERENCES

 1. Birren, J. E., editor: Handbook of aging and the individual, Chicago, 1973; University of Chicago Press, pp. 119, 177.
 2. Butler, R. N.: Why survive? Being old in America, New York, 1975, Harper & Row, Publishers, Inc., p. 254.
 3. Raskind, M. A., and Eisdorfer, C.: When elderly patients can't sleep, Drug Ther., August 1977, p. 44.
 4. Pfeiffer, E., Verwoerdt, A., and Wang, H. S.: The natural history of sexual behavior in aged men and women, Arch. Gen. Psychiatry 19:753, 1968.
 5. Kinsey, A. C., Pomeroy, W. B., and Martin, C. R.: Sexual behavior in the human male, Philadelphia, 1948, W. B. Saunders Co.
 6. Libow, L. S.: Interaction of medical, biologic, and behavioral factors on aging, adaptation, and survival, Geriatrics 29:75, 1974.
 7. Lehman, H. C., cited in Bromley, D. B.: The psychology of human aging, ed. 2, Harmondsworth, Eng., 1974, Penguin Books Ltd., p. 212.
 8. The employment problems of older workers, Bulletin 1721, U.S. Department of Labor, Bureau of Labor Statistics.
 9. Bromley, D. B.: The psychology of human aging, ed. 2., Harmondsworth, Eng., 1974, Penguin Books Ltd., p. 212.
10. Busse, E. W., and Pfeiffer, E.: Behavior and adaptation in late life (ed. 2), Boston, 1977, Little, Brown and Co., pp. 25, 48.
11. Comfort, A.: A good age, New York, 1976, Crown Publishers, Inc.
12. Busse, E. W., and Pfeiffer, E.: Mental illness in later life, Washington, D.C., 1973, American Psychiatric Association, p. 13.
13. Post, F.: The clinical psychiatry of late life, Oxford, Eng., 1965, Pergamon Press Ltd., p. 99.
14. Slater, E., and Roth, M.: Clinical psychiatry, London, 1969, Bailliere Tindall, pp. 548, 584.
15. Kay, D. W. K., Morris, V., and Post, F.: Prognosis in psychiatric disorders of the elderly, J. Ment. Sci. 102:129, 1956.
16. Roth, M.: Classification and aetiology in mental disorders of old age. In Kay, D. W. K., and Wall, A., editors: Recent developments in psychogeriatrics, Ashford Kent, Eng., 1971, Headley Brothers.
17. Butler, R. N.: Psychiatry and the elderly: an overview, Am. J. Psychiatry 132:893, 1975.
18. Libow, L. S.: Senile dementia and pseudosenility: clinical diagnosis. In Eisdorfer, C., and Friedel, R., editors: Cognitive and emotional disturbance in the elderly, Chicago, 1977, Year Book Medical Publishers, Inc. p. 77.
19. Kral, V. A.: Confusional states. In Howells, J. G., editor: Modern perspectives in the psychiatry of old age, New York, 1975, Brunner/Mazel, Inc., p. 356.
20. Terry, R. D.: Aging, senile dementia, and Alzheimer's disease. In Katzman, R., Terry, R. D., and Bick, K. L., editors: Alzheimer's disease: senile dementia and related disorders, New York, 1978, Raven Press.
21. Peck, A., Wolloch, L., and Rodstein, M.: Mortality of the aged with chronic brain syndrome. In Katzman, R., Terry, R. D., and Bick, K. L., editors: Alzheimer's disease: senile dementia and related disorders, New York, 1978, Raven Press, p. 299.
22. Libow, L. S.: Epidemiology—excess mortality and proximate causes of death. In Katzman, R., Terry, R. D., and Bick, K. L., editors: Alzheimer's disease: senile dementia and related disorders, New York, 1978, Raven Press, p. 315.
23. Kahn, R. L., Goldfarb, A. I., Pollack, M., and others: Brief objective measures for the determination of mental status in the aged, Am. J. Psychiatry 111:326, 1960.
24. Pfeiffer, E.: A short portable mental status ques-

tionnaire for the assessment of organic brain deficit in elderly patients, J. Am. Geriatr. Soc. **23**:433, 1975.

25. Basavaraju, N. G., Paraskevas, K., and Libow, L. S.: Primitive reflexes and perceptual sensory tests in the elderly: their usefulness in dementia. Unpublished paper.
26. Anderson, F.: Practical management of the elderly, ed. 2, Oxford, Eng., 1971, Blackwell Scientific Publications Ltd., p. 23.
27. Hachinski, V. C., Lassen, N. A., and Marshall, J.: Multi-infarct dementia: a cause of mental deterioration in the elderly, Lancet **ii**:207, 1974.
28. Wells, C. E.: Chronic brain disease: an overview, Am. J. Psychiatry **135**:1, 1978.
29. Charatan, F. B.: Depression in old age, N.Y. State J. Med. **75**:2505, 1975.
30. Folsom, J. C.: Reality orientation for the elderly mental patient, J. Geriatr. Psychiatry **1**:291, 1968.
31. Kubie, S. H., and Landau, G.: Group work with the aged, New York, 1975, International Universities Press, Inc.
32. Burrows, G. D., Vohra, J., Hunt, D., and others: Cardiac effects of different tricyclic antidepressant drugs, Br. J. Psychiatry **129**:335, 1976.
33. Hughes, J. R., William, T. G., and Currier, R. D.: An ergot alkaloid preparation (Hydergine) in the treatment of dementia: critical review of the clinical literature, J. Am. Geriatr. Soc. **24**:490, 1976.
34. Yesavage, J. A., Hollister, L. E., and Borian, E.: Dihydroergotoxin: 6-mg versus 3-mg dosage in the treatment of senile dementia, preliminary report, J. Am. Geriatr. Soc. **27**:80, 1979.
35. Frankel, F. H.: Electroconvulsive therapy, Task Force Report 14, Washington, D.C., 1978, American Psychiatric Association.

PROBLEM-SOLVING EXERCISES
Case one

Mr. J. B. is 68 and emotionally disturbed. He is a married certified public accountant who retired the previous year in good physical and mental health. Subsequently, he has suffered from loss of appetite, sinking sensations in his stomach, loss of interest, and lack of concentration. Sexual relations with his wife ceased several months ago. He has become increasingly depressed and preoccupied with his stomach; difficulty in sleeping has evolved into severe insomnia. He has lost about 22 pounds. He has been admitted to the hospital; and a full investigation, including all routine tests listed on p. 68, as well as an upper GI series, intermediate-strength purified protein derivative (PPD) test, and tests for malabsorption have not revealed any cause for his symptoms. A CAT scan is also negative.

Questions

1. Discuss the differential diagnosis in this case.
2. What additional tests might be helpful in establishing the diagnosis?
3. How would you treat this patient?

Case two

Mrs. F. T., a married woman aged 77, has been brought to the clinic by her husband, a retired machinist aged 80. He says that his wife has had a progressive loss of memory over the past 3 years and recently wandered from the house and was brought back by the police. For example, she forgets what she is going to say and does not complete sentences. She butters bread, then puts it in the toaster. She sometimes puts a pot on the stove and forgets about it, and once caused a fire in the kitchen. She neglects her personal hygiene, and is fecally incontinent, soiling her underwear. She does not sleep well at night and often gets up and wanders around the house. On at least one occasion she fell down and lacerated her scalp.

Her previous medical history was negative, and she has not been under the care of a physician. She was born in the United States, completed grade school education, married at age 20, and had three children. Her home and family are her life, according to her husband, and she has no outside interests. She takes no medications.

On examination, she is obese, poorly groomed, and untidily dressed. A mental status examination (see Chapter 5) reveals significant abnormalities in most parameters tested. Most impressive are errors in orientation and memory. She says that her husband, who is sitting next to her, is her father. Her talk is often rambling and irrelevant, with frequent references to her remote past. A neurological examination reveals no focal neurological deficit.

Questions

1. What is the differential diagnosis in this case? In your opinion, what is the most likely diagnosis?
2. What laboratory tests might you ask for?
3. What possible arrangements might you recommend to the family?
4. Discuss the prognosis in this case.

ANSWERS TO PROBLEM-SOLVING EXERCISES
Case one

1. The differential diagnosis would include depression associated with retirement and loss of role, SDAT or MID with insidious onset, and potentially reversible causes of organic brain syndrome (see pp. 65 and 66). Hidden malignant disease seems to be ruled out by the extensive physical workup, including ancillary investigations.

   If the patient's wife and other observers have been unable to document such features as memory loss, poor judgment, disordered behavior (wandering, getting lost, deterioration in habits and personal hygiene, and/or incontinence), there is little support for a diagnosis of dementia. However, all disease has to start somewhere, so dementia in its very early stages cannot be totally ruled out.

   The most likely diagnosis by far is depression. This often follows or accompanies some actual, threatened, or even fantasied loss in an older person. Many men, especially, invest the greatest amount of their libido in their work. Retirement, perhaps forced by the policy of Mr. B.'s employer, has left him with no role. He may believe he has lost his major reason for living and may be depressed as a result.

2. Additional tests: see recommended but not routine, and elective tests, pp. 68 and 69. An EEG in the case of depression would be more likely to show preservation of basic electrical rhythms of the brain, whereas, in dementia, there might be slowing or even beginning disorganization of rhythms.

A CAT scan might rule out cortical atrophy. Unfortunately there is no reliable correlation between a finding of cortical atrophy and the degree of mental impairment noted during life. The CAT scan would, nevertheless, rule out serious brain disease, such as a tumor, hematoma, or other space-occupying lesion.

3. Treatment could be psychodynamic. The physician should discuss with the patient his life situation with special reference to:

   • His feelings about retirement: what he plans to do with his time; what his avocations, hobbies, and recreational preferences are; whether he and his wife have interests in common.

   • His relationship with his wife now that he has more time with her, his sexual life with her, and her reaction to his loss of interest in sex. The following are possible topics that may emerge: dependence-independence; expressions of hostility; needs for nurturance; expectations and disappointments; money (its use and distribution); grandparenting; relations with the (usually married) children; and relations with other important figures (brothers, sisters, in-laws, etc.).

   Treatment could be psychopharmacological. The use of antidepressants should be considered. The choice would fall between the sedating antidepressants (amitriptyline, doxepin) and the nonsedating antidepressants (imipramine, protriptyline). It might be necessary, in the face of much tension and anxiety, to add a major tranquilizer, such as thiothixene, or possibly a combination of perphenazine and amitriptyline (Triavil). The dosage of imipramine or amitriptyline should begin at 10 mg 3 times a day and increase gradually up to 150 mg daily.

   Finally, if antidepressants are ineffective, ECT would have to be seriously considered. A course of 6 to 8 treatments given twice weekly with due precautions and after medical clearance can resolve a depressive illness, even where this seems to be primarily reactive (i.e., where there have not been previous attacks of depression during the patient's lifetime).

Case two

1. Depression can be practically eliminated because of the total and global impairment of all intellectual and personality functions without signs of weight loss, crying, or flattened affect. Thus, the differential diagnosis is that of dementia: primary dementia (SDAT) or secondary dementia. There is about one chance in eight that the patient suffers from some kind of secondary dementia.
2. Laboratory tests: see routine, recommended but not routine, and elective tests (pp. 68 and 69).
3. Arrangements to be suggested:
   - Keeping the patient at home with the help of aides or home help, together with a chief caretaker from the family
   - Placement in a state psychiatric facility or nursing home after or during diagnostic evaluation (for a state psychiatric facility, it would have to be an involuntary commitment, because the patient is not capable of expressing volition)
   - Placement in a private psychiatric sanitarium (but few families have the resources for this)
4. The prognosis depends on the cause of the dementia. If SDAT is the cause (diagnosed through elimination of other causes of secondary dementia), the patient's remaining life span will be reduced by 50%. If the dementia is secondary and the cause can be removed, then the prognosis may be better, particularly if the dementia is partially or completely reversible.

POSTTEST°

1. Objective evidence of aging is found in all the items below *except:*
   a. Slowing of responses

°Some questions may have more than one correct answer.

b. Lower IQ
   c. Nonprogressive memory impairment
   d. Reduction in sexual activity
2. The prevalence of chronic organic brain syndrome in the population above age 80 is:

   a. 5%   d. 30%
   b. 12%   e. 45%
   c. 22%

3. List the three major diagnostic groupings of the *psychoses* of old age.
4. The neurohistology of senile dementia of the Alzheimer type (SDAT) characteristically shows:
   a. Wallerian degeneration
   b. Inclusion bodies
   c. Giant cells
   d. Large numbers of senile plaques
   e. Basophil granules
5. In multi-infarct dementia, can the degree of mental impairment during life be correlated with the volume of infarcted brain observed at autopsy?
6. A causal relationship to so-called secondary dementia can be found in all of the following conditions *except:*
   a. Hypothyroidism
   b. Neurosyphilis
   c. Vitamin B_{12} deficiency
   d. Head injury
   e. Paranoia
7. Senile paranoid states respond exceptionally well to:
   a. Benzodiazepines
   b. Phenothiazines
   c. Antidepressants
   d. Anticonvulsants
   e. Amphetamines
8. List any five losses that occur in old age that may lead to depression.
9. The most important question in the psychiatric evaluation of elderly depressed patients is:
   a. Paranoid feelings
   b. Homicidal impulses
   c. Thought disorder

d. Suicidal feelings

e. Hallucinations

10. An early feature of parkinsonism associated with the use of the major tranquilizers is:

    a. Tardive dyskinesia

    b. Emotional incontinence

    c. Sleep reversal

    d. Cogwheel rigidity

    e. Akathisia

ANSWERS TO PRETEST AND POSTTEST

1. b. There is no evidence that the IQ is reduced in old age when the elderly subject is tested without being put under anxiety-increasing time pressure.

2. c.

3. Affective disorders, organic brain syndromes, and paranoid psychoses.

4. d. The senile plaque is regarded as the end stage of neuronal degeneration. Roth's work showed a correlation between plaque density and the degree of dementia during life.

5. Yes. The volume of infarction correlates with the degree of dementia measured during life.

6. e. Paranoid illnesses in late life are not related to secondary dementia except in a small minority of cases.

7. b. Senile paranoid states are very sensitive to phenothiazine and thioxanthene drugs. Both drugs are effective in suppressing hallucinations.

8. See p. 72 of text.

9. d. Suicidal feelings. Every depressed older patient should be specifically asked about his suicidal thoughts and feelings. The threat of suicide is greater in older white men than in older women or older black men.

10. e. Akathisia is generally regarded as the earliest sign of parkinsonism in phenothiazine use. The danger is that it may be mistaken for increased agitation and treated by increased dosages of the phenothiazine.

Chapter 5

A rapidly administered, easily remembered mental status evaluation: FROMAJE

LESLIE S. LIBOW

EDUCATIONAL OBJECTIVES
Attitudinal

The student should:
1. Realize that mental status testing is essential to a complete evaluation of many older persons.
2. Realize that formal mental status testing is often omitted from clinical evaluation of the elderly
3. Realize that many of the elderly who, at first glance, appear to have dementia ("to be senile") are suffering from pseudosenility syndromes and/or have communication disorders
4. Realize that ageism contributes to the overdiagnosis of dementia
5. Realize the serious implications of the diagnosis of dementia

Cognitive

The student should:
1. Know that speech, hearing, and/or language difficulties may contribute to the misdiagnosis of dementia
2. Know how to evaluate a patient who is suspected of having dementia

Skill

The student should:
1. Learn to do a mental status examination easily and rapidly
2. Recognize the clinical evidence of mental depression
3. Apply the mental status examination in all appropriate situations
4. Integrate the results of mental status testing with the history, physical examination, and appropriate laboratory tests

PRETEST
True or false

1. A command of mental status testing is essential only for psychiatrists.
2. There is a pathognomonic clinical sign leading to the diagnosis of dementia.
3. There is a pathognomonic laboratory or radiological test leading to the diagnosis of dementia.
4. Mental status testing is the same as a psychiatric interview.
5. Mental status testing in the elderly focuses on acute and/or chronic dementias.
6. Some dementias (perhaps 5% to 15%) are falsely interpreted as classic late-life, senile dementias, when, in fact, they reflect emotional depression, medication side-effects, metabolic disorder, or space-taking, central nervous system lesions.
7. The key to mental status testing is to use an easily remembered, easily administered technique that can be applied by the primary care clinician whenever appropriate.
8. FROMAJE is one such technique. The OMA refers to orientation, memory, and arithmetic.
9. An individual with normal responses to the FROMAJE questionnaire but whose

emotional state is quite disturbed, will score in the abnormal range without necessarily having dementia.

10. The scoring technique is crucial to the use of the FROMAJE test.

11. The score is of value for the inexperienced interviewer, in situations where different clinicians will be seeing the patient over time, or where research data are desired.

12. Mental status examination is of little use in a patient who has global aphasia.

13. When language and/or cultural barriers exist, a standard mental status examination will likely produce excessive false positive and/or false negative results.

14. Patients with dementia always need institutionalization.

15. It is necessary to repeat the FROMAJE test (or any other mental status test) on varying days and at varying times in order to achieve an accurate diagnosis.

The dementias* are major brain illnesses of late life. The serious social, medical, and prognostic implications of the diagnosis of dementia demand that the clinician utilize all available clinical skills in reaching the diagnosis. There is no one pathognomonic sign, symptom, or clinical or laboratory test for making the diagnosis of dementia. Thus, the history, physical exam, and appropriate laboratory tests must be used to reach an "impression" of the presence of dementia. A key element of the examination must be the inclusion of a mental status evaluation done by the primary care physician. Having an effective, sensitive, reliable, and easily administered and reproduced

---

*For the purposes of this text the term *dementia* is used synonymously with the term organic brain syndrome.

test is essential for the clinician. Such a test will assure that the evaluation of mental status is more than a passing, initial impression. It will also allow for follow-up comparison by the same, or as often happens, other clinicians.

One should remember that a mental status test focuses on dementia and is not equivalent to a psychiatric interview. A test that does not require source books and/or printed questionnaires and that is rapidly and easily administered by the clinician is one that is likely to be used. We have developed one such mental status evaluation approach, built around the acronym FROMAJE: F = function; R = reasoning; O = orientation; M = memory; A = arithmetic; J = judgment; E = emotional state.

The evaluation is sensitive, reproducible, and rapidly administered; and it does not require accompanying printed material. Students of medicine and other health professions, who have used this approach as well as graduate nurses, physicians, physician assistants, nurse practitioners, and physical and occupational therapists, have generally liked it and incorporated it into their clinical evaluations.

The importance of an accurate diagnosis extends beyond the seriousness of the disease. Approximately 5% to 15% of late-life dementias are actually masked presentations of other known and treatable illnesses. We refer to these as pseudosenilities or pseudodementias.[1-4] The underlying causes of these reversible dementias include mental depression, medication, metabolic disorders, head trauma, and primary or metastatic neoplasms. The complete differential diagnosis is discussed in Chapter 4. The FROMAJE mental status approach should be combined with the history, physical examination, and laboratory studies to arrive at the clinical diagnosis of dementia.

When used by medical students and lay interviewers, The FROMAJE test has proved to have an 80% to 90% concordance with the psychiatric diagnoses achieved independently by geropsychiatrists. The acronym provides an easily remembered approach, which is also one of breadth and brevity.

Other excellent mental status tests do exist, however, including those of Kahn and others,[5] Perlin and Butler,[6] Pfeiffer,[7] Blessed and others,[8] and Jacobs.[9]

The FROMAJE test is meant to serve as a guide for the primary care clinician, who may have little experience in formal mental status testing. The test emphasizes adequacy of overall mental function. The elderly person is becoming the major patient for most primary care physicians, and mental dysfunction is quite prevalent (4% to 10% of the elderly population). This regimented approach, not requiring a written text or form, is in the style of a medical approach to evaluation of clinical problems. The test may have to be repeated on different days and at different times of the day in order to reach a more reliable diagnosis.

The FROMAJE test (or any mental status examination) cannot be used well in the presence of aphasia. Similarly, language or cultural differences between patient and clinician will reduce the accuracy and meaningfulness of mental status testing. In addition, difficulties in hearing or vision may lead to mistaken diagnoses of dementia. The hurried interviewer may not allow adequate time (10 to 20 minutes) for the questions and answers and may inaccurately diagnose dementia.

Although the seven key parameters of mental function tested with FROMAJE are best administered as an organized test, some situations may require interspersing the questions throughout a general medical interview.

The test need not be scored, since an overall, global impression is of considerable value to the clinician. However, the inexperienced interviewer or those seeking quantifiable data may choose to apply the simple rating described. For example, the test score may be helpful in showing changes in mental status with changes in therapy. In addition, the score is helpful when multiple physicians are seeing the patient, as in a clinic setting.

The F = function parameter of FROMAJE needs special mention. Many patients with dementia (abnormalities in the ROMAJE parameters) are able to continue to function fairly well in the community and do not require institutionalization. More rarely, a patient will score quite normally on the ROMAJE questions but will be unable to function in the community.

The test is fully described as follows.

FROMAJE[*]

INSTRUCTIONS TO INTERVIEWERS
Approach to the interview

Spend some time with the patient in general discussion. State who you are and that you would like to spend about 15 to 20 minutes with the patient, asking him questions that will give you further understanding of how he is functioning. The initial familiarizing comments could center on how the patient is feeling and, most important, what his life has been like prior to this time. After es-

---

[*] F = function; R = reasoning; O = orientation; M = memory; A = arithmetic; J = judgment; E = emotional state.

tablishing some comfort and rapport, proceed with the interview with an approach such as: "I am going to ask you a series of questions, some of which are simple and some difficult, and the answers to these questions will help me understand how you are functioning." In the meantime, you will have noted the patient's hearing, vision, and manner of speech, and whether a communication problem exists between the two of you, such as dysarthria, aphasia, a hearing problem, or a language barrier.

The instructions that accompany FRO-MAJE allow for simple scoring, so that you can establish a 1-, 2-, or 3-point rating for all parameters, if you desire, rather than simply a global impression.

THE TEST
F = function

Function refers to an individual's *mental* ability to adequately maintain himself in the community and home. In the case of a patient in a nursing home, the question is whether the patient has the mental ability to return home and maintain himself. This includes matters of food, shelter, clothing, hygiene, and socially acceptable or unacceptable behavior. (Would the patient eat or starve, pay his rent, wander in the street, etc?) The F rating refers only to mental function and competence. An individual with adequate mental capabilities but who was physically incapable of maintaining himself at home (e.g., after a stroke) would score normally (1 point) for function.

To properly arrive at this rating, the interviewer must ask a relative, friend, and/or nurse about the patient's mental function in recent weeks or months and combine this information with the interviewer's own impression of the patient's ability to function.

Rating (points):

1 = Mental function is adequate, so that no at-home support is necessary.

2 = Because of mental impairment, patient will need some at-home support at least part of the day or week (from family, friends, visiting nurse service, etc.).

3 = Because of mental impairment, patient needs 24-hour at-home support and supervision, 7 days a week.

R = reasoning

Ask the patient to explain the meaning of a proverb. If you are unsure whether the request is understood or the proverb familiar, ask another one. If the patient's education or cultural background makes you believe that he does not comprehend the question (i.e., he may be non-English speaking), use another proverb or saying that is appropriate to this patient's education or culture (via an interpreter). Assign a rating based on the use of an appropriate proverb and language. Sample proverbs: "The early bird catches the worm," or "A stitch in time saves nine."

Rating (points):

1 = Patient explained proverb well; gave general connotations of proverb.

2 = Patient gave some semblance of meaning, but with some incompleteness or was unable to generalize.

3 = Patient was completely unable to ascribe any meaning or gave a totally incorrect explanation.

O = orientation

1. Time:
   a. "What day of the week is it?" (If necessary, present choices: "Is it Monday? Tuesday?")
   b. "What month is it?" ("Is it June? July?") "What is the date?"
   c. "What year is it?"
2. Place: "Where are you now?" ("Is this your apartment? Your house or hotel? A doctor's office or a hospital or nursing home?")
3. Self: "What is your name?"

Rating (points):

1 = Patient was generally accurate and made only minor errors in time, place, or self.

2 = Patient made a significant error in one area: time, place, or self.

3 = Patient made significant errors in two or three areas: time, place, or self.

M = memory

1. Distant:
   a. "Who was President of the United States during World War II and was in a wheelchair?"
   b. "What U.S. President was assassinated in the early 1960s?"
   c. "Where were you born? In what year were you born?"
2. Recent:
   a. "What did you have for breakfast today?"
   b. "Where were you yesterday?"
3. Immediate:
   a. "What did I ask you about the U.S. Presidents?"
   b. "Remember the numbers *4, 12,* and *18.* I will be asking you to repeat them in the next few minutes. (Minutes later.) What numbers did I ask you to remember?"

Rating (points):
1 = Patient was generally accurate and made only minor errors in distant, recent, or immediate memory.
2 = Patient made a significant error in one area: distant, recent, or immediate memory.
3 = Patient made a significant error in two or three areas: distant, recent, or immediate memory.

A = arithmetic

1. "Count back from 100 to 90."
2. "Subtract sevens from 100."
3. "Count from 1 to 20."

Rating (points):
1 = Patient was generally accurate and made only minor errors.
2 = Patient made one significant error.
3 = Patient made two or more significant errors.

J = judgment

1. "At night, if you need some help, how can you obtain it?"
2. "If you are having trouble with a neighbor, what can you do to improve the situation?"

3. "If you see smoke in a wastepaper basket, what should you do?"

Rating (points):
1 = Patient made a generally sensible response.
2 = Patient demonstrates some poor judgment.
3 = Patient shows extremely poor judgment.

E = emotional state*

Observe the patient's manner during the interview. Ask the patient about crying, sadness, depression, optimism, suspiciousness, delusions, hallucinations, mood swings, and future plans. Consider the patient's behavior in relation to his situation (some sadness or depression is quite appropriate for a significant illness or loss).

Rating (points):
1 = Emotional state seems reasonable and appropriate for patient's situation.
2 = Patient gives evidence of extensive or inappropriate depression, or grandiosity.
3 = Patient has extremely unreal or inappropriate ideas (delusional or hallucinatory behavior, extreme depression, and/or suicidal ideas).

TOTAL FROMAJE SCORE AND INTERPRETATION

All of the points are added together to form the total score:

Score (total points)

7 or 8 = Patient does not display significant abnormal behavior or mentation.

9 or 10 = Patient has mild dementia (organic brain syndrome) or depression.

11 or 12 = Patient has moderate dementia (organic brain syndrome) or depression.

---

*Depression is the mental illness that may closely resemble dementia and must be differentiated from it.

13 or more = Patient has severe dementia (organic brain syndrome) or depression.

Thus, a patient who had, for example, the following score (i.e., 10 points) would be rated as having mild dementia (organic brain syndrome):

F R O M A J E
2 1 2 2 1 1 1 = 10

A subjective overall rating of normal, or mild, moderate, or severe dementia is reached by the experienced clinician. The FROMAJE responses are recorded for later reevaluation with regard to the patient's response to therapy and/or time.

Patients with various types of aphasia (see Chapter 8) cannot be accurately evaluated by the FROMAJE scale or by any other mental status approach.

An E (emotional) rating of 3 points will produce a total score of 9 points, even if the patient scores normal (1 point) on all of the remaining FROMAJE ratings. Thus, a total score of 9 points or more may be a false positive for senile dementia, but it also serves to highlight depression:

F R O M A J E
1 1 1 1 1 1 3 = 9

REFERENCES

1. Libow, L. S.: Pseudo-senility: acute and reversible organic brain syndrome, J. Am. Geriatr. Soc. **21**:112, 1973.
2. Libow, L. S.: Senile dementia and pseudosenility: clinical diagnosis. In Eisdorfer, C., and Friedel, R. O., editors: Cognitive and emotional disturbance in the elderly, Chicago, 1977, Year Book Medical Publishers, Inc.
3. Wells, C. E.: Diagnostic evaluation and treatment in dementia. In Wells C. E., editor: Dementia, ed. 2, Philadelphia, 1977, F. A. Davis Co.
4. Lipowski, Z. J.: Organic brain syndrome: a reformulation, Compr. Psychiatry **19**:309, 1978.
5. Kahn, R. L., Goldfarb, A. I., Pollack, M., and Peck, A.: Brief objective measures for the determination of mental status in the aged, Am. J. Psychiatry **117**:326, 1960.
6. Perlin, S., and Butler, R. N.: Psychiatric aspects of adaptation to the aging experience. In Birren, J. E., Butler, R. N., Greenhouse, S. W., and others, editors: Human aging, biological and behavioral study, Pub. No. (HSM) 71-9051, Washington, D.C., 1971, U.S. Government Printing Office.
7. Pfeiffer, E.: A short portable mental status questionnaire for the assessment of organic brain deficit in elderly patients, J. Am. Geriatr. Soc. **23**: 433, 1975.
8. Blessed, G., Tomlinson, B. E., and Rota, M.: The association between quantitative measures of dementia and of senile change in cerebral gray matters of elderly patients, Br. J. Psychiatry **114**: 797, 1968.
9. Jacobs, J. W.: Screening for organic mental syndromes in the medically ill, Ann. Intern. Med. **80**:40, 1971.

POSTTEST
True or false

1. A command of mental status testing is essential only for psychiatrists.
2. There is a pathognomonic clinical sign leading to the diagnosis of dementia.
3. There is a pathognomonic laboratory or radiological test leading to the diagnosis of dementia.
4. Mental status testing is the same as a psychiatric interview.
5. Mental status testing in the elderly focuses on acute and/or chronic dementias.
6. Some dementias (perhaps 5% to 15%) are falsely interpreted as classic late-life, senile dementias, when, in fact, they reflect emotional depression, medication side-effects, metabolic disorder, or space-taking central nervous system lesions.
7. The key to mental status testing is to use an easily remembered, easily administered technique that can be applied by the primary care clinician whenever appropriate.
8. FROMAJE is one such technique. The OMA refers to orientation, memory, and arithmetic.

9. An individual with normal responses to the FROMAJE questionnaire but whose emotional state is quite disturbed, will score in the abnormal range without necessarily having dementia.

10. The scoring technique is crucial to the use of the FROMAJE test.

11. The score is of value for the inexperienced interviewer, in situations where different clinicians will be seeing the patient over time, or where research data are desired.

12. Mental status examination is of little use in a patient who has global aphasia.

13. When language and/or cultural barriers exist, a standard mental status examination will likely produce excessive false positive and/or false negative results.

14. Patients with dementia always need institutionalization.

15. It is necessary to repeat the FROMAJE test (or any other mental status test) on varying days and at varying times in order to achieve an accurate diagnosis.

ANSWERS TO PRETEST AND POSTTEST

1. False. All physicians and other health professionals should include a mental status evaluation in their examination.

2. False. Dementia is a clinical impression based mainly on mental status testing. There is no one sign or symptom that is diagnostic.

3. False. Thus far, no laboratory or radiological test is diagnostic of dementia. The computerized axial tomography (CAT) test, for example, cannot reliably diagnose dementia.

4. False. Mental status testing focuses primarily on dementia (organic brain syndrome). A psychiatric interview is a global evaluation of all mental function.

5. True. See answer 4.

6. True. The pseudosenilities (pseudodementias) must be sought out vigorously, since many are quite reversible with present-day treatments. See Chapter 4.

7. True. Experience indicates that clinicians are much more likely to employ tests that do not require written forms. The FROMAJE is a relatively easy test to administer.

8. True. Orientation, memory, and arithmetic are the most important and sensitive aspects of FROMAJE with regard to the diagnosis of dementia.

9. True. FROMAJE directs the clinician to focus on the emotional state (particularly mental depression). Depression is probably the most frequent cause of pseudosenility.

10. False. The format of FROMAJE serves as a *guide* to the clinician. It emphasizes essential areas of mental function. Scoring is not necessary, but it may prove helpful to the less experienced interviewer. It may also be helpful in situations where the clinicians change often, and/or in research situations.

11. True. See answer 10.

12. True. Global aphasia does not allow the clinician to reach the diagnosis of dementia.

13. True. The mental status test must be changed to suit special language and/or cultural backgrounds.

14. False. Many patients with dementia continue to live in the community.

15. True. Mental status may vary from day to night and from day to day. This may reflect the effects of sleep, fatigue, medications, and emotional depression. Thus, before the diagnosis of dementia can be made, the patient must be evaluated more than once.

Chapter 6

Pharmacology and medication

FREDRICK T. SHERMAN and LESLIE S. LIBOW

EDUCATIONAL OBJECTIVES
Attitudinal

The student should:
1. Confront his feelings that every symptom in the elderly requires a drug for treatment
2. Recognize that he may do more harm than good by giving an elderly patient a drug
3. Recognize that there may be different goals for drug therapy in late life, such as maximizing the quality of life through symptom relief rather than cure

Cognitive

The student should:
1. Understand how normal aging affects absorption, distribution, binding, metabolism, and excretion of commonly used medications in the elderly
2. Understand how common pathological processes found in the elderly affect drug metabolism
3. Know the most commonly prescribed and non-prescribed medications used by the community-residing elderly as well as the institutionalized elderly
4. Know the common side effects and drug interactions of these drugs
5. Know which medications require lower dosages in the elderly and which require normal adult dosages
6. Be aware of the most common clinical situations in the elderly wherein drugs are usually inappropriate means of therapy
7. Know the role of medication in the following common diseases or clinical situations of late life: diabetes mellitus, hypertension, stroke, dementia, depression, pain relief, and congestive heart failure (CHF)

Skill

The student should:
1. Be able to review an elderly patient's medication profile and comment on drug interactions and dosages
2. Be able to detect compliance problems and implement methods to correct them, including:
   a. Limiting the number of medications to as few as possible
   b. The use of non–child-resistant containers when indicated
   c. The use of other devices to ensure compliance (calendar schedule, Mediset, etc.)
   d. The use of large print on medication containers
   e. Training of the patient in self-medication prior to discharge from a skilled nursing facility or hospital, or within an office or other ambulatory setting
   f. Drug "clean outs" of home medicine cabinets
   g. Home visits by a visiting nurse service to ensure compliance
   h. The use of least expensive, equally bioavailable medications
   i. Patient and family education
   j. Involvement of a family member in the medication regimen of the elderly patient when appropriate
3. Be able to write and explain a prescription for an elderly patient, emphasizing:
   a. Generic medication when appropriate
   b. Large print of directions on the medication container
   c. Non–child-resistant medication containers when indicated
4. Be able to answer the following basic questions

about prescribing for the elderly patient:

a. Does the elderly patient really need the medication?

b. What is the appropriate dosage of medication for this elderly patient?

c. What will the drug do (therapeutically and side effects)?

d. How can the physician guarantee that the elderly patient will take the medication?

e. Is it necessary to continue the drug?

PRETEST*

1. Elderly patients (i.e., those over age 65) comprise (5%? 11%? 15%? 20%?) of the population and account for (5%? 10%? 15%? 20%? 25%?) of all prescriptions.

2. Drugs are handled by the following mechanisms: absorption, hepatic metabolism, distribution, binding, and excretion. What changes, if any, occur with each of these with age? Give an example of one drug in each category that is affected by the altered mechanism.

3. The elderly patient who cannot sleep may be suffering from:

a. Pain

b. Depression

c. Organic brain syndrome

d. Congestive heart failure (CHF)

e. Prostatism

4. Because SGOT, alkaline phosphatase, and total bilirubin values are normal in healthy elderly people, can it be assumed that hepatic metabolism of medication is also normal?

5. Drug interactions are common in the elderly patient. Put the drugs in "Drug A" with the drugs in "Drug B" to form the combinations that most commonly result in clinically significant drug interactions.

Drug A

____ a. Aspirin

____ b. Thiazide diuretics

____ c. Antacids

____ d. Phenothiazines

____ e. Tricyclic antidepressants

____ f. Insulin

Drug B

1. Digoxin

2. Tetracycline

3. Warfarin

4. Phenobarbital

5. Guanethidine

6. Propranolol

6. An 80-year-old, 40-kg woman requires gentamicin for a severe episode of urinary tract sepsis as well as aminophylline for bronchospasm. What information would you need to figure out the dosages of each?

7. What steps would you take to ensure compliance with an elderly individual in the following situations?

a. An elderly female patient is to be discharged from a hospital or skilled nursing facility in about a week. She is currently taking five medications simultaneously.

b. A 72-year-old insulin-dependent diabetic who has senile macular degeneration, diabetic retinopathy, and amyotrophy affecting her manual skills lives with her alcoholic husband. How would you ensure that the patient successfully self-administers her insulin?

Although elderly people make up 11% of the population in the United States, they receive more than 25% of all prescribed drugs and an unknown, but certainly much larger, percentage of nonprescribed medications. In 1978 the average community-residing older person spent approximately $100 for drugs, while his counterpart in a nursing home required $300 worth of medication. Nurs-

---

*Some questions may have more than one correct answer.

ing home residents take anywhere from three to seven different medications for their three or more chronic illnesses. In addition, the elderly patient is known to respond to many drugs differently from the younger adult, while he is able to handle other drugs without any special problems. Altered dosages, adverse drug reactions, drug interactions, and compliance become major issues that confront the physician when prescribing medications for the elderly patient.

Because of the serious implications of medication in the elderly, one must understand (1) the normal changes that occur with aging and how these changes may influence the way elderly people absorb, metabolize, distribute, bind, and excrete medication; (2) the frequent side effects of the commonly used medications in the elderly; (3) the common drug interactions that can be detrimental to the patient; (4) the problems of comprehension and compliance with a drug schedule; and finally (5) indications and contraindications for medication in an elderly individual.

Despite a clear need for an understanding of the clinical pharmacology and pharmacokinetics of the elderly, research has been limited for various reasons including[1]:

1. The expense and time required to keep laboratory test animals alive to evaluate the effects of drugs in old age (In addition, due to species variation, extrapolation to man of some age-related pharmacokinetic and pharmacodynamic alterations observed in experimental animals could be misleading.)

2. The lack of governmental regulations requiring testing of a drug specifically in the elderly (Clinical trials are usually done on young and middle-aged patients, and the elderly are included only by chance rather than by design. Seldom is the 70-to-85-year-old individual included in a drug trial.)

3. The complexity of the aging process and the difficulty of conducting careful clinical studies in elderly subjects

4. The lack of enthusiasm, until recently, on the part of many clinicians, pharmacologists, biochemists, and physiologists to study or research the aging process

One need only look at some commonly used drugs in the elderly to find clinical situations that must be considered when prescribing. Such situations include:

1. An increased incidence of digoxin toxicity in the elderly, in part because of a lack of awareness of the decreased glomerular filtration rate in the normal aged person

2. The prolonged hypoglycemic effect of chlorpropamide (Diabinese) because of the prolonged half-life of this drug in the elderly (Approximately 60% is excreted unchanged in the urine.)

3. The need for decreased maintenance dosages (by approximately 25%) of aminophylline given intravenously in elderly patients to achieve therapeutic serum levels (Even further reduction (by 50%) must be made in the elderly patient with congestive heart failure (CHF) or liver disease.[2])

4. The need for a decreased dosage (15 mg instead of 30 mg) of flurazepam (Dalmane) in the elderly because of the sedative side effect of the larger dosage[3]

PHARMACOLOGICAL CHANGES WITH AGE

Drugs are handled by the following mechanisms: absorption, distribution, protein binding, metabolism, and excretion. Because many changes occur with normal aging, the clinician should know what alterations in drug handling by the elderly patient have been shown to be clinically significant (Table 6-1).

Absorption

There are many changes in normal gastrointestinal function in late life. For example, decreased acid production and a resulting higher gastric pH may affect ionization and solubility of some drugs. Decreased intestinal blood flow may delay or reduce drug absorption. Despite these changes, however, little evidence exists that the gastrointestinal absorption

Table 6-1. Summary of factors affecting drug disposition and response in the elderly*

Effect	Altered physiology	Clinical importance
Absorption	Elevated gastric pH Reduced GI blood flow ? Reduced number of absorbing cells ? Reduced GI motility	Not sufficiently studied

Distribution	Body composition
	   Reduced total body water
	   Reduced lean body mass/kg
	      body weight; increased
	      body fat
	Protein binding
	   Reduced serum albumin
		Higher concentration of drugs
		   distributed in total body water
		? Longer duration of action of
		   fat-soluble drugs
		Higher free fraction of
		   protein-bound drugs

Elimination	Hepatic metabolism
	   ? Reduced enzyme activity
	   Reduced hepatic mass
	   Reduced hepatic blood flow
	
	Renal excretion
	   Reduced glomerular filtration
	      rate
	   Reduced renal plasma flow
	   Altered tubular function
		Apparently slower biotransformation
		   of some drugs
		Influenced by environmental
		   factors (e.g. nutrition and
		   smoking)
		
		Slower excretion of some drugs

Response	Multiple disease states Multiple drug use common Altered receptor sensitivity Organ specific age differences	More variation in dose response Adverse drug reactions common

*From Vestal, R.: Drug use in the elderly: a review of problems and special considerations, Drugs **16**:358, 1978.

of drugs is actually altered in any major way.[4,5]

There is some evidence that active transport of carbohydrates, lipids, and some vitamins from the gastrointestinal tract decreases with age. Examples include the absorption of galactose, 3-methylglucose, calcium, and thiamine. Most drugs, however, are absorbed by passive diffusion, and there appears to be little change in this mechanism with aging.

There are, however, some important drug interactions that can alter the gastrointestinal absorption of medication. For example, calcium, aluminum, and magnesium salts found in antacids, and iron salts found in nonprescription iron-containing preparations or ferrous sulfate, form inabsorbable complexes with tetracycline and thus decrease the absorption of this commonly used antibiotic. Withholding these preparations during tetracycline usage will allow proper therapeutic effect of the tetracycline. If necessary, the tetracycline can be given 1 to 2 hours before the antacid. Digoxin also complexes with antacids, so that the bioavailability of the digoxin is reduced with their use.

The anticholinergic effects of various drugs used in late life (e.g., propantheline bromide for the uninhibited neurogenic bladder of the stroke patient; or tricyclic antidepressants) may alter normal gastrointestinal function, resulting in delayed and/or prolonged drug absorption. The delayed gastric emptying, for example, can result in degradation of L-dopa and, hence, reduced bioavailability of this compound.[6]

In general, if an elderly patient does not respond to a medication, there is usually a compliance problem rather than impaired absorption. Other possibilities for a lack of response to a medication include:

1. Decreased sensitivity to the drug because of a pathological process (For example, the elderly patient with atrial fibrillation whose ventricular response does not slow with digoxin may have apathetic hyperthyroidism.)
2. Undermedication of the patient because of the physician's belief that elderly people require low dosages of all medications (Consequently, a therapeutic effect will not be achieved.)
3. Drug interactions, such as the digoxin-antacid example mentioned above

Liver metabolism

The ability of the liver to metabolize certain drugs appears to be altered with age. Hepatic metabolism of drugs may be affected by, or result from, the following changes with age:

1. The normal human liver decreases in size with age, with the main loss occurring after age 70.
2. Hepatic blood flow decreases with age; therefore, drugs that are extracted and metabolized by the liver may undergo a decreased rate of metabolic transformation.
3. Serum albumin decreases with age.[7]
4. There is conflicting data about the retention of sulfobromophthalein (BSP) in normal elderly individuals. Some studies show an increased retention of BSP with age, whereas others show no change.[8] Most other liver function tests, including alkaline phosphatase, SGOT, SGPT, and total bilirubin, however, are not altered in the normal elderly.

Animal studies show that microsomal enzyme activity and the rate of enzyme induction decrease with age. Studies in humans, which also show decreased hepatic metabolism, are complicated by other factors, such as changes in the volume of distribution. The half-life of antipyrine, (a drug that is rapidly absorbed and has minimal protein binding and extensive microsomal metabolism by the liver), for example, is 16% longer in older subjects when compared with younger ones.[9] Surprisingly, this 16% prolongation in half-life is more likely related to individual variation and smoking characteristics of the population studied rather than age differences.

For a number of drugs metabolized by the liver, it appears that there is a prolonged plasma half-life. Quinidine, acetaminophen, and desipramine (all metabolized, at least in part by the liver) have a prolonged half-life in the elderly. A longer half-life means that it takes longer to reach steady-state plasma levels and that the pharmacological effect may be prolonged after the drug is stopped. When total plasma clearance is also reduced, due to altered intrinsic metabolic capacity of the liver, higher plasma levels result in the elderly. For drugs that are highly extracted by the liver, a reduction in hepatic blood flow with age may result in an overall decrease in the rate of metabolic biotransformation.

There are many unknowns about the altered metabolism of drugs by the aged liver, and there are no clinical parameters to use to establish dosage alterations. Before prescribing a drug metabolized by the liver, however, the clinician should be aware of the route of metabolism of a drug and of any past history of chronic liver disease or impaired hepatic blood flow from CHF or portal hypertension. Starting at lower doses of hepatically metabolized drugs and gradually increasing the dosage are the preferred methods of drug administration.

Binding

The protein binding of certain drugs decreases with age. Because of the age-related fall in albumin, drugs that are primarily bound to it may have higher free concentrations, leading to greater concentrations at the receptor site as well as at the site of elimination. Reduced plasma protein also intensifies the competition among drugs for binding sites. Reduction in binding in the elderly has been found with phenylbutazone, phenytoin (Dilantin), warfarin (Coumadin), and meperidine (Demerol).

Clinically, the most important example is warfarin. It has been shown that in elderly patients with warfarin concentrations well above therapeutic levels, there is an increase in unbound warfarin that correlates with a fall in plasma albumin concentration.[10] At therapeutic concentrations of warfarin, however, there does not seem to be any age-related differences in bound or unbound warfarin.[11] A significant difference has been found between younger and older subjects in the synthesis of clotting factors at equal warfarin concentrations. Although clearly defined pharmacokinetic data are not yet available, warfarin should be used with particular caution in elderly patients because of the high risk of bleeding, which is approximately twice that of younger persons.

Heparin also causes an increased risk of bleeding complications in women over the age of 60.[12] Fifty percent of elderly women given intermittent doses of heparin will have such a complication. The reasons for the excessive bleeding in elderly women are unexplained, but obvious care must be taken in anticoagulating these patients. Pulmonary embolism and deep venous thrombophlebitis are the main reasons for anticoagulation with heparin and warfarin. Given the greater risks of an older patient bleeding from heparin (women) and warfarin (women and men), it is important to be aware of hematopoietic side effects when using these medications.

Because the list of drugs that interact with warfarin is endless, the physician working with elderly patients must be aware of those most commonly encountered. Aspirin (found in over 200 prescribed and nonprescribed drugs) displaces warfarin from its binding sites and increases the unbound warfarin concentration, with its potential serious consequences. Similarly, oral sulfonylureas taken to control hyperglycemia displace warfarin from albumin, resulting in a greater tendency for bleeding. Cimetidine, phenytoin, and trimethoprim-sulfamethoxazole have been reported to increase the effect of warfarin and prolong the prothrombin time.[13-15] Haloperidol inhibits the effect of warfarin and decreases the prothrombin time. When an elderly patient is taking warfarin, the physician should consult a list of drug interactions before altering, discontinuing, or initiating any drug therapy for that patient.

Renal function

The role of the kidney in the elimination of drugs is much better documented at this time than hepatic metabolism. Renal plasma flow, glomerular filtration rate, maximum reabsorptive capacity of the tubule for glucose (TmG), and the maximum excreting capacity of the tubule for diodrast and para-aminohippuric acid (PAH) all fall with normal aging. The glomerular filtration rate declines by about one third between ages 20 and 90, while renal plasma flow declines by 40% to 45% between ages 25 and 65. Despite decreases in the glomerular filtration rate, serum creatinine remains within normal limits as defined for healthy subjects because of the decreased production of creatinine that parallels the decreased muscle mass in elderly patients. A serum creatinine level above 1.5 mg/dl is rarely from age alone; rather, it implies a pathological decrease in renal function.[16] Therefore, relying on the serum creatinine or BUN values as indicators of renal function in late life can lead to serious errors. Monographs and formulas have been developed describing the change in creatinine clearance with age.[17]

Prescribing the aminoglycoside gentamicin on the basis of serum creatinine values can lead to inappropriately high serum levels of this drug in an elderly patient. The standard gentamicin regimen of 1.7 mg/kg (intramuscular intravenous) loading dose followed by 1.5 mg/kg every 8 hours modified for serum creatinine assumes that serum creatinine accurately reflects the glomerular filtration rate. If the serum creatinine level were 1.2 mg/dl in an 80-year-old women, she would receive the same dose of gentamicin or tobramycin per kilogram as her 20-year-old counterpart, even though the glomerular filtration rates differ by at least 30%. The nomogram shown in Fig. 6-1 is helpful in calculating the dosage schedule for elderly patients because it takes into account the relationship of age and sex to creatinine clearance. For example, the 80-year-old, 50-kg woman with a serum creatinine level of 1.4 mg/dl would receive a loading dose of 1.75 mg/kg of gentamicin for urinary tract sepsis. Her creatinine clearance, according to the nomogram, is about 28 ml/mm.

1. Select loading dose in mg/kg (lean weight) to provide peak serum level desired. Approximate peak levels from commonly used loading doses are indicated below:

LOADING DOSE	EXPECTED PEAK SERUM LEVEL BASED UPON ONE-HALF HOUR IV INFUSION
2.0 mg/kg	6-8 μg/ml
1.75 mg/kg*	5-7 μg/ml
1.5 mg/kg	4-6 μg/ml
1.25 mg/kg	3-5 μg/ml
1.0 mg/kg	2-4 μg/ml

*Recommended for most moderate to severe systemic infections.

2. Select maintenance dose (as percentage of chosen loading dose) to continue peak serum levels indicated above according to patient's creatinine clearance and desired dosing interval.

	PERCENTAGE OF LOADING DOSE REQUIRED FOR DOSAGE INTERVAL SELECTED:		
Cr clear	8 hr	12 hr	24 hr
90	90%	—	—
80	88	—	—
70	84	—	—
60	79	91%	—
50	74	87	—
40	66	80	—
30	57	72	92%
25	51	66	88
20	45	59	83
15	37	50	75
10	29	40	64
7	24	33	55
5	20	28	48
2	20	20	35
0	14	18	25
	9		

(Shaded areas indicate suggested dosage intervals.)

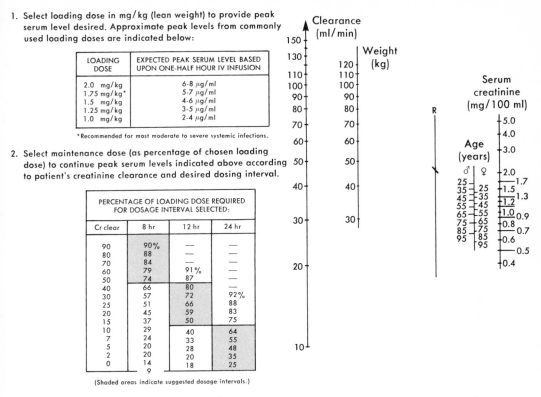

Fig. 6-1. Gentamicin nomogram; loading and maintenance doses as a function of age, sex, weight, and creatinine clearance. With a ruler, join weight to age. Keep ruler at crossing point of line marked "R." Then move the right-hand side of the ruler to the appropriate serum creatinine value and read the patient's clearance from the left side of the nomogram. (From Nielsen, S.: Letter to the editor, Lancet 1:1133, 1977.)

She should receive approximately 57% of the loading dose (1 mg/kg q 8 hours, or 50 mg q 8 hours) to maintain serum levels between 5 to 7 mg/ml. The 40-year-old, 60-kg woman would receive a similar loading dose (1.75 mg/kg), but her maintenance dose for the same serum creatinine value would be approximately 76% of the loading dose every 8 hours (1.33 mg/kg) or a total dose of 80 mg q 8 hours. Fig. 6-2 is a similar nomogram for intravenous aminophylline.

In any individual patient, the glomerular filtration rate may be measured from the endogenous creatinine clearance.

This may be difficult in the cooperative as well as in the confused elderly patient. Although one could catheterize the patient and risk the possibility of urinary tract infection, it would be better to begin using the nomograms and then draw plasma levels of the drug to determine the steady-state concentration.

In the case of digoxin, a drug used by 20% to 50% of nursing home patients, proper dosage is important because of the multiple incapacitating toxicities of the drug in the elderly patient. Digitalis toxicity was said to be present in 23% of all patients receiving this medication who

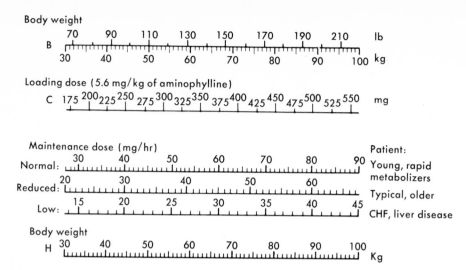

Body weight

B 70 90 110 130 150 170 190 210 lb
   30 40 50 60 70 80 90 100 kg

Loading dose (5.6 mg/kg of aminophylline)

C 175 200 225 250 275 300 325 350 375 400 425 450 475 500 525 550 mg

Maintenance dose (mg/hr)   Patient:

Normal: 30 40 50 60 70 80 90   Young, rapid
                                            metabolizers
Reduced: 20 30 40 50 60

Low: 15 20 25 30 35 40 45   Typical, older

                                            CHF, liver disease

Body weight

H 30 40 50 60 70 80 90 100 Kg

Fig. 6-2. Guidelines for intravenous aminophylline therapy in the elderly. Mark patient's weight in kg on Lines B and H. Use a ruler to connect these points. *Loading dose:* Line C provides a loading dose of 5.6 mg/kg. Give concentrated solution at a rate not exceeding 50 mg/min. Give 0 to ½ of this dose if patients have received theophylline within 12 hours. *Maintenance dose:* The infusion rate (in mg/hr) is obtained from the intersection on the following lines: normal—young patients expected to be rapid metabolizers; reduced—typical older patients (over 50 years); low—patients with CHF or liver disease. Begin infusion soon after injection of the bolus. The rate of infusion is critical and must be checked frequently by nursing personnel. (From Jusko, W., and others: Intravenous theophylline therapy: nomogram guidelines, Ann. Intern. Med. **86**(4):400, 1977.)

Fig. 6-3. Changes in plasma level and half-life of selected parenterally given medications. (From Bender, A.: Pharmacodynamic principles of drug therapy in the aged, J. Am. Geriatr. Soc. **22**:296, 1974.)

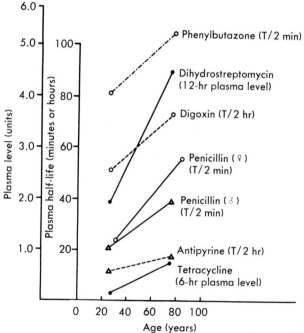

were admitted to a large city hospital, and the average age of the patients with digitalis toxicity was 73 years.[18] (Digitalis toxicity thus appears to be a disease primarily of the elderly.) The patients cited often had advanced heart disease, underlying atrial fibrillation, associated pulmonary disease, and abnormal renal function. Digitalis toxicity has also been reported to cause an altered mental status in elderly patients. Anorexia secondary to digoxin toxicity may be the most common reason for unexplained weight loss among the elderly. Beginning an elderly patient on a digoxin dosage of 0.125 mg daily by mouth will achieve a steady state in 8 to 10 days. In general, because of the altered metabolism and excretion of drugs in the elderly, it is better to start with low doses of medication and titrate the dosage upward in accordance with the therapeutic response or plasma drug level (Fig. 6-3).

SIDE EFFECTS

The elderly patient has a greater chance of having an adverse drug reaction because of altered excretion, altered metabolism, and/or altered receptor sensitivity or binding. Drug-induced illness was the reason for 3% of 6,000 admissions to a major teaching hospital.[19] Forty percent of these patients were over 60 years of age. Eight drugs accounted for one third of the admissions in all age groups: aspirin, digoxin, warfarin, sodium hydrochlorothiazide, prednisone, vincristine sulfate, norethindrone, and furosemide. In a hospital, the incidence of adverse drug reaction increases with age, being 15% for patients over age 60, 20% for those over age 70, and 24% for those over age 80.[20,21]

The following profile describes the typical patient at high risk for an adverse drug reaction:

1. Small elderly person (women more likely than men)
2. History of allergic illness
3. Previous adverse reactions
4. Multiple chronic illnesses
5. Renal failure
6. Too many physicians
7. Abnormal mental status
8. Patient living alone
9. Financial difficulties
10. Visual or audiological problems

Commonly used drugs and their side effects are listed in Table 6-2.

DRUG INTERACTIONS

Because the elderly patient takes multiple medications (both prescribed and nonprescribed), it is important to be aware of common drug side effects and potential drug interactions. To help the physician remember all possible drug interactions, a portable interaction chart (MEDISC*) can be used to determine common drug interactions at the bedside. The local pharmacist may keep a drug profile indicating all drugs the patient is currently taking and all known hypersensitivities. A few states require the pharmacist to keep such a record. Thus, if the pharmacist notices a potential drug interaction, he can call the physician, who in turn can alter the therapy.

Nonprescribed remedies, may also interact with prescribed medications. Therefore, in order to comprehensively assess the potential for drug interactions in an elderly patient, the physician must attempt to learn about all of the pa-

---

*MEDISC can be obtained by writing to Professionals Shopper, P. O. Box 696, 125 Elm St., New Canaan, Conn. 06840

Text continued on p. 107.

Table 6-2. Commonly used drugs in the elderly and their side effects*

Drug/class	Potential effect by aging	Possible mechanism	Suggested management
Warfarin	Elderly patients are twice as likely as younger patients to have a complication of warfarin therapy	Unclear; synthesis of vitamin K–dependent clotting factor, however, is less in the elderly taking warfarin than in the young	Firmly establish the need for warfarin; be aware of drug interactions and the obvious danger of bleeding
Phenytoin (Dilantin)	Increased incidence of neurological and hematological toxicity in elderly patients with hypoalbuminemia or renal disease	Phenytoin is 90% bound to albumin; elderly patients may have reduced plasma protein with subsequent reduction in binding of phenytoin; as a result, an increase in active free drugs may be expected	Reversal of toxic CNS symptoms has been reported with dosage reduction, while others have suggested that age-related dosage reduction will achieve only marginal improvement; note that plasma determinations of phenytoin may measure both bound and unbound drugs and may not explain manifestations of toxicity that are the result of an increased amount of free drug
Amitriptyline Imipramine	A higher number of geriatric patients receiving amitriptyline or imipramine experience confusional reactions, cardiotoxicity (quinidinelike effects and negative inotropic effects), orthostatic hypotension, and urinary retention	Possibly secondary to central anticholinergic effects of tricyclic antidepressants, a slowed metabolism, and higher serum levels of these drugs in the elderly[22]	Monitor for confusional reactions: orthostatic hypotension, resting tachycardia, and ECG changes

*Modified from Drug effects in the geriatric patient, Drug Intell. Clin. Pharm. **11**:597, 1977. Reprinted with permission. Copyright 1977 retained by *Drug Intelligence and Clinical Pharmacy, Inc.*, University of Cincinnati Medical Center, Cincinnati, OH 45267.

Table 6-2. Commonly used drugs in the elderly and their side effects — cont'd

Drug/class	Potential effect by aging	Possible mechanism	Suggested management
Thiazide diuretics	Elderly patients are more prone to orthostatic hypotension, hypo-kalemia, digitalis toxic-ity, hyponatremia, hy-perglycemia, and dehy-dration	Total body potassium decreases with normal aging, altered baroceptor response and peripheral venous disease may make the elderly more sensitive	Antihypertensive therapy in the elderly patient should be initiated with lower doses and the side effects monitored; antihypertensive agents may reduce cardiovascular mortality in patients over 65 with diastolic blood pressures between 90 and 104, and higher (not dem-onstrated for older white women)
Clindamycin	The incidence of diarrhea and pseudomembranous colitis appears to increase with age and is most common in middle-aged and older women	Common conditions in the elderly (inadequate diet, constipation) may predispose these patients to diarrhea or colitis	Monitor elderly patients receiving clindamycin therapy for diarrhea
Gentamicin	Enhanced drug toxicity (ototoxicity, nephrotox-icity); gentamicin ototoxicity is much more likely to present with vestibular symp-toms rather than hear-ing loss[23]	Renal excretion of gentamicin accounts for 98% of its elimination; elderly patients may have significantly reduced renal function, which will prolong the drug's half-life	Determine the actual or estimated creatinine clearance as a measure of renal function; several methods of adjusting the gentamicin dosage in renal failure are available (Fig. 6-1)
Penicillin G	Enhanced CNS toxicity; seizures, coma	Blood levels are elevated to toxic concentrations secondary to a prolonged half-life of the drug (the result of impaired renal elimination due to decreased active tubular secretion)	Elderly patients requiring multiple large doses of penicillin G should have their renal status established early in therapy and the dosage reduced or the dosing interval increased; elderly patients with mild to moderate renal failure may be treated with normal doses and dosing intervals, but with close observation

Continued.

Table 6-2. Commonly used drugs in the elderly and their side effects — cont'd

Drug/class	Potential effect by aging	Possible mechanism	Suggested management
Propranolol	Increased incidence of adverse reactions, including heart failure, bradycardia, pulmonary edema, and confusional syndromes	The mechanism is not yet clear; a prolonged half-life of the drug and elevated plasma levels have been reported in elderly patients, which may be related to reduced hepatic extraction	Carefully titrate the propranolol dosage in geriatric patients to the desired effect and monitor closely for adverse reactions
L-dopa	Elderly patients may be more likely to experience serious side effects, such as hypotension, syncope, anorexia, nausea, vomiting, and confusional states; L-dopa is also kaliuretic and therefore predisposes patients taking digoxin to digitalis toxicity[24]	An altered level of behavioral activation or arousal results from L-dopa therapy, possibly causing behavioral changes; no mechanism for this effect has been postulated	Elderly patients may require lower doses of L-dopa to avoid side effects; the behavior of geriatric patients must be carefully monitored for changes; if major changes do occur, drug discontinuation may be necessary
Benzodiazepine (diazepam, flurazepam)	Increased frequency of CNS depression in acute intravenous dosage for elective procedures and in chronic oral dosage	The half-life of diazepam is increased secondary to a marked increase in the volume of distribution[25]; the metabolic clearance rate is minimally affected; liver disease will also increase the drug's half-life	CNS depression is reported to decrease with dosage reduction; begin with lower doses of flurazepam (15 mg orally) and Diazepam (orally or intravenously)[3,26]; avoid alcohol, since the sedative effect may may be additive

Table 6-3. Some important drug interactions in the elderly

Drug A	Drug B	Interaction	Comments
Digoxin	Diuretics	Hypokalemia predisposes patients to digoxin toxicity	Add oral potassium supplement and monitor electrolytes frequently; the use of potassium-sparing diuretics should be done with caution and frequent monitoring of the potassium level
Tricyclic antidepressants	Guanethidine	The tricyclic blocks the norepinephrine pump, preventing the accumulation of quanethidine at its site of action, with a resulting decrease in hypertensive control	This interaction should seldom be encountered in the elderly population because of the infrequent use of guanethidine because of its serious side effects; if necessary, increase the dosage of guanethidine to overcome the tricyclic effect
Phenobarbital	Phenothiazine	The use of phenobarbital for sleep will cause induction of liver microsomal metabolism of the phenothiazine, decreasing the serum level of the phenothiazine	Reduced clinical effects of phenothiazine results from the addition of phenobarbital
Sulfonylurea	Warfarin	Displacement of warfarin from its binding site leads to increased free warfarin and increased anticoagulant effect; warfarin enhances the sulfonylurea hypoglycemic effects	Elderly patients on warfarin should be reviewed to determine: 1. Why they need the drug 2. If it is being monitored appropriately
	Phenybutazone	Phenybutazone displaces the sulfonylurea from its binding site, enhancing the hypoglycemic effect	3. Potential drug interactions

Continued.

Table 6-3. Some important drug interactions in the elderly—cont'd

Drug A	Drug B	Interaction	Comments
Methylphenidate (Ritalin)	Phenytoin	Methylphenidate retards liver microsomal metabolism, thereby increasing plasma levels of any of drug B	Increased possibility of phenytoin toxicity
	Tricyclic antidepressants		Increased tricyclic level leads to anticholinergic side effects
	Phenothiazine		Paradoxical increase in sedation caused by decreased metabolism
	Warfarin		Increased warfarin effect
Antacids containing magnesium trisilicate and aluminum hydroxide gel	Chlorpromazine Isoniazid	The antacid impairs the absorption of chlor- promazine and isonazid.	Recurrence of psychotic symptoms may result when antacids are added to the regimen
	Tetracycline	Formation of inabsorbable complexes	Discontinue antacids during the tetracycline course
Sulfonylurea/ insulin	Propranolol	Propranolol blocks the sympathetic response to hypoglycemia, elim- inating tremor, sweat- ing, and palpita- tions as helpful signs of hypoglycemia	The metabolic clearance of both propranolol and sulfonylureas is altered with age; because of the lack of signs, any change in mental status or a fall should suggest hypoglycemia
Thiothixene (Navane)	Alpha-methyldopa	Confusional state	
Chlorpro- pamide	Ethyl alcohol	Antabuse-type reaction with flushing and headache Hypoglycemic effect caused by ethyl alcohol (ETOH) can be severe in patients receiving chlorpropamide	A thorough history of ethanol use must be obtained; although wine can be used as a sedative hypnotic in the elderly, it should not be taken by the patient receiving chlorpropamide

tient's medications (past, present, nonprescribed, and prescribed). If the patient is homebound, the physician or visiting nurse should review the medication in the medicine cabinet, discard all those not needed or out of date, and review the most currently needed.

Table 6-3 lists some of the most common drug interactions experienced in the elderly patient.

COMPLIANCE

Comprehension of, and compliance with, a medication regimen are major problems in elderly patients taking medication on a short-term or chronic basis. Between 30% to 50% of all patients fail to comply with their physicians' prescriptions. One of the few studies of noncompliance among the elderly found that 59% of 178 elderly outpatients made errors in taking their medication.[27] A British study looking at noncompliance of recently discharged elderly patients (aged 65 and over) from an acute care hospital found that 50% deviated from the prescribed regimen; of these, 70% did not comprehend the regimen.[28] Patients who were prone to error were those who took three or more drugs or were taking the same drug before admission as at discharge (this suggests patients may have gotten confused with previous regimens). These patients either reverted to dosages operative before admission or to the actual medication used before admission.

There are many reasons for noncompliance among the elderly including (1) memory loss; (2) lack of written instructions; (3) environmental hazards, such as weather conditions or fear of crime, that may impede getting medication; (4) visual or hearing problems; and (5) lifelong personality patterns that include refusing to face illness or deal with medications.

Patients receiving medications for chronic diseases tend to comply less when poverty and unemployment are also problems. Since a significant percentage of the elderly are at or below the poverty level, the physician, in prescribing for the elderly patient, must consider cost factors and prescribe generically when equal bioavailability has been shown. Medicare has no outpatient drug benefit; thus, the physician must review the discharge medication regimen and prescribe only what is absolutely necessary. Other factors, such as the unpleasant taste of the medication, dissatisfaction with the physician visit, or lengthy waiting time with the physician and/or pharmacist, may contribute to noncompliance among the elderly.

The physician and team must not take for granted any aspect of compliance with the elderly patient. Specifically, efforts should be made to confirm that:

1. The patient fills the prescription
2. The patient and/or a family member understands and/or remembers the drug regimen
3. The patient is taking the medication that the physician has prescribed
4. The patient takes the prescribed medication for as long as the physician stipulates
5. The patient has been informed of pertinent, or disturbing side effects (orthostatic hypotension, dry mouth, urinary incontinence, etc.) and is capable of reporting adverse reactions

Since three simultaneous medications seem to be the most that many elderly patients can take without making significant errors, it is important to instruct the patient and/or family as to when, how, and for how long the medication is to be taken. Using common language, ("heart pill" for digoxin, "water pill" for diuretic) the physician should verbally explain the written prescription. In particular, a detailed explanation of the prescription must be given to a patient who has difficulty with communication caused by hearing or visual impairment. The physician must speak slowly, with proper illumination on his face, so that lipreading may be used to overcome any hearing deficiency. The physician must stipulate that the prescription be typed in large print so that the elderly patient can read it.[29]

Since elderly patients may see or have seen multiple physicians, it is important to determine that they are taking only those medications that are currently indicated. Asking the patient or family to bring in all medications at the initial visit can often eliminate many potential drug interactions. Similarly, when a home visit is made, the physician should inquire about and see all medications used in the past or currently.

Another factor with compliance in an outpatient setting is the ability of the patient to properly open and close the child-resistant medication container.[30] Some elderly people have difficulty with child-resistant medication containers. Thirty-three percent of community-residing elderly patients admitted to improper use of child-resistant packaging because of difficulty with the safety devices. In a survey of 120 community-residing elderly persons attending a senior citizens' seminar, 60% admitted to having difficulty opening medication containers with safety tops. In addition to the inability to properly use child-resistant containers, a large percentage of elderly patients are unaware that they can obtain their medications in non–child-resistant containers merely by asking the pharma-

cist or the physician. Elderly patients with no children at risk may opt to use non–child-resistant containers. Physicians should ask each patient about his ability to open child-resistant containers as well as his living situation, since only about 10% of the elderly live in three-generation households, where young children could regularly get the medication. Testing the patient's ability to open and close a typical container used by local pharmacists should be part of the evaluation of every elderly patient.

The task of ensuring compliance among the community-residing elderly is difficult, requiring patient education and follow-up.[31] Health care professionals working with elderly patients who are being discharged back into the community from hospitals or nursing homes must make attempts to ensure medication compliance. A self-medication program prior to discharge attempts to ensure that patients can properly take their medications once they are discharged.[32] The process, with varying time intervals, is as follows. Patients are selected in accordance with the nurse's and physician's assessment of their mental status. The patient is given a bottle of placebos, instructed to take one a day for 7 days, and told to mark down on a patient compliance card whether he took each one. At a designated time each day, the nurse counts the remaining tablets. After a week of successful administration, a second placebo on a twice or three-times daily schedule is added. If after 2 weeks a minimal amount of errors occur, the procedure is extended to include one of the patient's discharge medications. By this method it can be ensured that the patient is properly taking his medication at discharge. A modified evaluation system for self-administration can be used in the ambulatory care. Patients who fail to take their medications should be encouraged to use a medication calendar or diary. The Mediset* is a device that allows for a weekly loading of all medications and only one simple action to dispense all of the pills necessary for a given time.

INAPPROPRIATE USE OF DRUGS IN THE ELDERLY

The following are situations wherein drugs are often inappropriately used in the elderly.

Patients with a chronic indwelling urinary catheter should not be given continuous local or systemic antibiotics to prevent infection, because resistant bacteria will develop, leading to the ineffectiveness of the antibiotic.[33] Removal of the catheter and bladder training should be the primary goal.

Elderly patients with ankle edema should not universally receive a diuretic, because the edema may really be from dependency, disuse, or varicose veins. Ankle edema does not indicate heart failure unless other signs or symptoms are present. Elevation of the legs, ambulation, and compression stockings may be all that are required to eliminate the edema of dependency or venous disease.

Agitated, confused patients should not be treated with a tranquilizer until the cause of the confusion is found, if possible. Often the cause may be the other medications the patient is taking. If these medications are discontinued, the confusion may be resolved.

The normal elderly person experiences more frequent and longer nocturnal awakenings and sleeps less than his

---

*Information on this device may be obtained by writing to Drug Intelligence, Hamilton, Ill. 62341.

younger counterpart. Both rapid eye movement (REM) and stage 4 slow-wave sleep are decreased. Discussing the normal changes in sleep patterns may be all that is necessary to make the elderly patient feel comfortable. Other factors, however, may alter sleep patterns in late life. A history of the older person's daily habits may show frequent daytime naps and decreased physical activity leading to reduced nighttime sleep. Suggesting daytime activities, eliminating naps, and increasing physical activity may be the simplest prescription for establishing a more normal sleep pattern.

Medical or psychiatric problems may present with insomnia in late life. Nocturnal dyspnea from CHF can cause insomnia and is relieved by digoxin or diuretics. One must be careful to administer the diuretic early in the day to avoid another frequent cause for insomnia—diuretic-induced nocturia.

Pain from various arthritic compliants can cause insomnia and responds to proper diagnosis and therapy. Prostatism, uncontrolled diabetes mellitus, and any type of neurogenic bladder disturbance can cause nocturia. Hypoglycemia can cause nocturnal awakening. The patient may awake anxious and fearful, with signs of sympathetic overactivity. Pruritus, secondary to dry skin, can present with insomnia or difficulty in falling asleep.

Psychiatric illness, especially depression, may also present with insomnia. Classic symptoms or signs, such as weight loss and decreased appetite, may be absent. Constipation is not helpful in diagnosing depression, because it is a frequent complaint in the elderly. Insomnia, pessimism, loss of interest, decreased energy, impaired self-esteem, and somatic complaints are often major clues to depression that may be remedied by antidepressant therapy.

The "sundown syndrome" is nocturnal delirium seen in patients with mild to moderate organic brain syndrome. This abnormal behavior, thought to occur because of the lack of external stimuli that occurs with the coming of evening, presents with disorientation, bizarre behavior, and hallucinations. These episodes, if not handled properly, can result in institutionalization. Sedative antipsychotic medication is helpful.

Situational insomnia is transient and is associated with special life stresses. In these situations, diphenhydramine or chloral hydrate may be appropriate. A 4-oz glass of wine is also an adequate hypnotic for elderly people. Flurazepam given in low doses (15 mg) is also a satisfactory hypnotic but certainly not as enjoyable or inexpensive as a glass of wine. Higher doses of flurazepam (30 mg) can result in sedation and falls in elderly patients and should be avoided. Barbiturates are known to cause paradoxical excitation in the elderly and also induce microsomal enzymes, thus affecting the metabolism of other medications. However, if the barbiturates have been taken for years, there may be no good reason to discontinue them.

Many elderly individuals feel that they must have regular, daily bowel movements. To ensure this, they may take laxatives frequently; and this leads to a dependency on medication to have a bowel movement. Studies have shown that normal elderly people have anywhere from three bowel movements a day to three bowel movements a week. Increasing the amount of exercise and adding bran to the diet will eliminate constipation in most cases and prevent the inappropriate use of laxatives. A new complaint of constipation should always be investigated.

Although "hardening of the arteries" was once thought to be the predominant cause of dementia in late life, current thinking suggests that it is not. No drug has been shown to reverse this condition. Cerebral vasodilator drugs have not been shown to be effective in improving mental function in patients with dementia of any cause.

GENERAL PRINCIPLES FOR PRESCRIBING MEDICATION

Based on the altered handling of drugs in the elderly, we recommend that the following simple questions be asked in prescribing or reevaluating a medication for an elderly patient[34]:

1. Does the elderly patient really need the medication? Is the edema secondary to stasis (no diuretic, only elevation and ambulation) or CHF (digoxin and/or diuretic indicated)? Mild depression and loneliness should be initially treated by more frequent family visits, social work intervention, or appropriate physician discussions rather than by drug treatment of each symptom. Beware of treating symptoms in the elderly without an established diagnosis.

2. What is the appropriate dosage of medication for this elderly patient? Because of altered metabolism, excretion, binding, and volume of distribution in elderly patients, the following general rule applies with regard to dosage: *Start low, go slow (titrate), but be prepared to go high. Start low:* Loading doses are often not needed. *Go slow:* Titrate the dosage upward and look for therapeutic response or toxicity. *Be prepared to go high:* Large doses of diuretics may be used to treat CHF; antibiotics, excluding the aminoglycosides, can be prescribed in the usual "high" doses recommended for the 40-year-old, 70-kg man.

3. How can I guarantee that my elderly patient will take the medication?

a. Review all medications, looking for interactions, improper dosages, and toxicity.

b. Give the fewest medications possible (three or less).

c. Instruct the patient and/or family member, verbally and in writing, about the proper regimen.

d. Institute a self-medication program, if possible.

e. Make sure that the patient has access to the medication (order a non–child-resistant container) and can read the directions. Ask the pharmacist to type the label in large print.

f. Ask the visiting nurse service or relatives to monitor the patient's compliance. Perform a "drug cleanout" of the medicine cabinet and disgard all old and unneeded medications.

g. Discontinue medication whenever appropriate.

4. What will the drug do? Define what your expectations are. Is it the prolongation of life, the relief of a symptom (beware!), or improvement in the quality of life? Do not withold medication on the basis of the patient's age alone, especially when the quality of life can be improved.

5. Is it necessary to continue the drug? The entire drug regimen should be reviewed at each visit, whether it is in an outpatient department at a university teaching center, a nursing home, an acute-care hospital, or the patient's home. The focus should be on determining whether the drug is necessary. If it is not, it should be discontinued. In many cases, elderly patients have improved when all medications were stopped.

Summary of principles of drug prescribing in the elderly*

1. Is drug therapy required?
   a. Many diseases from which the elderly suffer do not require drug treatment.
   b. But, do not withold drugs on account of old age, particularly when appropriate drug treatment can improve the quality of life.
   c. Only use those drugs which the patient really needs.

2. Choice of appropriate drug and preparation
   a. Is a particular drug which is satisfactory for the younger patient suitable for the elderly? – e.g. increased likelihood of side-effects.
   b. Which preparation? – consider dosage form (syrup, effervescent tablet, suppository instead of capsule or tablet); its size, shape and colour.

3. Dose and dosage regimen
   a. In general, use smaller doses than are usually given to younger adults.
   b. Intermittent schedules should be avoided. Once-daily dosage is ideal.

4. Medication instructions
   a. Teach the patient to understand his drugs, especially their relative importance to his well-being.
   b. Drugs prescribed should be clearly labelled in large print and packaged in readily opened containers.
   c. Supervision of therapy may sometimes be desirable or necessary – e.g. a responsible and interested neighbour, relative or friend, or a community nurse.

REFERENCES

1. Hall, M. R.: Use of drugs in elderly patients, N.Y. State J. Med. 75:67, 1975.

*From O'Malley, K., Judge, T. C., and Crooks, J.: Geriatric clinical pharmacology and therapeutics In Avery, editor: Drug treatment, p. 123 (ADIS Press, Sydney/ Lea & Febiger, Philadelphia, 1976).

2. Jusko, W. J., and others: Intravenous theophylline therapy: nomogram guidelines, Ann. Intern. Med. **86**:400, 1977.

3. Greenblatt, D. J., and others: Toxicity of high dose flurazepam in the elderly, Clin. Pharmacol. Ther. **21**:355, 1977.

4. Gorrod, J. W.: Absorption, metabolism and excretion of drugs in geriatric subjects, Gerontol. Clin. **16**:30, 1974.

5. Crooks, J., and others: Pharmacokinetics in the elderly, Clin. Pharmacokinet. **1**:280, 1976.

6. Bianchine, J. R., and Shaw, G. M.: Clinical pharmacokinetics of levodopa in Parkinson's disease, Clin. Pharmacokinet. **1**:313, 1976.

7. Greenblatt, D. J.: Reduced serum albumin concentration in the elderly: a report from the Boston collaborative drug surveillance program, J. Am. Geriatr. Soc. **27**:20, 1979.

8. Kampmann, J. P., Sinding, J., and Miller, J.: Effect of age on liver function, Geriatrics **30**:91, 1975.

9. Vestal, R. E., and others: Antipyrine metabolism in man: influence of age, alcohol, caffeine, and smoking, Clin. Pharmacol. Ther. **18**:425, 1975.

10. Hayes, M. J., Langman, M. J. S., and Short, A. H.: Changes in drug metabolism with age: warfarin binding and plasma proteins, Br. J. Clin. Pharmacol. **2**:69, 1975.

11. Shepard, A. M., Hewick, D. S., Moreland, T. A., and Stevenson, I. H.: Age as determinant of sensitivity to warfarin, Br. J. Clin. Pharmacol. **4**:315, 1977.

12. Jick, H., and others: Efficacy and toxicity of heparin in relation to age and sex, N. Engl. J. Med. **279**:284, 1968.

13. Silver, B. A., and others: Potentiation of the hypoprothrombinemic effect of warfarin, Ann. Intern. Med. **90**:348, 1979.

14. Koch-Weser, J.: Hemorrhagic reactions and drug interactions in 500 warfarin-treated patients (abstract), Clin. Pharmacol. Ther. **14**:139, 1973.

15. O'Reilly, R. A., and Motley, C. H.: Racemic, warfarin and trimethoprim-sulfamethoxazole interaction in humans, Ann. Intern. Med. **91**:34, 1979.

16. Rowe, J. W.: Clinical research on aging: strategies and directions, N. Engl. J. Med. **297**:1332, 1977.

17. Rowe, J. W., and others: The effects of age on creatinine clearance in man: a cross sectional and longitudinal study, J. Gerontol. **31**:155, 1976.

18. Beller, G. A., and others: Digitalis intoxication, a prospective clinical study with serum level correlations, N. Engl. J. Med. **284**:899, 1971.

19. Caranasco, G. J., and others: Drug induced illness leading to hospitalization, J.A.M.A. **228**:713, 1974.

20. Seidl, L. C., and others: Studies in the epidemiology of adverse drug reaction. 3. Reaction in patients on a general medical service, Bull. John Hopkins Hosp. **119**:299, 1965.

21. Hurwitz, N.: Predisposing factors in adverse reactions to drugs, Br. Med. J. **1**:536, 1969.

22. Nies, A., and others: Relationships between age and tricyclic antidepressant plasma levels, Am. J. Psychiatry **134**:790, 1977.

23. Appel, G. B., and Neu, H. C.: Gentamicin, Ann. Intern. Med. **89**:528, 1978.

24. Granerus, A. K., and others: Kaliuretic effect of L-dopa treatment in Parkinson patients, Acta Med. Scand. **201**:291, 1977.

25. Klotz, U., and others: The effect of age and liver disease on the disposition and elimination of diazepam in adult man, J. Clin. Invest. **55**:347, 1975.

26. Reidenberg, M. M., and others: The relationship between diazepam dose, plasma level, age and central nervous system depression in adults, Clin. Pharmacol. Ther. **23**:371, 1978.

27. Schwartz, D., and others: Medication errors made by elderly, chronically ill patients, Am. J. Public Health **52**:2018, 1962.

28. Parkin, D. M., and others: Deviation from prescribed drug treatment after discharge from hospital, Br. Med. J. **2**:686, 1976.

29. Sherman, F. T.: "Geriatric" generic prescription form, N. Y. State J. Med. **78**:1292, 1979.

30. Sherman, F. T., Warach, J., and Libow, L. S.: Child resistant containers for the elderly, J.A.M.A. **241**:1001, 1979.

31. Wise drug use for the elderly: role of the service provider, Administration on Aging, U.S. Department of Health, Education, and Welfare, in press.

32. Libow, L. S., and Mehl, B.: Self administration of medications by patients in hospital or extended care facilities, J. Am. Geriatr. Soc. **18**:81, 1970.

33. Warren, J. W., and others: Antibiotic irrigation and catheter associated urinary tract infection, N. Engl. J. Med. **299**:570, 1978.

34. Hall, M. R. P.: Drug therapy in the elderly, Br. Med. J. **3**:582, 1973.

PROBLEM-SOLVING EXERCISES

Case One

Mrs. F. is an 82-year-old white women who has been admitted under your care to a skilled nursing facility from a nearby acute care hospital with the transfer information on pp. 114 to 115. You are unable to reach the referring physician until the next day. Mrs. F., although cooperative, is generally uninformed about her medical problems. She claims that her daughter knows her entire history. Her daughter, too, is unavailable until the evening. Review the transfer information form and answer the following questions.

Questions

1. What about this typical transfer application is inadequate, inaccurate, and/or inconsistent in terms of diagnosis, current therapy, or plans for the future? What information needs to be clarified, specifically with regard to the current drug regimen?
2. What drug side effects or drug interactions could have resulted in Mrs. F.'s suffering a fracture of her left femur?
3. The first three medications—digoxin, a diuretic, and a potassium supplement—are taken by many elderly patients, especially those who are institutionalized. What drug interactions, side effects, and compliance problems can you anticipate? What actions would you take to prevent any of these problems?
4. Mrs. F. is discharged on a regimen of the following medications: digoxin, 0.125 mg PO OD; chlorothiazide, 500 mg PO OD; potassium chloride elixir, 15 meq PO bid; pilocarpine hydrochloride 2%, 1 gtt OU O D; and Elavil, 25 mg PO tid. Write out the prescriptions for each of these medications and explain them to Mrs. F.

Case two

Mrs. S. is a 77-year-old white woman living alone in her own apartment who comes to the outpatient clinic because of lethargy and difficulty with sleep for 2 months' duration. She was seeing a local general practitioner but left his care because he did not spend enough

time with her, nor did he explain what he was recommending. She has a known history of hypertensive and arteriosclerotic heart disease for 10 and 5 years, respectively, and was hospitalized with a "heart attack" 2 years ago at another hospital. She denied pain at that time. She takes a small white pill under her tongue for chest pain that relieves her symptoms within minutes. She also has been labeled diabetic and has taken an oral hypoglycemic agent in the past. She mentions no specific dietary regimen, nor does she check her urinary glucose. She denies polyuria, polyphagia, and polydipsia. A review of systems is negative except for some nocturnal dyspnea. She claims that she is lonely and depressed since her husband died 3 years ago. She denies any suicidal thoughts.

Past medical history:

1. S/P total abdominal hysterectomy and bilateral salpingo-oophorectomy secondary to uterine fibroid tumors (age 38).
2. S/P cholecystectomy (age 43).
3. S/P cataract extraction, left eye (age 71).

Medication: Nitroglycerin, gr 1/150, sublingual, prn chest pain.

Family history:

1. One living sister in Cleveland who has hypertension and a history of breast carcinoma.
2. Cause of death of parents—"old age."
3. No children.

Social history: Mrs. S. had been married for 32 years before her husband's death from a heart attack 3 years ago. She was unable to have children. She worked as a housewife and had part-time employment in a dress factory. She is concerned about her sister's health and fears that she, too, will develop breast cancer. Her main income comes from her husband's pension and life insurance policies. She also receives Supplemental Security Income.

Physical examination: Mrs. S. is an obese white woman in no acute distress. She talks slowly and appears depressed.

BP: $\frac{190/105}{RA}$⟜ $\frac{190/100}{RA}$⟜ $\frac{190/105}{RA}$⟜

GERIATRIC NURSING HOME   Patient's Name: Frank, M
                                                            Age: 82
                                                            Referred From: Northside Acute
                                                                           Hospital
                                                            Date: 1/1/80

TO BE COMPLETED BY PHYSICIAN

1. BRIEF NARRATIVE SUMMARY:_____ S/P Fracture of left hip _____

    OTHER PERTINENT DIAGNOSIS:_____
                  1) CHF
                  2) Diabetes
                  3) Incontinence
                  4) Depression
    SPECIFY DATE OF CVA_____MI_____FRACTURE_11/1/79_AMPUTATION____
2. SURGICAL PROCEDURES: Specify Dates._____

3. MENTAL STATUS___ Confused _____
4. SPEECH_ Clear _____
5. RECOMMENDED MEDICAL ORDERS - PLEASE BE COMPLETE _____
    A: MEDICATIONS:_____

             1) Digoxin 0.25 mg P.O. O.D. x 5 day/week
             2) Chlorothiazide 500 mg P.O. B.I.D.
             3) Slow K ✚ Tab T.I.D.
             4) Diabinese 250 mg P.O. O.D.
             5) Warfarin 2.5 mg P.O. O.D.
             6) Pilocarpine
             7) Elavil 10 mg. P.O. T.I.D.

    B: DRUG CONTRA-INDICATIVE &/OR SENSITIVITIES_____
        ALLOPURINOL, TRIMETHOPRIM-SULFAMETHOXAZOLE, PENICILLIN_____
6. PHYSICAL REHABILITATION_____
    (Please Check) Weight Bearing - None_____ Partial _✓_____Full_____
    Prosthetic and/or Ambulation Devices:_Walker_____
    (Type of Fixating Device)__Richardson's Screw_____DATE_____
7. PERTINENT LABORATORY AND X-RAY DATA:_____TEST____DATE_4/1/79_
    LABORATORY_____HGB_10.1_____
    _____BUN_20.0_____
    _____BLOOD SUGAR 198_
    _____CALCIUM_10.1___
    _____OTHER_____
    EKG:__Old Inf Wall MI, NSR_____
    CHEST X-RAY__Cardiomegaly_____
    OTHER:_____

            F.M. DOCTOR   John Doctor   1/1/80
    (Print name of physician completing form)   (Signature) Date Form Completed

NURSING ASSESSMENT (To be completed by R.N.)
A. Please describe those nursing services which patient requires in response to
   primary and secondary diagnoses (include   Intake and Output,
   Dressings, Irrigations, Ostomy Care, Vital Signs, Monitoring Pain Factors,
   I.V.'s, etc.).
   Patient requires one person guarding while using walker.
   Needs pulse checked prior to digoxin.
   Urine for glucose twice weekly.

B. Is patient incontinent?
   Urine   Often   Seldom XXXX   Never   Foley
   Stool   Often   Seldom   Never XXXX
C. Please indicate presence or absence of Decubitus Ulcers. (If present, describe
   lesion as to size and outline present treatment regimen)
          NONE

D. Nutritional Factors (Describe special diet prescriptions, appetite, patient's
   ability to feed self, use of tube feedings, etc.)
          Diabetic Diet, Patient can feed self.

E. Mental Status
   1. Is patient confused or alert?   Alert usually
   2. Can patient make needs known?   YES
   3. Does patient participate in care, or require total assistance?
          Participates
   4. Please describe any other aspects of patient's functioning which are
      pertinent to care. (Include visual, hearing, or communicative impairments.)
          NONE

Signature: I.M. Nurse   *I.M. Nurse*   R.N.   Date: 1/1/80

SOCIAL SERVICE ASSESSMENT

SUMMARY OF PATIENT'S EMOTIONAL NEEDS: _____

  Mrs. Frank is a widow of 10 years who has been living in an apartment

  by herself. Her total monthly income is $350. Two hundred fifty

  dollars come from Social Security; the remainder comes from her

  husband's pension. Family does not want the patient to be advised

  about her transfer until the last minute.

SOCIAL WORKER'S NAME: *I. M. SOCIAL WORKER*   *I.M. Social Worker*
                              (PRINT)   (SIGNATURE)

Skin: Cold and dry without tenting. No ecchymosis. *Lymph nodes*—nonpalpable.

Head: Without abrasions, normocephalic.

Hair: Normal.

Eyebrows: Thinning of the lateral third.

Eyes: Pupils equal, round, reactive to light and accommodation. Extraocular movements intact. No exophthalmopathy, no nystagmus; left cateract, removal; right eye—disk flat. V—A-3:1; AV nicking present. No exudates or hemmorrhages. Left eye aphakic—otherwise same as right eye.

Ears: Impacted cerumen bilaterally; cannot have normal conversation without lipreading. Weber—no lateralizing. Rinne—bone conduction greater than air conduction.

Neck: No limitation of motion. No palpable thyroid or bruits. Carotids equal bilaterally without bruits. Positive neck vein distention at 30°. Positive hepatojugular reflux.

Chest: Clear to auscultation and percussion.

Heart: Heart rate—70 and regular. Point of maximum intensity (PMI) at sixth intercostal space, midclavicular line, and prominent. S_3 and S_4 heard.

Abdomen: Without palpable kidneys or spleen; liver is 13 cm in midclavicular line and is tender to percussion.

Rectal: Negative for masses. Hemocult ×1 negative.

Genitourinary: Labia, vagina, and cervix appear to be within normal limits. Pap smear taken. Bimanual—no uterus or adenexa palpable.

Extremities: Decreased hair on tibial areas and 1+ ankle edema.

Pulse: +1 bilaterally.

Neurological:

1. Mental status (FROMAJE score)—1 + 1 + 1 + 1 + 2 + 1 + 3 = 10 (see Chapter 5). Affect—depressed but no suicidal thoughts or plans.

2. Cranial nerves II to XII intact except for bilaterally decreased hearing.

3. Deep tendon reflexes (+ = normoactive; 0 = not present).

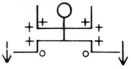

a. Palmar mental—negative.

b. Snout reflex—negative.

c. Babinski's reflex—bilaterally flexor (i.e., negative)

4. Motor—full strength bilaterally.

5. Sensory—intact to pinprick and light touch. Position sense equal bilaterally. Vibration sense decreased in lower extremities.

6. a. Cerebellar—finger to nose and heel to chin—both within normal limits.

   b. Rhomberg—within normal limits.

   c. No tremor.

7. Gait—uses no assistive devices. Not broad based and not at risk of falling.

Questions

1. What laboratory information would you like?

2. Do the laboratory tests help you make any diagnoses in this elderly patient?

3. What was peculiar about her "heart attack"?

4. What are your diagnoses?

5. How would you treat this 77-year-old white woman? What precautions should you take with her medications?

6. What would you ask her about her insomnia?

7. What illnesses have you considered as causes for her insomnia?

8. Why is a barbiturate a poor hypnotic in the elderly patient?

9. Should this patient be treated with a hypnotic at this time?

Case three

Mr. Y. is an 82-year-old white man with CHF, arteriosclerotic cardiovascular disease (ASCVD), and S/P left hemiparesis secondary to a cerebrovascular accident (CVA) with minimal residual weakness, who presented with urinary obstruction secondary to prostatic hypertrophy 2 years ago. Transurethral prostatectomy at that time revealed adenocarcinoma of the prostate gland. His acid phosphatase level and bone scan were normal. No therapy was started. He is mentally clear and ambulatory, and lives at home with his wife. He now has localized pain in the lower thoracic spine without a history of trauma. Aspirin has been used with moderate relief.

Question

1. What are your thoughts as to the etiology of Mr. Y.'s pain?

Physical and neurological examinations are unremarkable except for a minimal left hemiparesis and localized tenderness over the spinous processes of T-11 and T-12.

Questions

2. What tests would you order, and why?
3. What is the anemia caused by? What is your synthesis of the problem and what do you recommend?

Mr. Y. receives localized irradiation to T-11 and T-12 vertebrae with relief of pain. His aspirin is discontinued, and he is restarted on a regimen of diethylstilbestrol, 1 mg PO OD, which he had discontinued sometime in the past without notifying his physician.

He does well until 1 year later, when he comes to your hospital in a clearly deteriorated and wasted condition with diffuse spinal and rib pain. A bone scan confirms diffuse metastatic disease in these areas. Mr. Y. is mentally clear.

Question

4. What type of analgesic would you prescribe? What special considerations would you take with this 82-year-old white man in prescribing meperidine or morphine? How much meperidine would you give him, how often, and by what route of administration? What are your fears of addiction with him, considering his limited life span

at age 82? What other aspects of narcotic analgesics may be helpful in this patient?

Case four

Mrs. H. is an 85-year-old white woman who has been admitted to the acute-care hospital with a 2-day history of melena. A review of her medication, both nonprescribed and prescribed, reveals no medication-induced cause for her bleeding. Her hemoglobin and hematocrit values are unchanged from those of a previous office visit. Orthostatic changes in her blood pressure and pulse, not previously detected, are now present, suggesting significant intravascular blood loss. No medications that could cause orthostatic hypotension (diuretics, antihypertensive agents, phenothiazines, tricyclic antidepressants, L-dopa) can be implicated. A nasogastric tube reveals 300 ml of bright red blood. Mrs. H. is given 3 units of whole blood, after which her orthostatic changes are not present. Endoscopy reveals a large, bleeding gastric ulcer on the lesser curvature. Multiple biopsy specimens and brush cytology are taken. A urinary catheter inserted on admission measures her urinary output. She is placed on a regimen of antacids and cimetidine, and her bleeding subsequently stops. Five days after admission, she becomes confused and lethargic, with a temperature of 101° F. Physical examination is unremarkable except for her abnormal mental status. Microscopic examination of an unspun urine specimen aspirated from the catheter reveals multiple bacilli that are gram negative on staining.

Based on her presumed urinary tract sepsis that may be hospital acquired, you recommend that gentamicin be started.

Question

1. Based on the nomogram in Fig. 6-1, calculate the maintenance dose of gentamicin for Mrs. H. She weighs 45 kg and has a serum creatinine level of 1.3 mg/dl on the day of her acute confusion.

She responds to the gentamicin but develops acute pulmonary edema with wheezing after 2 days of therapy, probably secondary to volume overload from intravenous therapy. In addition to furosemide, she is given aminophylline to relieve the bronchoconstriction.

Questions

2. Calculate the loading and maintenance doses of aminophylline according to the graph in Fig. 6-2; take into account her current clinical condition(s).
3. Are there any other medication changes, additions, or deletions that you would consider?

ANSWERS TO PROBLEM-SOLVING EXERCISES
Case one°

1. Confusing and inadequate aspects of the transfer summary are as follows.

   Since incontinence, immobility, and dementia are the three most common reasons for institutionalization, and since Mrs. F.'s need for lifelong institutionalization is not clear, you must clarify her mental status. It is described as "confused," "depression," and "alert." Are these three observations consistent?

   Nothing is said about the cause of her left femur fracture. Is it from osteoporosis or osteomalacia? Can she be rehabilitated with this abnormal mental status?

   What is the cause of the nocturnal incontinence?

   Is the patient anemic? If so, why? Is the

°Although this chapter is on medication and the elderly patient, it is important to be introduced to the multiple problems in medical record transfer between the referring physician and the nursing home physician if these two are not the same individual. The referral information will serve as the basis for initial drug prescription. Numerous authors have commented on the inadequacy and inaccuracies of transfer information by physicians when sending their elderly patients to nursing homes or hospitals. It is clear that all transfer information should be reviewed thoroughly and questioned, and detailed records obtained from past hospitalizations and the referring physician. This information should be corroborated by the new information learned from the history and physical examination.

anemia secondary to blood loss from a major orthopedic procedure, or was the anemia present before the operation?

Why is Mrs. F. receiving warfarin?

2. Although many elderly patients slip in their homes as a result of poorly lighted stairs and inappropriately placed rugs or door sills, both physical illness and medications can lead to falls. At times, the falls appear to occur secondary to spontaneous fracture of the femur.

   This patient's fractured hip may have been medication induced, either from a drug side effect or a drug interaction. Emphasis should be placed on:

   • The use of multiple interacting medications in the elderly patient
   • The side effects of commonly used medications
   • How drug interactions and side effects can cause illness and institutionalization
   • Decreasing the number of medications to three or less and, certainly, to as few as possible
   • Obtaining all medications that the patient may have taken

   Each of the following medications could be implicated as a causative factor.

   Digoxin can cause digitalis toxicity leading to a cardiac dysrhythmia and subsequent hypotension and falling.

   Thiazide diuretics can cause orthostatic hypotension in elderly patients who, because of impaired homeostatic mechanism, are particularly susceptible to this complication. Checking blood pressure with the patient in the supine, sitting, and standing positions (after standing for 1 minute) will ensure that no orthostatic hypotension exists. Similarly, amitriptyline can cause orthostatic hypotension, especially when the drug is just begun. Telling the patient to rise slowly from a supine position can often prevent this unwanted side effect.

   Chlorpropamide (Diabinese) has a prolonged half-life in the elderly and consequently should be given only once a day.

Because of the drug's increased half-life due to reduced renal excretion, it may cause prolonged and serious hypoglycemia. Mrs. F.'s fall may have resulted from a confusional state related to prolonged hypoglycemia from the chlorpropamide or from hyponatremia resulting from a chlorpropamide-induced syndrome of inappropriate antidiuretic hormone excretion (SIADH).

Warfarin could have contributed to Mrs. F.'s fall, if she was taking it at the time. It is not clear from the summary why Mrs. F. is being given warfarin. Did she have a pulmonary embolism? Is she taking it as a prophylactic measure against possible thromboembolism following a major orthopedic procedure? Mrs. F.'s fall could have resulted from gastrointestinal bleeding resulting from the interaction of warfarin and aspirin. Elderly patients take nonprescribed preparations, many of which contain aspirin. Consequently, physicians must be particularly aware of these drugs and regularly review nonprescribed medications by asking the patient (or relative, when indicated) to bring all the drugs from the medicine cabinet to the hospital or physician's office.

Tricyclic antidepressants can cause acute confusional states in elderly patients, and although Mrs. F.'s dosage of amitriptyline is relatively low, her mental status may improve if this drug were discontinued; or, she may be depressed and need an increased dosage of the tricyclic antidepressant. It is important to emphasize that the withdrawal of drugs from an elderly patient may be more important than adding any, especially when mental status is compromised.

3. Digoxin toxicity is perhaps the most serious complication of this triad of medications, and is seen frequently in elderly patients receiving digoxin. The classic finding of nausea, vomiting, anorexia, and bradycardia may not be seen.

Elderly patients with atrial fibrillation may manifest digitalis toxicity by a regular nodal rhythm. An electrocardiogram (ECG) should confirm this change, and digoxin should be discontinued temporarily. Also, digitalis toxicity may manifest itself by a worsening of CHF accompanied by a rise in pulse rate.

A change in mental status (confusion, depression, and/or psychosis) may be a presenting sign of digoxin toxicity in an elderly patient. Certainly, digoxin toxicity may be causing Mrs. F.'s confused behavior. The diuretic can only make the possibility of digitalis toxicity more likely because of hypokalemia. Therefore, intermittent measurement of electrolytes should be done to determine whether there is a need for increased potassium supplement.

Mrs. F.'s dosage of digoxin is 0.25 mg PO OD ×5 days/week. Since renal function decreases with normal aging and since digoxin is mainly excreted by glomular filtration, you must be cautious about a maintenance dose of 0.25 mg PO. A more reasonable maintenance dose would be 0.125 mg PO OD in this 80-year-old woman whose glomular filtration rate is approximately 30% less than that of a younger adult despite normal serum BUN and creatinine values. Taking medication on a once-daily basis is preferable to skipping days, because of problems that some elderly patients have with recent memory. Therefore, giving digoxin, 0.125 mg PO OD, is probably the best approach to providing Mrs. F.'s cardiac glycoside. Also, the possibility of discontinuing her digoxin altogether should be raised. It has been shown that nearly 70% of geriatric patients can have their digitalis glycoside stopped without detrimental effect. This appears to apply particularly to those patients who are in sinus rhythm. Since 20% of patients receiving digitalis have side effects, many often serious, the physician needs to continually evaluate whether his elderly patient needs digoxin. Contrariwise, CHF has occurred on discontinuation of digoxin.

Mrs. F. is receiving a twice-daily diuretic that could be causing her nocturnal incontinence. Changing to a once-daily regimen may restore continence and improve her functioning. Also, because of her diabetes, the potential diabetogenic effect of the thiazide must be considered. Slow-K tablets, an oral slow-releasing potassium supplement, are rather large for some elderly patients to swallow, and compliance may decrease. A suitable alternative would be an effervescent potassium chloride solution or elixir. These, too, have disadvantages in terms of taste.

4. Writing prescriptions and explaining them to Mrs. F., who can be played by another student, will give the student practice in dealing with multiple prescriptions and their oral and written explanations. The student should write the prescription emphasizing the following: generic medications, typing of instructions in large print, and requesting non−child-resistant containers for patients who either live alone or have no children in the house (otherwise patients should be tested in opening and closing child-resistant containers).

Case two

1. The following data is available:
   - Hgb: 13.0; Hct: 40; WBC: within normal limits
   - Na: 133; Cl: 97; K: 4.5; CO_2: 26; BUN: 36; glucose: 175
   - Chest x-ray − PA and last chest film: cardiomegaly with left ventricular prominence; cephalization of blood
   - ECG: normal sinus rhythm; 1° AV block; left ventricular hypertrophy; old inferior wall myocardial infarction
   - Urine analysis: unable to obtain (poor cooperation)
   - CA
     PO$_4$
     Albumin
     Total protein
     Total bilirubin } within normal limits
   - T_4 by RIA: 4.5μg/dl to 12.0μg/dl
   - T_3 resin uptake: 15% (N = 25% to 35%)
   - TSH: 60 (N = 0 to 10/ml)

- T_3 by RIA: result available in future
- Hemocult slides ×6: negative

2. Mrs. S. appears to be a depressed woman with heart disease presenting as CHF (nocturnal dyspnea, ankle edema, hepatomegaly, S_3 gallop, and neck vein distention at 30°). She is also hypothyroid. The diagnosis of hypothyroidism in the elderly based on clinical presentation may be very difficult. Many of the signs and symptoms of the disease, such as cold intolerance, dry skin, hoarseness, deafness, ataxia, constipation, and confusion are all nonspecific and may be attributed to other concurrent illnesses. Because hypothyroidism in an elderly patient may go unsuspected even after a thorough history and physical examination, it is recommended that all elderly patients suspected of thyroid disease be evaluated with tests of thyroid function, such as a T_4 by radioimmunoassay (RIA) and T_3 resin uptake. This combination of tests will reveal those patients with unsuspected hypothyroidism and hyperthyroidism as well as abnormalities of binding proteins, so common among the elderly.

3. Painless myocardial infarctions are frequently seen in the elderly population. In a study of Rodstein,[1] only 20% to 30% of myocardial infarctions in an elderly population were typical; 30% presented entirely silently, and the remaining 40% presented in an atypical fashion.

   Sudden onset or worsening of dyspnea in elderly patients with and without a history of CHF was the initial symptom in 20% of the patients studied by Pathy.[2] Thirteen percent of this elderly population presented with an acute confusional state as the initial symptom of their myocardial infarction. Syncopal episodes, hemiplegia (due to cerebral infarction following hypotension or cerebral embolism), embolic occlusion of noncerebral arteries, and faintness are other frequent manifestations of myocardial infarction among the elderly. Therefore, the physician should consider myocardial infarction as a possible diagnosis in an older person whose general condition suddenly worsens, especially if dyspnea, confusion, hemiplegia, and/or syncope are prominent features, with or without chest pain.

4. Diagnoses are as follows:
   - *Etiological:* Arteriosclerotic cardiovascular disease (based on angina history); hypertensive cardiovascular disease (based on eyegrounds, BP, ECG). *Anatomic:* Old inferior wall myocardial infarction—left ventricular hypertrophy (ECG). *Physiological:* CHF, stable angina, normal sinus rhythm. *Cardiac status and prognosis:* To be determined.
   - Primary hypothyroidism based on laboratory diagnosis and psychiatric presentation. Loss of the lateral third of the eyebrows is commonly seen in the elderly. Similarly, the ankle jerk is lost in 50% of all geriatric patients. The ankle jerk may be helpful in the diagnosis of hypothyroidism if it shows a delayed relaxation phase. Mrs. S.'s lethargy and abnormal mental status should raise the possibility of a reversible form of dementia secondary to hypothyroidism. A heart rate above 70 is as likely as one below 70 in the elderly hypothyroid patient.
   - Depression and/or dementia secondary to hypothyroidism or reactive to the situation.
   - Insomnia secondary to the above diagnoses or other cause.
   - Diabetes mellitus, adult onset by history, noninsulin dependent.
   - S/P cholecystectomy.
   - S/P total abdominal hysterectomy and bilateral salpingo-oophorectomy.
   - Bilateral hearing deficit secondary to cerumen and/or other etiology. A hearing deficit may also be the reason for a patient appearing demented. Removal of the cerumen may greatly increase the patient's ability to communicate.

5. Treatment of this particular patient with both coronary artery disease and hypothyroidism is a therapeutic dilemma. Elderly patients with hypothyroidism and coronary artery disease are particularly sensitive to the cardiac effects of thyroid hormone, manifested by increasing angina, heart failure, and occasionally sudden death. Thyroxine (T_4) should be started with a low dosage (0.025 mg) and gradually titrated upward with dosage increments of 0.025 mg at 10 to 14-day intervals. A single dose of thyroxine begins to work in 4 days and reaches its maximum effect in 9 days. Few older patients need more than 0.20 mg per day. Clinical response, T_4 by RIA and thyroid-stimulating hormone (TSH) should be monitored. Triiodothyronine (T_3) should not be used in the elderly, because it is erratically absorbed and can cause high T_3 serum levels that may lead to serious cardiovascular effects such as dysrhythmias.

Although Mrs. S. has been labeled diabetic in the past, we have little evidence to document it. A random blood glucose determination of 175 is not helpful in establishing a diagnosis. A fasting blood sugar value greater than 110 or a 2-hour postprandial blood glucose value greater than 200 would be abnormal, even for her age. Therefore, before Mrs S. is labeled diabetic, fasting and 2-hour postprandial blood glucose determinations are indicated. A glucose tolerance test is often difficult to perform and interpret in ill elderly patients because of the conditions imposed by multiple medications, illnesses, and exercise limitations. A glucose tolerance test is seldom needed in the diagnosis of diabetes mellitus in the elderly.

Mrs. S. has both systolic and diastolic hypertension. Her eyegrounds are consistent with hypertension and her PMI is displaced laterally, suggesting cardiomegaly. Treatment should be instituted initially with a thiazide diuretic to bring her diastolic blood pressure to safer levels. Potassium supplement is needed only if the patient demonstrates hypokalemia. Checking the blood pressure with the patient in the supine and standing position will determine whether orthostatic changes are developing from the diuretic. Mrs. S.'s CHF may be controlled by her diuretic as well as her thyroid replacement. Digoxin should be withheld until these two drugs have had time to take effect.

6. Further discussion with the patient regarding her insomnia is indicated. Does she have difficulty in falling asleep, frequent nocturnal awakenings, or early-morning wakefulness? Are her frequent awakenings from nocturia, dyspnea, or pruritis? Does her insomnia result from a confusional state, or is she depressed?

7. Illnesses causing her insomnia might include CHF, leading to nocturnal dyspnea or hypothyroidism, leading to confusion.

8. Elderly patients often respond paradoxically to barbiturates, with restlessness, agitation, or frank psychosis. Barbiturates should be avoided in the treatment of elderly patients as well as hypothyroid patients because of the possibility of myxedema coma.

9. No. Although insomnia is one of Mrs. S.'s chief complaints, patients with hypothyroidism are extremely sensitive to sedatives and can slip into a coma. Her drug regimen should be limited to hydrochlorthiazide, 50 mg PO OD; thyroxine, $25\mu g$ PO OD; and nitroglycerin, 1/150 sublingual, prn, chest pain.

Case three

1. Although metastatic disease is certainly high on the list, other noncancerous causes of back pain should be considered. Not all pain in cancer patients is from cancer. Pain associated with cancer is usually a late symptom of disease and is not present at the time of diagnosis in most cases. Other possible causes of back pain in this elderly individual include osteoporosis and osteoarthritis. Few elderly persons reach old age without the development of either of these conditions. Despite the prevalence of osteoporosis and osteoarthritis in the elderly, it is unwise to attribute new or severe back pain to these entities. Osteoporosis can be implicated as a cause of

back pain only when a history of trauma or recent acute vertebral collapse can be elicited, or when steroids have exacerbated the process. Painless vertebral collapse is commonly seen on spinal films of elderly patients (either partial, as shown by a "codfish vertebrae," or more severe collapse with wedging). Clinical examination of the abdomen will often reveal a transverse abdominal skin crease in patients with vertebral collapse.

Osteoarthritis, radiographically demonstrated by disc degeneration and narrowing, sclerosis of bone margins, and osteophyte formation, commonly will cause back stiffness with little or no pain. Acute low back pain, simulating a sciatica secondary to a disc lesion, may result from trauma to an osteoarthritic sacroiliac joint. Pain on movement or palpation of the sacroiliac joint confirms the diagnosis, and treatment with local infiltration of hydrocortisone and/or an anesthetic agent is often beneficial.

A prolapsed intervertebral disc is an uncommon event in the geriatric population above age 75. Other causes of back pain include multiple myeloma, Paget's disease, bacterial or mycobacterial osteomyelitis, pancreatitis, penetrating gastric ulcer, and aortic aneurysm.

2. Assume you have ordered the following tests, with these results:
   • CBC to rule out anemia of any etiology in a patient with cancer
     Hct: 30.0
     Hgb: 10.0 g/dl
     WBC: 7,500
   • Sodium, chloride, potassium, carbon dioxide, glucose, and BUN: all within normal limits
   • Calcium, phosphorus, and alkaline phosphatase specifically because of metastatic disease: all within normal limits
   • Acid phosphatase: increased
   • Bone survey: osteoblastic lesion of T-11 and T-12 with osteophytes formation of lower lumbar vertebrae
   • Bone scan: increased uptake at T-11 and T-12

- Hemoccult slides ×6; positive on three slides

3. Once again, multiple pathology is the rule rather than the exception in late life. Clearly, Mr. Y. has a metastatic deposit on his thoracic spine. In addition, he has anemia probably secondary to blood loss from the ingestion of aspirin. Long-term aspirin ingestion can lead to occult bleeding in 70% of patients using the drug, but only a small percentage develops iron deficiency anemia. Elderly patients with low dietary iron intake may be particularly susceptible to iron loss from aspirin-induced bleeding. There does not appear to be a relationship between the occurrence of occult bleeding and dyspeptic symptoms. Therefore, the absence of dyspepsia in an elderly patient taking aspirin does not exclude chronic gastrointestinal blood loss. Although Mr. Y. does have a complication of aspirin therapy, it has been shown that aspirin is superior to all other oral agents (including codeine) in the short-term control of mild to moderate pain from unresectable cancer.[3] Acetaminophen is also effective, but less so than aspirin. The latter drug does not have the complication of gastrointestinal bleeding and should be the drug of choice for pain in the elderly patient when an oral nonnarcotic analgesic is indicated. In Mr. Y.'s case, other alternatives must be considered. Specifically, radiotherapy to bony metastasis has been successful in subjective pain relief in 65% to 75% of patients with metastasis from primary prostate, thyroid, or renal carcinoma.[4] Radiation can produce rapid relief of pain as well as local cytotoxin effect and prevention of tumor spread.

4. Although nonnarcotic analgesia should be tried, narcotic analgesia may be required. Although addiction is possible, this potential problem must be balanced against the limited life span of this seriously ill but mentally clear individual. The liability of a patient becoming addicted to meperidine after a 10-day course of 100 mg intravenously every 4 hours is less than 1%. In a study, almost 40% of house physicians at university hospitals believed that the liability was greater than 1%; 22% considered the liability to be greater than 6%. In addition, less than 1% of the narcotic addicts in the United States become addicted while in a hospital setting.[5] A large percentage of patients (73%) receiving narcotic analgesics continue in significant pain because the physician fears addiction or misunderstands the pharmacology of the drug. Addiction, an unlikely possibility, may occur with terminal elderly patients receiving narcotics. This, however, should not deter a physician from offering them. Furthermore, the analgesia should be given prior to the development of the pain. Close observation of the patient will determine how frequently the medication needs to be given.

In the treatment of chronic pain, emphasis should be on preventing the recurrence of the pain rather than treating the pain once it has occurred. In the control of pain related to surgery, elderly patients have been shown to have greater pain relief after an intramuscular injection of 10 mg of morphine or 20 mg of pentazocine than younger patients.[6] The side effects of these drugs were not influenced by age despite the increased pain relief experienced by the older individual. Therefore, it is recommended that the dosage of morphine to patients be based not on their height, weight, or other variables, but on their age. From a given dose of morphine, greater pain relief should be expected in an older person than in a younger person.

The side effects of narcotic analgesia are important in the elderly and include:

- Sedation, especially with morphine and oxycodone (a component of Percodan). Meperidine has less sedative side effects.
- Suppression of the cough reflex, especially with codeine and oxycodone. Elderly patients have a decreased protective airway reflex, and the addition of analgesia with antitussive effect may

predispose the patient to aspiration and resulting pneumonia.

- Constipation, which may be further aggravated in an immobile patient by the use of narcotic analgesics. Usually meperidine and methadone are less constipating than morphine.
- Urinary incontinence, which may re-result from increased smooth muscle tone of the bladder itself or of the vesical sphincter. Urinary retention may result in patients with prostatic hypertrophy.
- Orthostatic hypotension secondary to peripheral vasodilation. This effect is further exacerbated by the concomitant use of a phenothiazine, which has alpha-adrenergic blocking activity. Narcotics, with the exception of meperidine, usually decrease the heart rate and may exacerbate existing bradyarrthymias in the elderly patient.

Important drug interactions that occur in elderly patients are the potentiation of narcotics by phenothiazines and the potentiation of barbiturates, benzodiazepines, and tricyclics by narcotics

It would be preferable to start Mr. Y. on an oral narcotic analgesic. Oral meperidine is only one third to one half as effective as intramuscular or subcutaneous meperidine. Therefore, one should be prepared to use a higher dosage for oral administration of this drug. Studies have shown that the usual length of action of intramuscular or subcutaneous meperidine is 2 to 4 hours, with an average of 3 hours. Therefore, a starting dosage of 50 mg intramuscularly every 3 hours or 75 to 100 mg orally every 3 hours unless refused would be acceptable. The writing of prn pain orders allows the patient to develop pain, call the nurse, wait, and develop further anger, anxiety, and cyclical pain. To prevent this cycle, the next dose of analgesic should be given before the previous one has worn off.

The dosage may have to be increased as needed by Mr. Y.'s pain. One hundred mg of meperidine is within the therapeutic range for treatment of severe pain, and higher doses are required in many instances.

Case four

1. Follow the instructions on Fig. 6-1.
2. Connect the two weight scales by a vertical line at 45 kg. The loading dose is 250 mg. If Mrs. H. were a normal elderly person, her maintainance dose would be 30 mg/hr. Since she has pulmonary edema, her maintainance dose should be 20 mg/hr.
3. The dosage of cimetidine should be lowered or stopped, since it, in addition to her fever, may be causing the confusional state.

REFERENCES

1. Rodstein, M., The characteristics of non-fatal myocardial infarction in the aged, Arch. Intern. Med. **98:**84, 1956.
2. Pathy, M. S. Clinical presentation of myocardial infarction in the elderly, Br. Heart J. **29:**190, 1967.
3. Moertel, C. G., and others: A comparative evaluation of marketed analgesic drugs, N. Engl. J. Med. **286:**813, 1972.
4. Murphy, T. M.: Cancer pain, Postgrad. Med. **53:** 187, 1973.
5. Marks, R. M., and Sachar, E. G.: Undertreatment of medical inpatients with narcotic analgesics, Ann. Intern. Med. **78:**173, 1973.
6. Bellville, J. W., and others: Influence of age on pain relief from analgesics, J.A.M.A. **217:**1835, 1971.

POSTTEST*

1. Elderly patients (i.e., those over age 65) comprise *(5%? 11%? 15%? 20%?)* of the population and account for *(5%? 10%? 15%? 20%? 25%?)* of all prescriptions.
2. Drugs are handled by the following mechanisms: absorption, hepatic metabolism, distribution, binding, and excretion. What changes, if any, occur with each of these with age? Give an example of one drug in

---

*Some questions may have more than one correct answer.

each category that is affected by the altered mechanism.

3. The elderly patient who cannot sleep may be suffering from:
   a. Pain
   b. Depression
   c. Organic brain syndrome
   d. Congestive heart failure (CHF)
   e. Prostatism

4. Because SGOT, alkaline phosphatase, and total bilirubin values are normal in healthy elderly people, can it be assumed that hepatic metabolism of medication is also normal?

5. Drug interactions are common in the elderly patient. Put the drugs in "Drug A" with the drugs in "Drug B" to form the combinations that most commonly result in clinically significant drug interactions.

Drug A

_____ a. Aspirin

_____ b. Thiazide diuretics

_____ c. Antacids

_____ d. Phenothiazines

_____ e. Tricyclic antidepressants

_____ f. Insulin

Drug B

1. Digoxin
2. Tetracycline
3. Warfarin
4. Phenobarbital
5. Guanethidine
6. Propranolol

6. An 80-year-old, 40-kg woman requires gentamicin for a severe episode of urinary tract sepsis as well as aminophylline for bronchospasm. What information would you need to figure out the dosages of each?

7. What steps would you take to ensure compliance with an elderly individual in the following situations?
   a. An elderly female patient is to be discharged from a hospital or skilled nursing facility in about a week. She is cur-

rently taking five medications simultaneously.

   b. A 72-year-old insulin-dependent diabetic who has senile macular degeneration, diabetic retinopathy, and amyotrophy affecting her manual skills lives with her alcoholic husband. How would you ensure that the patient successfully self-administers her insulin?

ANSWERS TO PRETEST AND POSTTEST

1. 11% of the population; 25% of all prescriptions. In addition, the elderly use an unknown and probably much larger percentage of nonprescribed medication. Future projections show that by the year 2020, when the elderly makeup approximately 16% of the population, they will receive 38% of all prescribed drugs.

2. *Absorption:* This does not appear to be affected in any major way by normal aging. Drug interactions can affect absorption (e.g., antacids taken with digoxin can affect absorption of digoxin; anticholinergic medications taken with L-dopa can affect absorption of L-dopa. *Hepatic metabolism:* Microsomal enzyme activity and the rate of enzyme induction decrease with age in animals. Studies in humans show a prolonged half-life of drugs partially metabolized by the liver, such as quinidine or desipramine. *Distribution:* Changes in distribution of drugs vary with aging, depending on whether they are distributed in both fat, lean body mass, or both. The percentage of body fat increases with age, while lean body mass decreases. The volume of distribution of diazepam, for example, has increased approximately fourfold by age 80 from what it was at age 20. *Binding:* Since albumin concentration decreases with normal aging, there may be more free drug available to interact at the receptor site. There is a higher fraction of unbound phenytoin in the elderly, for example. *Excretion:* Renal function decreases by 30% as one ages from 20 to 90. Consequently, aminoglycoside antibiotics and digoxin, both predominantly excreted by the kidney, have longer half-lives and higher serum levels in the elderly when given in the usual adult dose.

3. All of these. Arthritic or anginal pain may affect the patient's ability to fall asleep or remain asleep. CHF may lead to nocturia or paroxysmal

dyspnea. Prostatism may also lead to nocturia. Both depression and organic brain syndrome can affect sleeping patterns in the elderly.

4. No. Although SGOT, alkaline phosphatase, and total bilirubin values are unchanged in the normal aged, there is evidence that hepatic metabolism of drugs in animals and humans is slowed.

5. a,3; b,1; c,2; d,4; e,5; f,6.

6. The patient's weight, age, and creatinine clearance are important in determining the dosage of aminoglycoside. Serum creatinine remains within normal limits in the healthy elderly, while the glomerular filtration rate progressively falls. Consequently, serum creatinine in the elderly is not an adequate indicator of creatinine clearance. Associated diseases (CHF or liver disease) are critical to determining the correct dosage of aminophylline. Nomograms are available for determining the gentamycin and aminophylline dosages (Figs. 6-1 and 6-2).

7. *Situation a:*
   - Does the patient need all five medications? Three medications may be the upper limit that can be taken without compliance errors in many elderly patients.
   - Institute a self-medication program while the patient is still in the hospital or skilled nursing facility.
   - Assess her financial status and ability to purchase drugs.
   - Dispense the drugs in non-child-resistant containers if indicated.
   - Make sure that the patient has written instructions.

Situation b:
   - Assess whether the patient actually needs insulin or whether she can take an oral hypoglycemic agent in addition to dietary management.
   - If insulin is needed, determine whether the patient can manipulate a preset syringe. If so, seven preset syringes can be placed in her refrigerator by a relative or the visiting nurse service each week. Adaptive devices that magnify the scale of the syringe or preset the dose are also available.

Chapter 7

Stroke, fractured hip, amputation, pressure sores, and incontinence: principles of rehabilitation treatment

RAMON VALLARINO and FREDRICK T. SHERMAN

EDUCATIONAL OBJECTIVES
Attitudinal
The student should:
1. Deal with the prejudice that rehabilitation efforts in the elderly are usually unsuccessful
2. Confront his possibly negative feelings toward elderly people with major disabilities and develop a positive attitude toward their rehabilitation
3. Recognize that treatment is completed not only when signs and symptoms of the illness have abated, but when functional restoration has occurred
4. Recognize that what seems like minimal therapeutic gains to the observer may actually be major functional changes for elderly patients, whether they reside in the community or in an institution
5. Recognize that the elderly patient must be looked at as a "whole" beyond the organ system diseases
6. Recognize that a team approach utilizing the skills and input of many professionals is usually needed in the rehabilitation of the elderly

Cognitive

The student should:
1. Be able to define the basic techniques and principles of rehabilitation medicine
2. Be able to define dysfunction and disability and list the dysfunctions and disabilities most commonly found in the elderly
3. Be able to define the scope of responsibility and the capabilities of a rehabilitation service and its staff with regard to disabilities seen in the elderly
4. Be able to state the main differences between rehabilitation of the young and rehabilitation of the old
5. Be able to define activities of daily living (ADL) and know when and how to refer patients for assessment of self-care needs
6. Be able to outline the major rehabilitation steps in dealing with the elderly patient who has:
   a. Loss of mobility
   b. A stroke
   c. A fractured hip
   d. An amputation
   e. A pressure sore
   f. Urinary and/or fecal incontinence
   g. A gait disorder
   h. Loss of independence in ADL

Skill

The student should:
1. Be able to assess the functional ability of the patient as a whole in addition to each organ system
2. Be able to assess the major functional deficits and outline therapy for the elderly patient who has:
   a. Loss of mobility
   b. A stroke
   c. A fractured hip
   d. An amputation
   e. A pressure sore
   f. Urinary and/or fecal incontinence

g. A gait disorder

h. Loss of independence in ADL

PRETEST°

1. Rehabilitation of the elderly differs from that of the young in the following way(s):
   a. The goals are often different.
   b. The rehabilitation process is more likely to be interrupted by a medical problem in the elderly.
   c. The rehabilitation process is often slower in the elderly.
   d. The elderly can only expect relief of pain and discomfort.
   e. The most common rehabilitation problems encountered in the elderly are due to trauma.

2. A physiatrist is a:
   a. Paramedical technician
   b. Nurse certified in physical therapy
   c. Physician
   d. Physical therapist

3. A rehabilitation program for the elderly individual is extremely difficult, perhaps futile, when the patient:
   a. Is a bilateral below-knee (BK) amputee secondary to peripheral vascular disease
   b. Lacks the ability to follow instructions
   c. Lacks the ability to move both his right arm and right leg from a stroke
   d. Lacks the motivation to participate in a rehabilitation program because of depression

4. Occupational therapy:
   a. Provides assessment of, and training for, perceptual disorders resulting from stroke
   b. Provides exercises for the patient using functional activities for therapeutic purposes

c. Assesses the patient's ability to eat, to dress, and to toilet by himself

5. An assessment of the elderly stroke patient's ability to perform activities of daily living (ADL) is made during the following stage(s) of stroke rehabilitation:
   a. The acute stage, encompassing the first few days following the stroke
   b. The intermediate stage, when the patient is medically and neurologically stable
   c. The late stage, when the patient stops making progress

6. In the elderly unilateral BK amputee with arteriosclerotic cardiovascular disease manifested by angina and compensated congestive heart failure (CHF), which of the following methods of ambulation would consume the least amount of energy and, therefore, stress the cardiovascular system least?
   a. Hopping using crutches
   b. Hopping using a standard walker
   c. Walking using a BK prosthesis
   d. Hopping using a platform walker

7. Phantom pain (a painful sensation perceived by the patient in the nonexistent amputated limb) can be aided by:
   a. Helping the patient adjust psychologically to the amputation
   b. Deferring the prescription of an artificial limb until the pain subsides or at least improves
   c. Expediting the prescription of an artificial limb
   d. Giving liberal doses of analgesics

8. Two days ago, an 80-year-old woman had a transmetatarsal amputation of the right foot. The most probable etiological factor is:
   a. An automobile accident
   b. Osteogenic sarcoma
   c. Peripheral vascular disease
   d. Embolism

9. A 72-year-old woman sustained a frac-

ture of the left subcapital area of the femoral neck, which was surgically treated with an endoprosthesis of the Austin Moore type. By the end of the third week, her ambulatory status should be:

a. Non-weight bearing (NWB)

b. Partial weight bearing (PWB)

c. Full weight bearing (FWB)

10. The most crucial measure for the prevention of pressure sores is:

a. Adequate nutrition

b. Systemic antibiotics

c. Changing the position of the patient every 2 hours

d. Prevention of urinary and/or fecal incontinence

e. The use of a water bed

BASIC DEFINITIONS AND CONCEPTS

The knowledge and skills of rehabilitation medicine are a key element of the comprehensive approach to the geriatric patient. An alternate name for the discipline is *physical medicine and rehabilitation.* This alternate name underscores the use of physical agents (heat, water, ultrasound, electricity) and mechanical modalities (exercise) for diagnosis and therapy.[1,2] Rehabilitation medicine is focused on correcting the patient's disability. *Disability* is defined as the functional loss experienced by the individual, including physical, psychological, social, and vocational losses. The functional loss at the level of a limb, an organ, or a system may be called a *dysfunction.* (For example, Mr. J. D.'s right upper and lower limbs are dysfunctional as a result of a stroke. Mr. D. is a disabled individual who cannot feed himself.) Major dysfunctions or the sum of multiple minor ones may render a person disabled. The terms *impediment, impairment,* and *handicap* are used in the literature to refer to either dysfunction or disability. One should not become confused by these semantic inconsistencies.

Examples of dysfunction, disability, and rehabilitation procedures are given in Table 7-1.

In order to eliminate or minimize the patient's disability, rehabilitation medicine must (1) treat the dysfunctions if they have potential for improvement; (2) implement ways that the patient can compensate for his disability (i.e., train him to enhance his residual skills, provide him with adaptive tools [Fig. 7-1],

Table 7-1. Common dysfunctions, disabilities, and rehabilitation procedures in the elderly

Dysfunction	Disability	Rehabilitation procedure
Amputated leg	Inability to walk	Fitting of prosthesis and training in its use
Hemiplegia	Inability to dress	Teaching one-handed dressing
Subluxed metacarpophalangeal joints	Inability to tie shoelaces	Attaching self-adhering (Velcro) closures to shoes
Fractured hip	Inability to bear weight on the affected limb	Teaching partial weight-bearing ambulation with a walker

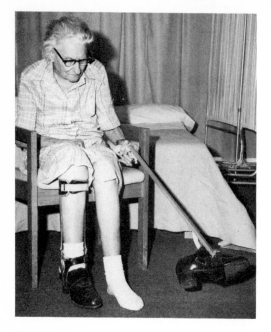

Fig. 7-1

Question: Mrs. P. M. is a 92-year-old woman. What is her dysfunction, and what are her disabilities? What assistive device is she using?

Answer: Her dysfunction is right-sided hemiplegia. Her disabilities include difficulties in ambulation and dressing. She is shown using a reacher, which allows her to get articles from a distance.

and adjust the environment in which he will function to his reduced capabilities); (3) help the patient and family adjust psychologically to the patient's residual limitations; and (4) contribute to a team effort to develop a supportive approach that will permit the elderly patient to return to a fulfilling, dignified existence.

Geriatric rehabilitation as a special discipline

Rehabilitation of the elderly differs from that of the young in three major ways: in its goals, in its potential obsta-

cles, and in the special physiological and psychological characteristics of the patients.

Rehabilitation goals

Rehabilitation assists the patient in returning to a normal life. The meaning of the word *normal* varies with age and with the individual patient. Familial obligations and responsibilities, employment status, income, taxation, and leisure-time activities all change with aging.[3] The older individual will usually lead a less vocationally oriented life than the younger individual. In general, the younger individual will need to return to work, whereas the older individual will usually be satisfied to return to living independently in the community.

The majority of older women and more than one fourth of older men live alone. For them, independence in mobility and the ability to perform daily basic self-care needs (activities of daily living [ADL]) are of paramount importance.[4] ADL consists of any activity necessary or desirable for each individual, including transfers (in and out of bed or chair), ambulation, cooking, feeding, dressing, bathing, toileting, homemaking, shopping, or traveling. The ability to perform ADL will often mean the difference between independent living in the community; dependent living in the community with the support of family, friends and/or community agencies; or institutionalization.

Obstacles to successful rehabilitation

Lack of vigor or energy. In contrast to younger individuals, older individuals (particularly those over the age of 75) may lack reserve vigor or energy because of an acute or chronic illness (often multiple), disuse, bed rest, or normal loss of muscle strength.

Lack of motivation. As a consequence of depression or other emotional stresses, including loss of job, loss of spouse or friends, or inadequate funds, the older patient may be disinterested in participating in therapy, or even refuse therapy.

Poor mentation. The elderly patient suffering from an acute or chronic organic brain syndrome (reversible or irreversible) may be unable to cooperate, follow directions, or learn instructions.

Tendency for disabilities to recur. The disabilities of the elderly, more than those of the young, tend to recur when new stresses are present.

Tendency to lose mobility. Approximately 20% of the elderly population have some problems with mobility. Five to eight percent are homebound. Other individuals who have no problems with mobility tend to stay at home because of lack of motivation, dislike of cold weather, fear of falling, or fear of crime. Both minor and major illnesses may immobilize the elderly individual. Viral gastroenteritis or a urinary tract infection may lead to immobility in the elderly while causing relatively minor symptoms in the younger individual. Major illnesses of late life, such as stroke, amputation, hip fracture, arthritis, and Parkinson's disease, usually affect the patient's ability to ambulate. Immobility, regardless of the cause, can be the beginning of a relentless downhill course characterized by disuse, muscular atrophy, pressure sores, thrombophlebitis, pulmonary embolism, pneumonia, constipation, urinary retention, and/or mental depression. Finally, immobility may lead to joint contractures that may be impossible to correct.

Difficulty in establishing a therapeutic relationship. Since the rehabilitation process requires the patient's cooperation, it is essential to establish rapport with him. Usually the patient is at least one generation older than the interviewer and has markedly different life experiences. While the interviewer may want to get specific health-related information from the patient, the patient may have different priorities. The health care professional may experience fear, anxiety, apathy, and/or pessimism in the presence of the disabled elderly. These feelings are heightened if the patient is confused. The clinician must confront his negative feelings toward the disabled elderly patient in order to form a therapeutic relationship. Encouraging reminiscence is a useful method of developing good rapport.

The younger health care professional has to accommodate himself to the slower pace of the ill elderly. Instructing a patient in doing a task and then assisting him in order to speed up the process is a frequent error. For example, pushing the wheelchair of a patient who is able to propel it independently merely satisfies the professional's hurried pace. Similarly, dressing a patient who can dress himself impedes his independence.

Physiological characteristics of the elderly

Most isolated physiological processes, such as cardiac output and nerve conduction velocity, decline with age.[6] Integrated functions, which are the summation of these individual physiological processes, show a more pronounced decline. Consequently the rehabilitation process will be slower than in younger individuals.

Team approach to rehabilitation

Since rehabilitation deals with all aspects of an individual's life, it is natural that the effort be shared by representatives of many disciplines, whether the patient is in the community, an acute care hospital, or a skilled nursing facility. The physiatrist, a physician specializing in physical medicine and rehabilitation, is primarily responsible for treating the patient's disability. The physical and occupational therapists perform daily therapy while nurses and nurse's aides are responsible for maintaining patient gains. A rehabilitation nurse acts as a liaison between the physical, occupational, and speech therapists and the nurse, the nurse's aide, and the patient's family, so that therapy can continue when the patient returns to his unit or home. The activities therapist offers the patient a variety of leisure-time activities that provide social and intellectual stimulation. The social worker counsels the patient and family and negotiates with agencies in developing supportive care and economic assistance when needed. Psychologists and members of the clergy can also counsel elderly rehabilitation patients. The geriatrician or other primary care physician shares leadership with the physiatrist.

Case history

A 75-year-old woman is admitted from a university hospital acute care service to a skilled nursing facility for rehabilitation following a stroke. The physician in charge of the case finds mild congestive heart failure (CHF) and prescribes a thiazide diuretic. On the following day, while performing his routine evaluation, the physiatrist finds that the patient is confused and unable to participate actively in physical or occupational therapy. He reports the patient's condition to the physician, who confirms a deteriorated mental status. Metabolic and endocrine causes are sought. Meanwhile, the nursing service continues passive

range-of-motion exercises and proper positioning of the patient, which began immediately after the stroke occurred. With control of the heart failure and gradual hormonal replacement for newly diagnosed hypothyroidism, the patient's mentation improves, and physical and occupational therapy are started. A few days later, the physical therapist reports that the patient lacks motivation and seems upset. The social worker discovers that the patient is depressed because she has not been visited by her only daughter and has not received her Social Security check.

The social worker makes arrangements for the Social Security check to be mailed directly to the patient's room and contacts the daughter, who has been busy with her own child's illness. The daughter's visits are resumed; the patient's motivation increases, and she becomes more involved in her physical and occupational therapy.

EVALUATION OF THE PATIENT

The clinician should know how to evaluate a geriatric patient from a rehabilitation viewpoint. The process includes the following four components: diagnostic assessment, prognosis, goals, and prescription.

Diagnostic assessment

The diagnostic assessment consists of the history and physical examination, including accurate measurement of range of motion, manual muscle testing, and assessment of ADL, and gait. When indicated, electrodiagnostic studies may be needed in addition to the usual laboratory tests and x-ray studies.

History

The following specific rehabilitation-oriented questions, often not included in the routine medical history, must be answered in order to make a proper diagnosis:

1. Is the patient disabled? In what sense? Which ADL are affected? For how long?
3. Is the disability due to the dysfunction?
4. Are there other factors in addition to the present dysfunction that contribute to the patient's disability?
5. Is the patient able to participate actively in therapy?

Special emphasis should be placed on:

1. *The duration of the dysfunction and disability:* The prognosis and the type of therapy prescribed depend on when the dysfunction and disability occurred. For example, bipedal full weight–bearing ambulation training is usually not suitable for a patient with a recently fractured hip. Similarly, a patient who suffered a stroke 1 year previously will usually not benefit from muscle reeducation but will more likely benefit from a program of ADL training using substitution techniques and special devices.

2. *The relationship between the current illness and the observed dysfunctions and disabilities:* Perhaps the patient was already disabled by arthritis for many years preceding the recent stroke. Similarly, a gait abnormality may not be due to the recent hip fracture but to an antecedent extrapyramidal syndrome.

3. *Complicating factors:* In addition to the dysfunction(s) caused by the patient's left hemiparesis or contracted left knee, for example, are there other factors contributing to the patient's disability? Depression, domestic conflicts, loss of social interest, and/or obstacles in the home that may prevent safe and efficient ambulation must be identified. Lack of vigor, endurance, and/or motivation are the most common complicating factors.

Physical examination

The basic physical examination should emphasize the:

1. Performance of the patient as a whole (The examiner must look at the patient's ability to change position in bed or in a chair, ability to maintain sitting balance, ability to transfer [get out of bed into a wheelchair or stand from a sitting position], standing balance, and ability to ambulate.)
2. Nervous and musculoskeletal systems (Dysfunctions in these two systems are the most frequent causes of disability in the elderly.)
3. Skin (Pressures sores and scars that might limit range of motion must be searched for.)
4. Mental status (see Chapter 5)
5. Cardiopulmonary status
6. Visual and hearing acuity

Additional examinations

Additional examinations used for evaluating the disabled geriatric patient are goniometry, muscle testing, and electrodiagnosis. These two types of examinations should be part of the standard physical examination.

Goniometry is the documented measurement of the range of motion of the joints. The examiner uses a goniometer to measure the motion of the joint in degrees. The axis of the goniometer should be positioned as accurately as possible over the axis of rotation of the joint. The joint is then moved throughout its range, actively and passively, and stretched as tolerated. Although it is unrealistic to expect that every joint be examined with a goniometer, it is important to manually and visually examine the range of motion of all joints and, if any abnormality is suspected, to perform goniometry to accurately document the loss of joint motion.

Muscle testing is the manual evaluation of the strength of the muscles. Thorough testing of each muscle is a laborious, time-consuming task that demands sufficient knowledge of morphological and functional anatomy. Initial and successive muscle testing should be performed by the same examiner. The findings are recorded using the following classifications:

Zero (0): No contraction is felt or seen.

Trace (1): The muscle tightens but cannot produce movement even with gravity eliminated (working on a horizontal plane).

Poor (2): The muscle produces movement with gravity eliminated, but not against gravity.

Fair (3): The muscle produces movement against gravity but does not overcome any resistance.

Good (4): The muscle produces movement against gravity plus some manual resistance.

Normal (5): No deficit is detected.

Electrodiagnosis (electromyography and measurement of the nerve conduction velocity and evoked potential) can help determine whether paralysis or paresis is due to either a muscular or a neurological abnormality. If it is due to a neurological abnormality, for example, electrodiagnosis will help determine whether the lesion is central or peripheral and, if peripheral, where the lesion is located.

Prognosis

In rehabilitation, a prognosis has to be established for both the dysfunction and the disability. The prognosis of a dysfunction follows rules that are general in medicine (i.e., the natural history of an illness, its severity and duration, and the effects of therapy). The prognosis of a disability greatly depends on the prognosis of the dysfunction, as well as such factors as vigor, mentation, motivation, the effect of concurrent illness, and the expected benefit from a rehabilitation program.

Goals

Without goals, therapy is not directed, continues indefinitely, and may support false expectations. One must clearly define the aim of the rehabilitation program by answering the following questions: What can the patient achieve? What can realistically be expected? An assessment of the patient's dysfunction(s) and disability will lead to the establishment of short- and long-term goals. Frequently, only tentative goals can be set at the initial assessment, because the patient's mentation, vigor, or motivation may change. An elderly patient who is participating in rehabilitation and becomes ill with pneumonia will need to have new goals established while he regains his strength. On the other hand, the initially confused patient may become mentally clear and require the establishment of higher goals.

Rehabilitation prescription for treatment in an institutional setting or home

The rehabilitation prescription includes any or all of the following: (1) physical therapy; (2) occupational therapy; (3) speech therapy; and (4) special requests or warnings to the staff or family, such as precautions against seizure, respiratory, or cardiovascular problems.

An example of a rehabilitation prescription follows:

Mrs. T. K. is a 72-year-old woman who suffered left-sided hemiplegia from a stroke 3 weeks ago.

Physical therapy:
1. Instruct the nursing staff and/or family in proper positioning in bed.
2. Reeducate muscles in the left upper and lower extremities.
3. Apply passive range-of-motion exercises to the left extremities.
4. Train the patient in sitting balance, progressing to standing balance in the parallel bars.
5. Treat daily.

Occupational therapy:
1. Have the patient use the upper limb in functional activities to improve strength and coordination.
2. Provide ADL evaluation and training.
3. Provide perceptual evaluation and training.
4. Treat daily.

Notice: Please observe redness of the left heel. (There is an impending pressure sore).

Warning: Take cardiac precautions. (The patient had a myocardial infarction 3 months ago).

The therapist is expected to administer the prescription by selecting a specific technique from those available. For example, during ambulation training, the therapist will decide how much assistance to give to the patient and what appliance (walker, cane, or crutches) to use. Therapy can be given in the gymnasium, at the hospital bedside, or in the home.

The rehabilitation effort must not be limited to the therapy sessions. What is taught in formal therapy must be practiced in the ward or at home. In the hospital or nursing home, nurses and nurse's aides have the responsibility of encouraging and assisting the patient in using his newly learned skills. In the home, the family and/or community agencies, such as the visiting nurse service, have the responsibility of providing ongoing therapy.

The primary care physician and the physiatrist must remain involved throughout the dynamic, often lengthy, process of rehabilitation. Reevaluation on a scheduled basis is necessary to assess results of therapy, make adjustments in the program, and confirm or revise the prognosis and goals.

STRUCTURE OF A REHABILITATION PROGRAM

A rehabilitation medicine service provides two types of therapy: physical and occupational. Speech therapy is usually a part of the service. Important additional components of the rehabilitation service are recreational therapy and counseling. Counseling may involve the services of a psychologist and/or a social worker. The director of rehabilitation should be a physiatrist, although it is not unusual for this position to be held by an orthopedic surgeon, a neurologist, a geriatrician, or, in small facilities, a senior physical or occupational therapist. In a developed geriatric program the rehabilitation staff is integrated into a team approach that includes the primary care physician, physician assistant and/or nurse practitioner, nurse, and social worker.

Physical therapy

Physical therapy is the use of physical modalities for therapeutic purposes. Physical modalities used in geriatric rehabilitation are (1) exercise (active, passive); (2) heat (hot packs, paraffin, diathermy); (3) ultrasound; and (4) hydrotherapy; and (5) electric transcutaneous nerve stimulation.

The physical therapy staff consists of registered physical therapists, assistant physical therapists, and aides.

No equipment can substitute for the abilities of a therapist. On the other hand, some modalities cannot be delivered without equipment; and this machinery may efficiently assist the rehabilitation process. Basic equipment for a physical therapy gymnasium consists of:

1. *Walkers:* These provide balance and shift weight bearing to the upper limbs. Walkers are the most frequently used equipment in geriatric rehabilitation for ambulation and stair-climbing training. Specific types of walkers include the standard walker, platform walker, wheeled walker, reciprocal walker, and stair-climbing walker.

2. *Canes and crutches:* These devices partially support the patient's weight and help maintain balance for safe ambulation (Fig. 7-2).

3. *Parallel bars:* These supportive bars are adjustable to different heights and are used in standing and ambulation training.

4. *Treatment tables:* Often the patient must exercise and receive treatment lying prone or supine.

5. *Pulleys, shoulder wheel, and hand ladder:* These devices help the patient actively exercise the upper limbs.

6. *Hot packs:* A hot pack is a canvas pack filled with a hydrophilic substance that delivers superficial wet heat after being soaked in hot water. It may be helpful in relieving some types of musculoskeletal pain, mild superficial inflammatory conditions, and muscle spasms.

7. *Paraffin baths:* A paraffin bath is a warm, melted wax that conforms to irregular surfaces, such as the arthritic hand. The effect is the same as that of hot packs.

8. *Diathermy:* By means of short waves

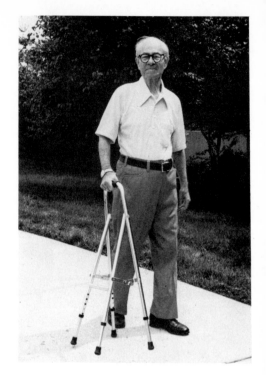

Fig 7-2

Question: Mr. H. S. is an 89-year-old man. What type of ambulation aid is he using?

Answer: He is demonstrating the use of a hemi-walk cane, a device that combines features of a walker and a cane. This ambulation aid is used in the rehabilitation of the stroke or fractured hip patient. It provides a source of support when balance is impaired and distributes weight bearing between the affected lower limb (the left in this case) and the cane. Other types of canes (quadripod ["quad"], tripod, single-axis canes) can be used by patients whose balance is more stable. Canes are held with the hand that is opposite the affected lower limb.

or microwaves, heat develops under the area of exposure to a depth of 2 cm. Diathermy may be helpful in the treatment of fibrositic pain, painful osteoarthritic joints, and ligament sprains.

9. *Ultrasound:* The electrically in-

duced vibration of a quartz crystal generates an acoustic vibration of a frequency too high to be heard. This vibration is transmitted by the tissues to a depth of approximately 5 cm from the surface and produces heat and agitation of the tissues. It may be helpful for relief of pain and, to some extent, for loosening contractured joints.

10. *Hydrotherapy:* The buoyancy, heating effect, and massaging action of a jet stream of warmed water are combined in this modality. Hydrotherapy is most frequently used (1) for exercising limbs that have lost range of motion; (2) for the painful swollen upper limb that results from the shoulder-hand syndrome; and (3) as a vehicle for antiseptic agents in the treatment of infected incisions, diabetic ulcers, pressure sores, and burns.

Heat may be detrimental and even lead to a burn under the following circumstances, which are frequently present in the elderly[2]:

1. When the patient cannot dissipate heat because of the physiological loss of normal sweating associated with aging or impaired local circulation, a burn can occur.

2. When the patient does not perceive or complain about pain because of hypoesthesia from a cerebrovascular accident (CVA), neuropathy, or confusion, a burn can occur.

3. In the presence of cardiac illness, the systemic effects of heat can cause heart failure.

4. Metal implants, such as hip prostheses, can retain large amounts of heat and damage surrounding tissue. Ultrasound and diathermy are contraindicated in this instance.

5. Electronic cardiac pacemaker output may be affected by shortwave and microwave heating appliances.

6. Malignant tumor growth may be accelerated by heat, particularly ultrasound.

7. Acute inflammation may progress with the application of heat.

Exercise used in physical therapy[7]

Exercise, defined as therapeutic motion, has both systemic and local effects. Systemically, exercising improves the functioning of the cardiovascular and respiratory systems. Inappropriately performed exercise may overtax a system that has little reserve, resulting in complications, such as angina, dysrhythmias, or cardiac failure. Locally, exercising adds strength and endurance to the muscles, maintains the range of motion of the joints, and improves local circulation. Exercise also improves coordination and motor skills. It is important that exercises be graded to the patient's condition, with the therapist bearing in mind that they may cause harm. Exercises must be implemented with the concurrence of a physician and performed under the direction of a skilled professional.

Exercises are classified as active (when the motion is performed by the patient) or passive (when the motion is performed by the action of the therapist). Active exercise is classified, in reference to motion around a joint, as follows:

1. *Isometric:* The muscle contracts, but there is no motion around the joint (e.g., contracting the quadriceps while holding the knee extended).

2. *Isotonic:* The muscle contraction produces movement around the joint (e.g., bending the elbow).

Active exercise can also be classified in reference to the amount of resistance encountered, as follows:

1. *Active resistive:* Resistance is ap-

plied by means of the therapist's hand or weights.

2. *Active isokinetic:* A constant resistance is supplied by a machine throughout the whole range of motion.

3. *Active assistive:* The debilitated limb is assisted by the therapist in completing a motion.

4. *Active with elimination of gravity:* The action of a debilitated muscle is facilitated by having it work on a horizontal plane.

Special techniques used in physical therapy

Some specific techniques widely used by physical therapists in geriatric rehabilitation are described in later sections dealing with the disorders they aim to treat. These techniques are muscle reeducation, balance training, ambulation training, stair climbing, and prosthetic training.

Occupational therapy

Occupational therapy is the use of therapeutic activity to restore, improve, and maintain physical function. The staff of an occupational therapy department consists of registered occupational therapists, certified occupational therapy assistants, and aides.

The services provided by occupational therapy are functional activities, perceptual evaluation and training, sensory evaluation and training, assessment and implementation of ADL, and the fabrication and fitting of upper-limb splints.

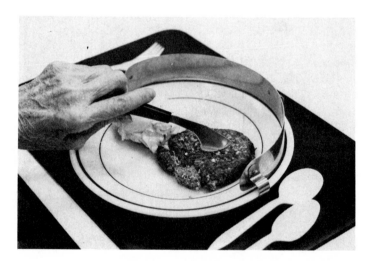

Fig. 7-3

Question: Why is Mrs. J. B. using the assistive devices shown above, and what are they?

Answer: Mrs. B. suffered a stroke with residual right-sided hemiparesis. She is unable to use her right hand to eat. The assistive devices are:
  1. A rocker knife, which allows her to cut her meat one-handed with a rocking motion rather than a sawing motion, which requires another utensil to secure the meat
  2. A metal plate guard, which prevents food from falling off the plate
  3. A self-adhering mat, which prevents the plate from slipping

Tools and materials for leathercraft, weaving, carpentry, gardening, needlecraft, typing, and painting are used in occupational therapy. These functional activities, organized in the form of projects, are given to the patient on the basis of whether they are appropriate for his dysfunction and challenge his interest. They will improve strength, range of motion, dexterity, coordination, and sensory perceptual skills. A simulated home or apartment environment, including utensils for eating, kitchen appliances, furniture, and a toilet and bathtub, are used for training the patient in ADL. The following are the most important of these activities: (1) changing position in bed, (2) transferring in and out of bed, (3) transferring to and from a chair, (4) toileting, (5) dressing and undressing, (6) feeding oneself, and (7) wheelchair propelling.

Training in ADL may include the use of assistive devices to compensate for permanent dysfunctions, such as a rocker knife to cut meat with one hand, a sockdonning appliance to put on socks when the patient cannot reach his foot, or utensils with a swivel mechanism to compensate for hand tremor (Fig. 7-3). Occupational therapy also assesses and trains the patient in the use of safety devices in the home, such as grab bars, rails, and raised toilet seats.

COMMON PROBLEMS AND THEIR REHABILITATION

Twenty percent of the elderly population have serious limitations of mobility.[8] Forty percent of the elderly population, however, are limited in their ability to perform activities, such as work or housekeeping.

The following major disabling conditions seen in elderly patients may lead to hospitalization or long-term institutionalization:

Amputation
Arthritis
Cardiac conditions
Chronic obstructive pulmonary disease
Deconditioning (unfitness)
Dementia
Depression
Fracture of the hip
Hearing and visual impairments
Incontinence (urinary and/or fecal)
Parkinson's disease
Stroke

Stroke, fracture of the hip, amputation, gait disorders, pressure sores, and incontinence are discussed as follows, mainly from the point of view of physical rehabilitation, rather than medical or surgical diagnosis and management.

Stroke

Stroke and *cerebrovascular accident (CVA)*, are terms generally applied to the sudden, often catastrophic, development of a focal neurological deficit caused by a vascular disorder.

Epidemiology

Incidence. Although the incidence of stroke, especially in the elderly, is declining, approximately 500,000 persons suffer a stroke in the United States every year.[9]

Prevalence. Approximately 2,500,000 persons living in the United States have suffered a stroke.

Age. Three quarters of all CVAs occur in those over 65 years of age.[10] The incidence of stroke is three times higher in those over 75 than in those aged 65 to 74. Clearly, stroke is a disease predominantly found in the elderly population.

Sex. While stroke affects the younger man more frequently than the younger woman, there is no sex-related difference in incidence in late life.

Etiology. Ten percent of strokes are due to subarachnoid hemorrhage; 15% are due to intracerebral hemorrhage; and 75% are due to cerebral infarction

Thrombosis, usually on the basis of arteriosclerosis, is the most common cause of cerebral infarction. Embolism emanating from an ulcerated plaque or a thrombosis in the heart is a less frequent cause.

Outcome. One third to one half of all stroke victims will die during the first 30 days after the episode. Eighty percent of patients with intracerebral hemorrhage, 50% of patients with subarachnoid hemorrhage, and 40% of patients with cerebral infarction will die within the first 30 days. Of 100 persons surviving a stroke, 10 will be left without any dysfunction, 40 will have mild dysfunction for which they can compensate, 40 will have significant dysfunction and will require special services to cope with their partial disabilities, and 10 will need institutional care.

Assessment

In each stroke patient, it is useful to clinically classify the etiology of the stroke with reasonable accuracy, localize the lesion, and determine the time that has elapsed and the severity of the dysfunction. Invasive techniques are not usually necessary. A computerized axial tomogram of the head may be helpful. Stroke in the elderly is most frequently due to occlusion of portions of the middle cerebral artery. The resulting syndrome is characterized by homonymous hemianopia, contralateral hemiplegia, and/or hemianesthesia, with the upper limb more affected than the lower and aphasia occurring most frequently when the dominant hemisphere is involved.

Prognosis

The patient and family will be concerned about the prognosis. The prognosis for rehabilitation of the older stroke patient depends on (1) the prognosis for neurological return; (2) mentation, including perceptual accuracy; (3) motivation; (4) vigor; and (5) the availability and implementation of a sound program of rehabilitation.[11-13] The sooner the program is implemented, the sooner the patient will be rehabilitated. Programs implemented late after the stroke, however, are still valuable and may improve the level of function and quality of life of the patient.[14,15]

The prognosis for neurological return depends on (1) the time that has elapsed (the earlier it is after the stroke, the greater the hope for neurological return) and (2) the severity of dysfunction (the less severe the dysfunction at the time of examination, the more likely the possibility for neurological return).

Currently, a lost neurological function cannot be reinstated by opening new pathways or by enhancing the function of damaged or undamaged neurons. Consequently, rehabilitation of the stroke patient depends largely, but not completely, on spontaneous neurological return. Spontaneous neurological return is the best ally of rehabilitation.

In general, most neurological return occurs during the first month after the stroke. By the end of the third month, no further return of significance is to be expected. Muscular tone can be a relatively valuable indicator of the chances of neurological return. Persistent lack of tone (flaccidity) for a number of weeks suggests poor future neurological return. Early return of tone with or without some degree of spasticity brings hope for further neurological restoration.

Especially disabling dysfunctions

Not all of the dysfunctions that result from a stroke weigh equally in producing disability. Motor loss, the most common dysfunction, is perhaps the least disabling of all. Perceptual loss, sensory loss, aphasia, loss of balance, hemicorporal neglect, hemianopia, and, of course, cognitive damage from multi-infarct dementia (MID) are causes of severe, often untreatable disabilities. It may be impossible to rehabilitate a vigorous, motivated, and mentally clear patient, because perceptual losses or hemianesthesia renders him unaware of a major portion of his body. This patient may remain a disabled individual in need of permanent support.

These highly disabling dysfunctions are predictive factors when groups of stroke patients are surveyed. No one indicator, however, has definitive value when one is looking at the individual patient. Each patient runs his own course and deserves a trial of rehabilitation.[18]

Rehabilitation prescription

The student should recognize three different stages in stroke rehabilitation. The prescription is different at each stage.

Immediate stage. The immediate stage is the time when the patient is densely hemiplegic, immobile, and perhaps comatose. If not treated appropriately, he will develop complications, such as pressure sores, contractures, phlebitis, pulmonary embolism, aspiration pneumonia, and bowel impaction, all of which contribute to the high morbidity and mortality of the immediate stage, which lasts approximately 7 to 14 days.

The physical therapy prescription during the immediate stage includes (1) instructions to nurses to change the position of the patient at least every 2 hours to prevent pressure sores, to properly position the patient's joints to prevent contractures, and to position the patient to prevent aspiration pneumonia; and (2) range-of-motion exercises to all joints — passive to the paralyzed limbs and active to the nonparalyzed limbs to prevent joint contractures and muscle wasting.

The occupational therapy prescription includes instructions to assist nursing personnel in implementing efficient ways of transferring the patient.

Intermediate stage. The intermediate stage begins when the patient is medically and neurologically stabilized (approximately 7 to 14 days from onset). During this stage, he may or may not show spontaneous neurological return. If some return is present, therapy should be aimed at intensifying the return by means of muscle reeducation. If there is no return, the goal is to enhance the remaining capabilities in an attempt to compensate for the dysfunction. The physical therapy and occupational therapy prescription during the intermediate stage includes (1) sensory perceptual evaluation and training; (2) muscle reeducation exercises; (3) functional activities to prevent neglect of the affected side and to improve the skills of the returned movements; (4) ambulation training, beginning with parallel bars; (5) ADL evaluation and training; and (6) training in transfer technique with or without assistance (Fig 7-4).

Late stage. The late stage is reached when approximately a month has elapsed and no return has occurred or when, after intensive therapy, the patient stops making progress. Patients enter this stage at different levels of function. Some are totally disabled, whereas others exhibit minimal or no disability. The goal is to find ways to cope with the dysfunctions

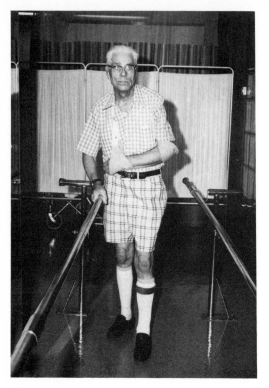

Fig. 7-4

Question: Mr. E. H. is a 75-year-old man. What device is he using to assist him during ambulation training? Why is he wearing a sling?

Answer: He is training in ambulation in the parallel bars. These bars give him firm support while ambulating. The sling partially prevents subluxation of the left shoulder by counteracting the force of gravity, and it prevents his flaccid left arm from swinging freely, interfering with his gait and hitting objects in the environment.

by means of substitution techniques, including braces and assistive devices. It is also the time when special counseling efforts are made to help the patient adjust to residual disabilities and to mobilize the supportive elements that will provide long-term assistance to the patient.

The physical therapy prescription during the late stage includes (1) maintenance exercises and ambulation on a long-term basis, administered by properly trained unskilled persons, such as relatives, friends, or home attendants; and (2) an assessment of the need for a brace or a cane. Usually, a short leg brace, constructed in plastic or with two metal bars, compensates for foot drop and/or instability of the ankle. If a cane is needed for balance, the patient should be trained to use one (quadripod, hemi-walk cane, or regular cane).

The occupational therapy prescription includes teaching substitution techniques so that the patient can perform ADL as independently as possible. The need for appliances to facilitate ADL (reachers, donning devices, utensils, elastic shoelaces, special clothing) and adaptive equipment for the home (wheelchair, grab bars, bathing stool, lifters) should be assessed (Figs. 7-5 to 7-7). Relatives and/or attendants (home health aides) should be taught efficient ways of helping the patient.

• • •

It is often difficult to separate the three stages of stroke rehabilitation. The physical and occupational therapists introduce the previously described therapeutic elements at the appropriate times. For example, wheelchair self-propelling may be taught very early if the therapist feels that the patient is going to be left with serious disability in ambulation.

Speech therapy, although discussed in detail in Chapter 8, must be stressed. As soon as a disorder in communication, such as aphasia or dysarthria is detected, the speech pathologist should be consulted. Although speech therapy cannot hasten the return of a lost function, it can enhance spontaneous return.

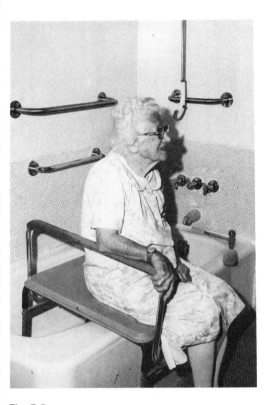

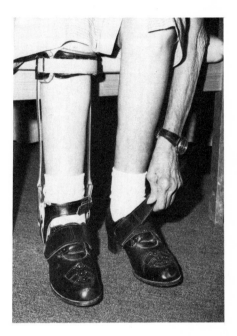

Fig. 7-6

Question: What type of brace is Mrs. P. M. wearing on her right lower limb?

Answer: She is wearing a conventional double-bar, short leg brace to facilitate ambulation by preventing "foot drop" and stabilizing her ankle. She is using her functional left hand to fasten the self-adhering (Velcro) closure on her shoe. These closures take the place of laces, which are difficult to tie with one hand.

Fig. 7-5

Question: Is this scene in an institutional setting or the individual's home? What pieces of adaptive equipment have been provided to assist Mrs. S. S., a 75-year-old woman who suffered a stroke, in bathing herself?

Answer: Assistive equipment used in bathing can be provided to patients whether they are in their own home, a nursing home, or an acute care hospital. Mrs. S. is shown sitting on a tub transfer bench, which allows her to slide from her wheelchair into the tub for bathing. Grab bars, a long-handled bath brush, and a flexible shower hose are devices that allow her to be independent in bathing with one hand.

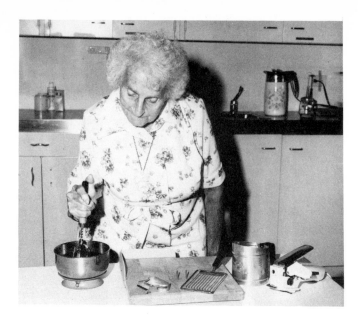

Fig. 7-7

Question: What is your diagnosis?

Answer: Mrs. S. B., a 79-year-old woman, suffered a stroke 1 year ago and was left with a nonfunctional, flaccid left upper extremity. She was trained in the use of adaptive equipment to facilitate homemaking in the kitchen.

Question: What section of the department of rehabilitation trained Mrs. B. in the use of the devices shown in the figure?

Answer: The occupational therapy section. One of the roles of this section is to assess and train the patient in the self-care activities of daily living (ADL). For a woman with the potential for remaining at home, kitchen activities are an important element of the program.

Question: List the appliances you see in front of Mrs. B. and describe them.

Answer: The appliances from left to right are:

1. A one-handed egg beater
2. A suction base that holds the bowl to the table
3. A wooden cutting board with a food guard and nails to hold the food while it is being cut with one hand
4. A one-handed vegetable peeler
5. A one-handed tomato slicer
6. A one-handed flour sifter
7. A one-handed electric can opener

With coordinated rehabilitation effort, elderly patients who survive a stroke can return to the community.

Fracture of the hip

Fracture of the upper end of the femur (hip fracture) is typically an illness of the elderly.[16]

Of the 200,000 hip fractures that occur in the United States every year, 74% occur in individuals over 65 years of age. Elderly white women sustain a fractured hip three times as often as elderly white men. Blacks are rarely affected. Therefore, the fractured hip is mainly a condition of elderly white women.

Osteoporosis, resulting from aging, menopausal hormonal deficits, or disuse, has classically been implicated as the etiological factor of the fractured hip in advanced ages. Much attention, however, is being given to the study of the pathophysiology of the fractured hip, especially with regard to racial, genetic, and occupational factors. Trauma is being questioned as the immediate cause of the fracture, even though it is well-known that recurrent falls are often the harbinger of a fractured hip. It is unclear whether the fracture is caused by uncoordinated muscle contraction during the act of falling to the ground or by the force of impaction.[17,18] Further biomechanical research is needed to resolve this question.

Classification and management

For practical purposes, fractures of the upper end of the femur can be divided into two classes: subcapital fractures[19] and trochanteric fractures (intertrochanteric and subtrochanteric). *Subcapital fractures* are those which occur right under the femoral head, somewhere in its neck. They are intracapsular (inside the tenoligamentous capsule of the hip joint) and if displaced may cause impaired blood supply to the proximal fragment by disrupting the lateral and medial circumflex arteries that enter the capsule at its distal attachment. This lack of blood supply often leads to aseptic necrosis of the femoral head.

Two frequent complications of the subcapital fracture are nonunion and post-traumatic degenerative joint disease secondary to avascular necrosis or to damage to the cartilage. Five percent of subcapital fractures are impacted and, therefore, more stable. Impacted subcapital fractures exhibit a lower rate of complications.

The *trochanteric fracture* (intertro-chanteric and subtrochanteric) is extracapsular. The blood supply to this area is abundant; consequently, there are fewer complications than with the subcapital type. An intertrochanteric fracture may be unstable if it is comminuted or if the fracture line approaches the vertical plane.

It takes approximately 12 weeks for femoral fractures to heal. During this period of time, the fragments must remain approximated and held in place by means of internal fixation devices (pin, nails, screws), immobilization, or a combination of both. When internal fixation has been used, a progressive schedule of weight-bearing ambulation occurs, depending on the type of fixation device used. Table 7-2 is a commonly accepted weight-bearing schedule for ambulation training following a fractured hip. Each case, however, is to be handled individually in accordance with the patient's ability to cooperate and the surgical and radiological circumstances.

The nondisplaced or slightly displaced subcapital fracture may be adequately treated by internal fixation with pins after a closed reduction under radiographic control (no exposure of the fracture).

The displaced subcapital fracture is usually managed by replacing the supra-trochanteric area by an endoprosthesis (e.g., Austin Moore prosthesis).[21] For the elderly, this procedure has the advantage of permitting immediate ambulation after surgery if the patient's general level of motivation and vigor permits it. An endoprosthesis is indicated when the fracture is so unstable that malunion (healing in an abnormal position) is foreseen or when the displacement is so severe that vascular damage must have occurred and aseptic necrosis is foreseeable.

Table 7-2. A commonly used weight-bearing schedule for different devices

Device	Non-weight bearing*	Partial weight bearing*	Full weight bearing
Fixation pins (e.g., Knowles or Hagie)	First 8 weeks	After 8 weeks	After 12 weeks
Hip fixation implant (e.g., Jewett nail and plate)	First 8 weeks	After 8 weeks	After 12 weeks
Compression hip screw system (e.g., Richard's compression screw)	Not necessary	As tolerated‡	As tolerated (approximately after 1 week)
Femoral hip prosthesis (e.g., Austin Moore type)	Not necessary	As tolerated	As tolerated

°Non-weight–bearing (NWB) ambulation (ambulation without weight on the affected limb) and partial weight–bearing (PWB) ambulation (ambulation with some weight placed on the affected limb) often present problems in ambulation training for the older patient because hopping requires strength, coordination, balance, and an understanding of what is being taught. Therefore, it may be difficult or impossible for the confused elderly patient to learn non-weight– or partial weight–bearing ambulation.
‡"As tolerated" means that the patient can begin ambulation as soon as he has sufficient vigor and is reasonably free from pain.

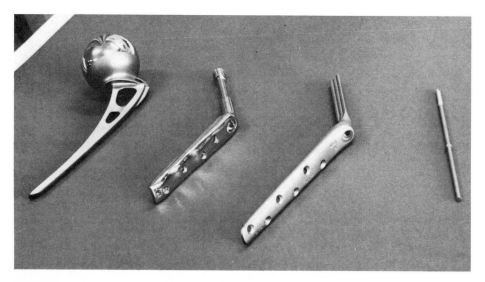

Fig. 7-8
Question: Name the devices pictured above that are used in the surgical treatment of a fractured hip.
Answer: From left to right:
   1. A femoral hip prosthesis (endoprosthesis), used to replace the femoral head
   2. A compression hip screw system
   3. A hip fixation implant (nail/plate)
   4. A fixation pin

To reduce the time of immobilization, intertrochanteric fractures frequently are handled surgically by open reduction and fixation with a nail and plate.[20] Only after the bone is partially or totally healed, is partial or full weight bearing allowed. A collapsible screw (e.g., Richard's compression screw) causes the distal and proximal segments of the fracture to impact into each other while the device collapses on itself. This device permits earlier weight bearing; the tip of the screw seldom penetrates into the acetabulum.

Devices used in the surgical treatment of a fractured hip are shown in Fig. 7-8.

Assessment

Assessment is based on the history, the physical examination, and radiological assessment.

The *history* includes the circumstances of the fracture, the type of fracture, and the orthopedic procedure. Orthopedic treatment possibilities include (1) closed reduction and no surgical procedure (conservative management), used in many demented patients, in patients not ambulating prior to the hip fracture, and in patients unable to undergo an operation[22]; (2) surgical insertion of a fixation device, such as pins or a nail; and (3) surgical insertion of an endoprosthesis. Because the schedule of weight bearing is a function of the type of device used and of the time since the operation, it is important to know the date of the operation and the device used.

The *physical examination* includes (1) the mental status of the patient, because it will influence future rehabilitation efforts; (2) the state of healing of the surgical wound; (3) the status of the skin (pressure sores may have developed); (4) neurological assessment of the patient's

limb with the clinician looking for quadriceps palsy secondary to injury of the femoral nerve during surgery and for foot drop caused by compression of the common peroneal nerve at the upper end of the fibula by improperly fitting splints; (5) range of motion of the hip, knee, and ankle; and (6) measurement of the length of the legs to detect any difference resulting from surgery.

Radiological assessment includes both anteroposterior and lateral views of the fracture to determine the alignment of the segments, the position of the fixation device, and the status of healing as shown by the callous formation.

Rehabilitation goals

Usually, the goal of rehabilitation is to restore the prefracture level of ambulation and function, either unassisted or with a walker or cane.

Rehabilitation prescription

The rehabilitation prescription may include general conditioning exercises, progressively resistive exercise for the upper-extremity muscles in preparation for ambulation, bilateral quadriceps and gluteus isometrics, active exercises, range-of-motion exercises, and progressive ambulation at the appropriate level of weight bearing. Ambulation will usually start with the parallel bars and progress to the use of an ambulation aid. Eventually, most elderly people achieve independent ambulation without assistive devices. Stair climbing should be practiced when indicated.

An ambulation aid, such as the standard walker, is often prescribed for the elderly patient in the non-weight–and partial weight–bearing stages. Many patients who achieve an efficient, safe gait with a walker may want to use this device permanently. Except for the inappropriateness of its size when public or private transportation is being used (buses, subways, cars), a walker adequately fulfills the needs of the older ambulator. Even stair climbing can be performed with specially designed walkers. A cane, while less bulky than a walker, also gives much less support. Elderly patients usually have difficulty ambulating with crutches. The difficulty may be attributed to minor deficits in coordination, to slowness of righting reflexes, and to proprioceptive impairment.

Complications

Immobility. All of the previously described complications of immobility can affect the elderly patient with a fractured hip; they can prolong the acute hospitalization and the rehabilitation effort and lead to institutionalization.

Painful postoperative hip. The soreness of a postoperative hip should progressively subside in a few weeks. Steady or increasing pain should prompt immediate physical and radiological examination.[23]

The differential diagnosis of the painful postoperative hip fracture includes:

1. Separation of the bone fragments
2. Subluxation of an endoprothesis
3. Osteomyelitis
4. Aseptic necrosis
5. Displacement of the fixation device with protrusion into the acetabulum or pain-sensitive soft tissues
6. Traumatic periarthralgia, such as bursitis or capsulitis
7. Myositis ossificans (deposits of bone in muscle)
8. Referred pain from the spine or pelvis
9. Fibrositis
10. Septic arthritis with or without absess formation

Leg shortening and deformities. Hip fractures may lead to a discrepancy of length in the lower limbs; malunion and impaction of the segments are the main causes. A lift in the shoe is all that is needed to compensate for this discrepancy. Deformities of the affected limb can result from either subcapital or trochanteric fractures. Typically, the deformity is an external rotation of the whole lower limb caused by displacement of the segments or by poor positioning of the immobilized limb after surgery, resulting in a contracture of the hip joint.

Prognosis

Early postoperative mobilization, including getting the patient out of bed, general conditioning exercises, range-of-motion exercises, and ambulation training will prevent complications and expedite the patient's return to the community. The majority of elderly people with hip fractures will return to their homes and will ambulate without assistive devices.

Amputation

The loss of part of a lower limb most frequently affects elderly individuals. Three fourths of all amputations are performed on patients 65 years of age or older.[16]

Etiology

At least 85% of amputations performed in the elderly are secondary to ischemia of the limb, commonly caused by arteriosclerosis. In more than one half of these cases, diabetes mellitus is detected and is thought to have enhanced the arteriosclerotic process. Less frequently, ischemia is due to embolism, thromboangiitis obliterans (Buerger's disease), or other vasculitis. Amputations secondary to trauma, neoplasia, and infection account for the remaining 10% to 15% of amputations.

Site and level of amputations

The presence of arteriosclerotic-induced ischemia is almost exclusively limited to the lower extremities. The level of the amputation is determined by the viability of the tissues and the amount of blood supply immediately above the surgical line. As a rule, the more distal the amputation, the more useful the remainder of the limb and the easier the prosthetic replacement. The more distal the amputation, however, the more difficult it is for the remaining stump to heal because of insufficient blood supply.

Distal amputations are now performed more frequently because of the establishment of more accurate ways of determining the amount of the blood supply (e.g., by using the Doppler ultrasound technique) and because of recognition of the importance of preserving the knee joint, if prosthetic ambulation is to be achieved.

Consequently, the proportion of below-knee (BK) to above-knee (AK) amputations has greatly changed. In the past, the elderly patient was usually subjected to an AK amputation; the trend now is to perform BK procedures and preserve the knee joint. More distal amputations (such as those of toes, and transmetatarsal, tarsometatarsal, and transtarsal amputations) heal slowly in the elderly and produce serious deformities of the foot. The supramalleolar amputation has more chance to heal, but the gains over the standard BK amputation are not sufficient to very often justify this type of amputation. For prosthetic purposes, the ideal length of the BK stump is midcalf. The AK stump should be as long as possible to facilitate prosthetic fitting, allowing ambulation to be more efficient.

The preservation of the knee joint is important at any age and is crucial to the elderly amputee. Preserving the knee joint increases the mechanical advantages, thereby saving energy and reducing cardiac work, and leaves proprioception intact. Absence of the knee joint is a major barrier to prosthetic ambulation in the elderly.[24]

It has been shown repeatedly that more BK than AK amputees become prosthetic ambulators.[25-27] The increased energy required to walk with an AK prosthesis is one reason for this. Approximate figures for energy consumption indicate that in the young, ambulating with one BK prosthesis increases energy consumption by 10%, whereas ambulating with one AK prosthesis increases energy consumption by 20%. In the elderly, there is a 20% increase in energy consumption with one BK prosthesis and an increase of up to 100% with one AK prosthesis. Consequently, the AK ambulator has to cope with a significantly increased demand on his cardiovascular reserve. Fortunately, the elderly individual with an amputation reduces the energy consumption and the stress on his cardiovascular system by choosing his own comfortable pace. Otherwise, the elderly individual could seldom tolerate the demand on cardiac output that is required by prosthetic ambulation. Table 7-3 shows the degree of difficulty and energy consumption of prosthetic ambulation.[28-30]

Assessment

In addition to the routine considerations applicable to every disabled older individual, special areas of concern in the elderly amputee include the following.

Table 7-3. Degree of difficulty and energy consumption of various types of prosthetic ambulation

Most difficult (most energy consumption)	Bilateral: AK and AK Bilateral: AK and BK Unilateral: AK Bilateral: BK and BK
Least difficult (least energy consumption)	Unilateral: BK

1. Mental status
2. The status of the opposite lower limb and of the upper limb
3. Cardiovascular status
4. Auditory and visual status
5. The presence of diabetes and the stability of the blood glucose level
6. The presence of an accompanying neuropathy
7. The characteristics of the wound, including the skin, interstitial tissue (edema), sensation, muscle strength, and range of motion of the joints
8. The presence of preamputation disorders of ambulation, such as fractures, arthritis, stroke, ataxia, Parkinson's disease, and other neurological dysfunctions
9. A previous history of successful prosthetic rehabilitation in the opposite limb or in the same limb at a lower level
10. The patient's social situation (living alone or with an ill spouse)

Problems associated with prosthetic ambulation

Systemic problems. Prosthetic ambulation may unduly stress the cardiovascular system and thereby exacerbate dysrhythmias, angina, or congestive heart failure (CHF). Electrocardiographic monitoring while the patient is ambulating with the prosthesis may reveal ischemic changes or dysrhythmias. Hypoglycemia may occur in the diabetic patient who is receiving a fixed dose of insulin or oral agent, because of increased glucose utilization for energy during the period of prosthetic rehabilitation. Monitoring the 2-hour postprandial blood glucose level, as well as hypoglycemic symptoms, will determine the need for reduction of the insulin or oral agent. A peripheral neuropathy may leave areas of hypoesthesia or anesthesia on the stump or a proprioceptive deficit that may make the patient unaware of trauma, thereby impairing healing of the stump.

Status of the opposite limb and upper extremities. The opposite limb must be reasonably healthy for prosthetic ambulation to be successful. The presence of ischemia in the remaining extremity may prevent ambulation because of pain. Hair loss, a temperature gradient, and the absence of a pulse are clues to the health of the opposite limb. The upper limbs must have normal strength and be free of significant dysfunction (pain, contractures, paralysis), since they will partially support the weight of the body during prosthetic ambulation training. Previous dysfunctions affecting ambulation that occurred prior to the amputation must be evaluated to establish realistic goals.

Local problems. The interstitial tissue of the stump may be swollen secondary to surgical trauma, infection, panniculitis, lymphedema, or systemic fluid retention. Shrinking of the stump will be necessary until it decreases in size and can fit into the socket of the prosthesis. Shrinking is accomplished by wrapping the stump with an Ace bandage or a one-piece elastic bandage (shrinker). Muscle strength and range of motion of the knee and hip joints will be impaired by disuse or inappropriate positioning of the stump.

Rehabilitation goals[31]

If the patient is mentally clear, well motivated, and sufficiently vigorous, he should benefit from a rehabilitation prescription.

It is sound practice to establish tentative goals for the prosthetic program. "We will learn together" is a satisfactory answer to the patient's question about ultimate outcome when the outcome is unknown. When the outcome is predictable, sensitivity to the patient's ability to cope with the information is crucial. Realistic goals will be based on what is learned from the patient's performance in the gymnasium, in occupational therapy, on the ward, and at home.

Overall, there are two possible goals for the elderly amputee: rehabilitation with prosthetic ambulation or rehabilitation with a wheelchair (with or without a cosmetic prosthesis). Between these two extremes, there are multiple combinations in which either the wheelchair or the prosthesis is used more frequently.

The question of whether or not to fit an elderly amputee with a prosthesis is perhaps the most difficult question in geriatric rehabilitation. A prosthetic lower limb should be prescribed for any of the three following purposes:

1. To permit bipedal ambulation (Walking with a well-fitted prosthesis consumes less energy than hopping on one leg with a walker or crutches.)
2. To permit or facilitate transfers (Most elderly amputees can be trained to transfer even without prostheses: the unilateral amputee by pivoting on the remaining limb

and the bilateral amputee by lifting his body with his upper limbs or by sliding on a board. Some amputees do not develop sufficient power in their remaining limbs and cannot transfer without a prosthesis.)
3. To help the patient adapt psychologically and socially to his condition (A feeling of completeness constitutes an important gain, and confidence in one's cosmetic appearance encourages social participation.)

There are three types of patients for whom a prosthesis has limited value. These are:

1. Most of the chronically demented, who may not realize they have lost a limb, nor experience the benefits of a prosthesis (These patients are unable to participate in active rehabilitation.)
2. The bedridden or those with terminal illness
3. The already rehabilitated who have, without a prosthesis, achieved all of the wheelchair mobility, ADL independence, and psychological adjustment that they need or desire

The indications for a prosthesis are less clear for a large group of mildly confused elderly amputees. When it is questionable whether a patient will be able to use a prosthesis, he should be fitted with a temporary prosthesis and given a trial of ambulation. A temporary prosthesis is a relatively inexpensive artificial limb made of a prefabricated or plaster socket, artificial foot, and connecting pieces. The patient and his rehabilitation team will "learn together" whether wearing an artificial limb will help him become rehabilitated. If ambulation training with the temporary prosthesis is successful, a permanent prosthesis can be made.

Whatever the decision regarding a prosthesis, the patient must receive a rehabilitation prescription with the idea that prosthetic ambulation is just one factor in the overall outcome. Improvement in strength, the ability to transfer, wheelchair mobility, ADL independence, and psychosocial adjustment should be stressed to the patient as realistic goals. He should be discouraged from putting all his hopes and expectations on being able to walk with a prosthesis.

Rehabilitation prescription

The rehabilitation prescription includes two aspects: (1) preprosthetic training and stump preparation, and (2) fitting of a prosthesis and ambulation training. Before a prosthesis is prescribed, physical therapy must improve the patient's general strength through general conditioning (calisthenics) and resistive exercises. During these progressive exercises, the patient's cardiopulmonary status should be monitored. Simultaneously, the stump should be shrunk by the constant wearing of an Ace bandage or a shrinker. The range of motion of the hip and knee joints must be maintained while the surgical wound heals. Complete healing, however, is not an absolute prerequisite for the use of a prosthesis.

BK prosthesis

The BK prosthesis consists of (1) a specially contoured socket into which the stump is placed so that the majority of the weight is borne by the patellar tendon, (2) a suspension device that holds the artificial limb to the stump, (3) a shank portion (usually made of a laminated synthetic material) equivalent to the portion between the knee and the foot, and (4) a wooden foot with or without an ankle joint.

AK prosthesis

The AK prosthesis includes an artificial knee joint in addition to the other four components described for the BK prosthesis. The AK socket has four sidewalls that follow the muscular contours of the stump. The weight, although borne mostly by the ischial bone as it makes contact with a small platform in the posterior edge, is distributed over the entire surface of the socket (total contact socket). The elderly AK amputee may walk more safely with the prosthetic knee fixed in extension. A locking device, which the patient must unlock in order to sit, is used for this purpose. The prosthesis is usually suspended by a metal band around the pelvis, linked to the prosthesis by a hinge at the level of the hip (Fig. 7-9).

Other appliances for the amputee

It is unusual to see an older amputee ambulate a significant distance without any supportive device. For transferring or ambulating, almost every elderly amputee needs a cane or canes, crutches, or a walker. It is necessary to provide a wheelchair for most unilateral amputees and virtually all bilateral amputees to assure mobility when they are not wearing the prosthesis. To facilitate transfers, the leg rests of the wheelchair must be of the "swing away," removable type. If the patient is to transfer by means of a sliding board, the arm rests of the wheelchair must also be removable (Fig. 7-10). The rear axle of the wheelchair must be in an "amputee-type" position, approximately 4 inches further back than a standard wheelchair axle. This reduces the chance of the wheelchair tilting backward as a result of the lack of counterweight applied by the lower limbs.

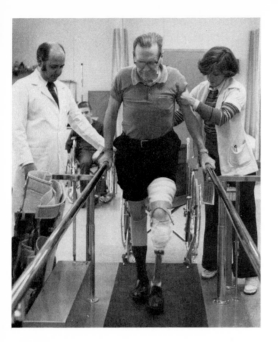

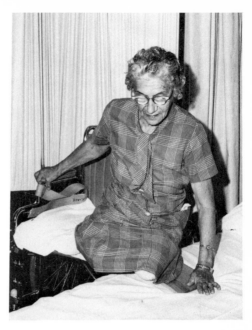

Fig. 7-9

Question: What are the most likely medical diagnoses? What are your rehabilitation diagnoses?

Answer: Mr. C. W., a 71-year-old man, has suffered bilateral lower-extremity amputations resulting from peripheral vascular disease and diabetes mellitus. He is shown training in ambulation in the parallel bars, using a left BK pylon and a right AK prosthesis.

Phantom limb sensation and phantom pain[32]

The presence of a nonpainful perceptual representation of the removed limb (phantom limb sensation) is an extremely common phenomenon. This is not necessarily an annoying feeling, except when pain accompanies it (phantom pain). Phantom limb sensation can cause falls (and fractures) when the patient tries to walk on his phantom leg. Phantom limb sensation usually disappears over a period of weeks to months.

Fig. 7-10

Question: What is Mrs. J. M., a bilateral AK amputee, doing?

Answer: She is using a sliding board for transferring from the wheelchair to the bed. The board bridges the space between the wheelchair and the bed. It can also be used in transferring from an automobile to a wheelchair and vice versa. In order for Mrs. M. to use a sliding board, the wheelchair must have removable arm rests.

Persistent phantom limb sensation or phantom pain may be alleviated by replacing it with a new sensation from the stump. During the prosthetic rehabilitation program, the stump is given an abundance of superficial and proprioceptive stimulation. Satisfactory psychological adjustment to the amputation seems to be a positive factor that promotes the early waning of phantom limb sensation or pain. Depression tends to aggravate and perpetuate the condition.

Prognosis

Prosthetic ambulation is achieved by the elderly patient in 70% to 80% of unilateral BK amputees, in 50% of bilateral BK amputees, in less than 50% of unilateral AK amputees, and in an unknown small percentage of bilateral AK amputees.

Overall, the majority of mentally clear elderly patients who survive amputation of a lower extremity will ambulate with a prosthesis. Many will return to their communities.

Gait disorders

Efficient bipedal ambulation requires normal musculoskeletal and nervous systems. Defective functioning of either system increases in prevalence in the elderly because of physiological changes (increased sway, impaired ability to decrease sway with visual cuing and to recover balance once it is lost). "Once you're going, you've got to go" refers to this inability to recover balance and the subsequent fall.[33] Accumulated pathological events (hemiparesis, parkinsonism, peripheral neuropathy, muscle disuse, visual loss) also affect ambulation. Consequently, a fall is a frequent outcome of gait disturbances in the elderly.

Diagnosis

The differential diagnosis of an impaired gait includes:

1. *Neurological causes:* These include Parkinson's disease, normal-pressure hydrocephalus, hemiparesis, peripheral neuropathy, demyelinating disorders, anterior horn disease, ataxia, sensory disorders, perceptual disorders, medication side effects, and poor vision. A neurological examination should be performed.

2. *Muscular causes:* Included in this category are myopathies, myositis, and simple disuse. Muscle testing should be performed.

3. *Pain in the musculoskeletal system:* Such pain can limit ambulation and joint mobility. Gait analysis, mobilization of the joints, and palpation of muscles as well as articular and periarticular areas will determine whether pain is causing the impaired gait.

4. *Contracture of joints involved in ambulation:* The joints of the hips, knees, and ankles should be examined and moved through their full range of motion. Goniometry should be performed.

Two frequent gait disturbances are the idiopathic gait disorder of some older individuals and the gait of the parkinsonian patient. Although different in etiology and pathogenesis, both gaits have in common a hesitant, shuffling, unsteady pattern. The patient with the idiopathic disorder exhibits normal muscle tone, whereas the muscle tone of the parkinsonian patient is increased. One could speculate that the parkinsonian patient is forced to shuffle because of rigidity (Fig. 7-11), whereas the patient with the idiopathic disorder may choose to shuffle to maximize his safety.

Treatment

The gait dysfunction should, if feasible, be corrected with medication (e.g., L-dopa for parkinsonism), physical modalities for pain (e.g., heat), and exercises for muscle weakness and joint contractures.

For the idiopathic and the parkinsonian gait disturbance, a program of training should be prescribed, including the following techniques:[34]

1. Teach the patient to think of his toes during ambulation and bring them up with every step. By using this simple

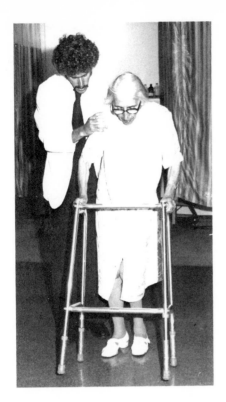

Fig. 7-11

Question: Mrs. B. K. is an 82-year-old woman. What ambulation aid is she using, and why?

Answer: She is using a standard walker during the assessment of her ambulation capability. Her gait is unsafe as a result of her advanced Parkinson's disease. Eventually she was trained in using a wheeled walker. The parkinsonian patient has difficulty with a standard walker because of rigidity and the shuffling gait. The wheeled walker provides constant support while allowing the patient to proceed at a greater pace.

technique, the patient is often able to break the feeling of being glued to the floor and develop a safer gait.

2. Teach the patient to spread his legs apart while walking to get a wider, more secure base.

3. Teach the patient to turn using small steps and keeping a wide base. The legs must not be crossed while turning.

4. Provide the patient with a walker. If the patient has a shuffling gait, a wheeled walker is most appropriate because it provides constant support while allowing the patient to proceed at a quicker pace.

5. Gently push the patient from different directions to give him practice in standing balance. Obviously, appropriate precautions must be taken to prevent falls.

Under supervision, the patient should practice these techniques frequently during the day (Figs. 7-12 and 7-13).

Pressure sores

The skin and underlying tissues may ulcerate if sufficient pressure is applied continuously. This pressure will cause ischemia and eventually tissue necrosis. The resulting lesion is called a pressure sore. *Decubitus ulcer* and *bedsore* are other terms used to describe the same phenomenon.

The normal intracapillary pressure is 32 mm Hg. The weight of the body on a bony prominence creates a pressure of 40 to 75 mm Hg. Consequently, the capillaries over bony prominences will normally collapse when a patient lies supine. If the capillary collapse lasts for a period of 2 hours, irreversible tissue necrosis will occur.

Ninety-six percent of all pressure sores occur in the lower part of the body, 67% around the hips and buttocks and 29% on the lower limbs. Any area subjected to sustained pressure over a bony prominence is at risk.

Etiology

Immobility is the primary cause of pressure sores. Normal elderly individuals feel discomfort, perceive it, and re-

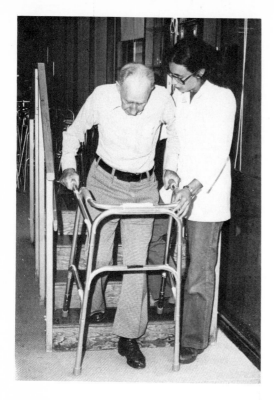

Fig. 7-12

Question: Mr. H. H. is a 75-year-old man. What is he doing, and what ambulation aid is he using?

Answer: He is using a stair-climbing walker while descending a flight of training stairs. The stair-climbing walker is specially designed so that it can be tilted and still remain stable.

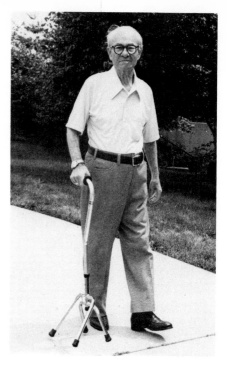

Fig. 7-13

Question: What device is Mr. H. S. demonstrating?

Answer: He is demonstrating the use of a "quad" cane. While this appliance is less stable than the hemi-walk cane he is using in Fig. 7-2, it is small and can be used in more crowded environments.

act by frequently changing the position of their trunk and limbs. Sensory, perceptual, or motor dysfunctions impair the ability of the elderly patient to perceive discomfort and react. Elderly patients with poor mobility, especially those who are bedridden or wheelchair-bound, are prone to develop pressure sores. The weakened and disabled older individual confined to bed during the immediate postoperative or post-CVA period or while awaiting transfer from the acute care hospital to a long-term care facility is also at high risk.

Prevention

Mobility will prevent pressure sores. The patient must actively or passively change the position of his limbs and trunk every 2 hours. Many different pads, cushions, and mattresses have been developed to distribute the weight of the body over a larger area, thereby reducing the amount of pressure over a given point. The sheepskin, foam pad, gel pad, air cushion, air mattress, sand bed, water mattress, alternating pressure mattress, and rotating frame are devices that will assist personnel in preventing pressure sores. If these devices are not properly monitored, however, they may fail and pressure sores will occur.

Each patient should be assessed to determine whether he is prone to develop pressure sores. The following preventive measures should be implemented in those who are at a risk: (1) changing the position of the patient every 2 hours day and night, (2) keeping the skin dry and clean, (3) placing pads or cushions under bony prominences, and (4) periodically reinspecting high-risk areas.

Treatment

The following four principles apply to the healing of a pressure sore: (1) removal of pressure, (2) removal of any necrotic tissue, (3) control of any local infection, and (4) maintenance of an adequate nutritional status.

Removal of pressure. Pressure is removed primarily by changing the position of the patient. The patient's weight can also be distributed over a larger area by using devices such as a water bed or a ripple mattress, which alternately inflates and deflates certain segments on a timed cycle.[35] Obviously, every device will fail unless it is continually monitored.

Removal of necrotic tissue. The necrotic tissue must be debrided to let new tissue grow. With a pair of scissors and a scalpel, the black eschar can be removed and the ulcer debrided to the point of minor pain or bleeding. Small areas of necrosis can also be debrided by means of enzymatic agents.

The extent of the pressure sore must be determined. Large sinuses or pockets of purulent material can be hidden underneath a small sore. Sinography, the injection of radiographic dye into a draining pressure sore, will delineate sinus tracts that may communicate with the bowel. Discharge, erythema around the opening, tenderness, fluctuation, or simply lack of improvement may suggest that the wound is much more extensive. Surgical consultation must not be delayed in these cases, since extensive debridement may be necessary. When large amounts of tissue are involved, skin grafting will promote healing once the base of the sore is clear of eschar and free of infection.

Control of local infection. Multiple anerobic and aerobic bacteria will undoubtedly colonize the base of a hospital- or nursing home–acquired pressure sore. Unless there is surrounding cellulitis or evidence of systemic infection, there is no need to culture the sore or prescribe systemic antibiotics.

The pressure sore should be debrided and cleansed with peroxide, saline, a providone-iodine solution, or proteolytic enzymes. After cleansing, antibacterial powders or ointments can be applied, such as those containing polymyxin B, neomycin and bacitracin, or nitrofurazone.

Osteomyelitis is a threat, however, whenever a pressure sore occurs. Routinely x-raying all bones beneath developed pressure sores or even areas of redness may show osteomyelitis. If osteomyelitis is present, appropriate antibiotic therapy, usually intravenous, and local surgical measures must be considered. Long-term intravenous therapy can be given in the home setting.

Maintenance of an adequate nutritional status. In addition to normal hemoglobin values and albumin concentrations, an adequate protein-vitamin-caloric intake is necessary for the healing of an ulcer.

• • •

The healing of a pressure sore is a time-consuming effort that requires the coordinated effort of the nurse, physician, and other members of the rehabilitation team. The process may take months. Clearly, prevention is the easiest approach.

Incontinence

Incontinence is the lack of voluntary control of the evacuation of urine (urinary incontinence) or feces (fecal incontinence). It may be either transient or chronic. Urinary or fecal incontinence is a tragedy for the elderly individual. Embarrassment may lead to loss of self-esteem, despair, dependence, and even institutionalization unless a thorough investigation is undertaken and proper therapy initiated.

Urinary incontinence
Epidemiology

Urinary incontinence is more prevalent in women than in men, the ratio being approximately 1.5 to 1. Of the institutionalized elderly, 25% to 33% suffer from urinary incontinence, whereas only 15% of the community-residing elderly have this disorder.[36]

Approximately 70% of patients with fecal incontinence also have urinary incontinence. It is rare to find fecal incontinence without urinary incontinence, unless a local proctological process is the cause.

Basic physiology of urination

Emptying of the bladder is controlled by local and distant actions of the nervous system. Three neuronal centers can be recognized:

1. In the bladder wall, isolated inefficient neuromuscular actions can autonomously contract the bladder.

2. Autonomic centers of the sacral cord establish a direct reflex arc that automatically empties the bladder when it is adequately filled, unless the reflex is inhibited by higher centers.

3. Neuronal centers in the brain can voluntarily inhibit the sacral reflex and keep micturition as a socially acceptable act.

Normal micturition requires the integrity of these three neuronal centers together with a normal bladder, urethra, and pelvic perineal muscles.

Etiology

Nonneurogenic causes. Transient incontinence may accompany acute illness in the elderly and be resolved after the illness is successfully treated. Any mental, emotional, or physical stress affecting the elderly person may be accompanied by incontinence of short duration. Fecal impaction and senile vaginitis may also lead to transient incontinence in the elderly. If the elderly patient is unable to get to the toilet because of high bed rails, restraints, or poor gait, then incontinence may result.

Inefficient perineal musculature may lead to weakness or elongation of the muscular structures that hold the bladder and urethra in a normal position. These muscles have a sphincterlike action over the urethra, and through them voluntary control of micturition is achieved. Inefficiency of this muscular structure may lead to internal prolapse and cystocele, resulting in stress incontinence.

Urethral or periurethral pathology in the form of inflammation, infection, cystocele, urethrocele, tumors, or trauma may produce urgency incontinence.

Local bladder pathology in the form of calculus, carcinoma, or infection may produce urgency incontinence. Infection, however, is much less likely to cause incontinence in the elderly than in younger individuals. Infection usually results from residual urine secondary to either prostatic disease or a neurogenic bladder disturbance.

Neurogenic causes. Disorders of the nervous system are the most common cause of urinary incontinence in the elderly. The four types of neurogenic bladder disturbances and their characteristics are as follows: (1) the autonomous neurogenic bladder, (2) the atonic neurogenic or sensory paralytic bladder, (3) the reflex neurogenic bladder, and (4) the uninhibited neurogenic bladder.

The *autonomous neurogenic bladder* is caused by the interruption of both afferent and efferent fibers of the sacral reflex. The sacral cord, the cauda equina, or the peripheral nerves are affected by tumor, a congenital defect, or vascular pathology. The sensation of fullness is absent, and the emptying of the bladder is inefficient and must be done by manual compression.

The *atonic neurogenic or sensory paralytic bladder* is due to the interruption of afferent input of the reflex arc and occurs when the posterior sacral roots are impaired by tabes dorsalis, diabetes mellitus or vitamin B_{12} deficiency. Since the motor tracts and fibers are not interrupted, the ability to voluntarily micturate remains; but because the sacral and brain centers cannot register bladder filling, the bladder becomes overdistended, leading to chronic retention and overflow.

The *reflex neurogenic bladder* results

from the loss of connections between the brain and the sacral center. The elderly individual with a spinal cord lesion due to metastatic cancer, vascular accident, infection, etc., may develop paraplegia and a reflex neurogenic bladder. There is a loss of sensation and voluntary control. Consequently, the bladder episodically empties with a variable degree of efficiency.

The *uninhibited neurogenic bladder* is the most frequent neurological cause of incontinence in the elderly. Sensation is retained, but the ability to voluntarily inhibit the spontaneous contractions of the bladder is lost. Consequently the patient feels the urge to urinate but must do so quickly; otherwise urgency incontinence results. Ill-defined, probably diffuse lesions in the cortex or its efferent pathways interfere with the cortical inhibiting role. This kind of incontinence can occur as well in partial lesions of the spinal cord affecting the motor efferent inhibitory pathways.

Investigation of bladder function

History of bladder function. The following must be ascertained: (1) the number of micturitions during the day and night; (2) the presence or absence of urgency, dribbling, and incontinence; (3) the precipitation of incontinence by physical or emotional stress; (4) the duration of the condition; (5) whether the pattern varies under given circumstances; (6) the relationship with the fluid intake pattern and medications, specifically diuretics; and (7) illnesses that may relate to urinary incontinence (CVA, local prostatic disease).

Clinical examination. A complete pelvic and rectal examination should be performed, including inspection of the vulva, urethral orifice, vagina, rectum, prostate gland, and perineum. The bladder should be percussed and palpated to determine overdistension. A thorough neurological examination should follow.

Cystometry. The pressure changes occurring within the bladder as it is filled with water will identify the type of neurogenic bladder disturbance. The cystometrogram will give information on the following: (1) residual urine, (2) bladder capacity, (3) intravesical pressure at various stages, (4) the presence or absence of uninhibited bladder contractions, and (5) the point at which the desire to void is first felt. The procedure can be done at the bedside with a portable unit.

Micturating cystogram. X-ray examination of the bladder after it is filled with a radiopaque fluid is a method of recording bladder pathology and changes in the urethral flow during micturition. In the elderly, this procedure may help differentiate between neurogenic and nonneurogenic causes.

Cystoscopy. Cystoscopy will identify inflammation, trabeculations, diverticula formation, and less frequent causes of incontinence, such as papilloma, stone, or carcinoma.

Treatment

For the incontinent patient with a non-neurogenic bladder, the treatment should be directed at the removal of the causative factor(s), namely tumor, pelvic diaphragm inefficiency, and, less commonly, infection. For the neurogenic bladder, a combined approach using incontinence charting, bladder training, and medication is often effective in elderly patients. The numerous complications of catheterization are thus avoided.

Incontinence chart. The treatment of the uninhibited neurogenic bladder, the most common cause of incontinence in the elderly, should include the use of an incontinence chart. The incontinence chart allows the recording of the patient's status (incontinent or not incontinent) every 2 or 4 hours. The bed linens are changed, if needed, and/or the patient is taken to the toilet to urinate. The chart will show the incidence and pattern of incontinence and permit evaluation of the treatment. It will also promote consistent nursing attention. Initially, the patient should be monitored every 4 hours. If a considerable proportion of episodes of incontinence are present, then toileting and charting should be done every 2 hours.

Once charting has shown the pattern of incontinence, appropriate measures should be taken. These include (1) having the nurse or relative assist the patient in toileting at a regular interval, before he becomes incontinent; (2) providing accessibility to the toilet by using a portable toilet; (3) altering the amount and timing of fluid intake in the evening in a patient who is incontinent during the night; and (4) adjusting the diuretic schedule when indicated. If incontinence persists, medication should be used.

Medications. Anticholingeric drugs will produce a pharmacological blockage of the uninhibited sacral micturition reflex. Atropine, and belladonna have been used in the past, but almost any drug that produces urinary retention as a side effect may be used. Propantheline bromide (Pro-Banthine) and orphenadrine hydrochloride (Disipal) are also suitable. The following three factors are important when treating incontinence with anticholinergic medications.

1. The administration of the drug should anticipate the periods of incontinence in accordance with the incontin-

ence chart. If incontinence is widespread, the drug should be given at appropriate intervals (throughout the 24 hours). If incontinence occurs only at night, then the drug should be administered before the patient retires.

2. The use of these drugs is aimed only at increasing bladder capacity by diminishing uninhibited contractions. They will be successful only in the uninhibited bladder and when they are combined with meticulous nursing care.

3. The possibility of side effects, particularly the exacerbation of an attack of acute angle-closure glaucoma and/or cardiovascular complications must always be kept in mind, although these side effects are rare with the dosages used in treating incontinence.

The treatment for incontinence associated with urinary retention and overflow (atonic and autonomous neurogenic bladders) should aim to reduce the residual urine to less than 100 ml. Comfortable positioning for urination and voluntary contraction of the abdominal musculature or manual compression of the abdominal wall (Crede's method) are used together with cholinergic medication (e.g., bethanechol chloride) that pharmacologically stimulates the contraction of the bladder. Medication may be needed indefinitely. Incontinence and retention caused by a reflex neurogenic bladder are treated through intermittent catheterization and maneuvers oriented to stimulate the triggering of the reflex arc, such as perineal massage. These techniques aim to establish a socially acceptable and comfortably timed pattern of urination while maintaining a low residual volume.

Urinary collectors. Urinary collectors (Texas catheter, Uro-sheath rubber collectors) can help the incontinent man who is mentally clear and who can properly apply the device and keep it clean. The confused male patient, however, requires considerable nursing attention to use a urine collector. He may not recognize the purpose of the collector, tubing, and bag, and pull them off. For the female patient, no satisfactory device has yet been developed. Specially manufactured incontinence pads, however, are capable of absorbing limited amounts of urine. The indication for them is mostly with stress incontinence, wherein the patient suffers from minor losses of urine.

Fecal incontinence

While less frequent than urinary incontinence, fecal incontinence is more annoying for the patient, his family, and nursing personnel. The causes of fecal incontinence are multiple and include carcinoma of the colon or rectum, fecal impaction, and neurogenic causes. Whatever the cause, fecal incontinence requires a prompt etiological diagnosis and therapy.

Etiology

The following is a classification of the causes of fecal incontinence:

A. Diseases that affect the colon, rectum, or anal sphincter
   1. Carcinoma
   2. Diverticulitis
   3. Colitis of various causes
   4. Surgical disruption of the anal sphincter
   5. Rectal prolapse
   6. Inappropriate use of purgatives
   7. Malabsorption syndrome
B. Diarrhea of various causes; including iatrogenic
C. Fecal impaction with paradoxical mucous diarrhea flowing around the hard fecal mass

D. Neurogenic fecal incontinence
  1. Loss of local sensation and/or loss of the ability to voluntarily close the external sphincter secondary to neurological involvement from diabetes, for example, or a sacral cord lesion
  2. Uninhibited defecation, seen commonly in patients with multiple cerebral infarcts or dementia (These patients usually have one or two formed stools a day, soon after a meal, because of the stimulation of the gastrocolic reflex.)

Treatment

Identifying the cause of fecal incontinence is paramount. Incontinence secondary to impaction is amenable to total cure. Initially, the impaction must be removed by digital examination and/or small-volume enemas. Further constipation can be prevented by appropriate fluid intake; ambulation; high-residue food; and laxatives, suppositories, or enemas.

When the cause of incontinence is neurogenic, the problem is handled by inducing programmed constipation and evacuation. The patient can be constipated with kaolin and paregoric and be evacuated on a weekly or biweekly basis through the use of a laxative, suppositories, or enemas.

A modern approach to fecal incontinence is the implantation of electrodes in the area of the external sphincter in order to keep it contracted by means of the passage of a tetanic current. This method is far from being accepted for general use, but it may well be a promising development. Biofeedback is also being used somewhat successfully in mentally clear elderly patients.

• • •

Small objective improvements, whether they be in ambulation, transfers, stair climbing, or toileting, may have large subjective meaning for the elderly patient, his family, and the team of health care professionals. While the rehabilitation process may be slow and complicated by acute and chronic physical and mental disabilities, it is crucial in maximizing the functional independence of the elderly individual.

REFERENCES

1. Rusk, H. A.: Rehabilitation medicine (ed. 3), St. Louis, 1971, The C. V. Mosby Co.
2. Krusen, F. H., Kottke, F. J., and Ellwood, P. M.: Handbook of physical medicine and rehabilitation, ed. 2, Philadelphia, 1971, W. B. Saunders Co.
3. Butler, R. N., and Lewis, M. I.: Aging and mental health: positive psychosocial approaches, ed. 2, St. Louis, 1977, the C. V. Mosby Co.
4. Willard, H. S., and Spackman, C. S.: Occupational therapy, ed. 4, Philadelphia, 1971, J. B. Lippincott Co.
5. Brickner, P. W.: Home health care for the aged, New York, 1978, Appleton-Century-Crofts.
6. Goldman, R.: Decline in organ function with aging. In Rossman, I., editor: Clinical geriatrics, ed. 2, Philadelphia, 1979, J. B. Lippincott Co.
7. Darling, R. C.: Exercise. In Downey, J. A., and Darling, R. C., editors: Physiological basis of rehabilitation medicine, Philadelphia, 1971, W. B. Saunders Co.
8. Fact book on aging: a profile of America's older population, Washington, D.C., 1978, The National Council on the Aging, Inc.
9. Garraway, W. M., and others: The declining incidence of stroke, N. Engl. J. Med. **300:**449, 1979.
10. Sahs, A. L., and others, editors: Guidelines for stroke care, DHEW Pub. No. (NRA) 76-14017, U.S. Department of Health, Education, and Welfare, Public Health Service.
11. Anderson, T. P., and others: Predictive factors in stroke rehabilitation, Arch. Phys. Med. Rehabil. **55:**545, 1974.
12. Lehmann, J. F., and others: Stroke rehabilitation: outcome and prediction, Arch. Phys. Med Rehabil. **56:**383, 1975.
13. Feigenson, J. S., and others: Factors influencing outcome and length of stay in a stroke rehabilitation unit, Stroke **8:**651, 1977.
14. Lehmann, J. F., and others: Stroke: does rehabilitation affect outcome? Arch. Phys. Med. Rehabil. **56:**375, 1975.

15. Anderson, T. P., and others:Stroke rehabilitation: a reconsideration of some common attitudes, Arch. Phys. Med. Rehabil. **59:**175, 1978.
16. National Center for Health Statistics: Unpublished data.
17. Lender, M., and others: Osteoporosis and fractures of the neck of the femur, Isr. J. Med. Sci. **12:**596, 1976.
18. Brocklehurst, A. N., and others: Fracture of the femur in old age: a two-centre study of associated clinical factors and the cause of the fall, Age Aging **7:**2, 1978.
19. Arnold, W. D., and others: Treatment of intracapsular fractures of the femoral neck with special reference to percutaneous Knowles pinning, J. Bone Joint Surg. **56-A:**254, 1974.
20. Jacobs, R. R., and others: Treatment of intertrochanteric hip fractures with a compression hip screw and a nail plate, J. Trauma **16:**599, 1976.
21. D'Arcy, J., and Devas, M.: Treatment of fractures of the femoral neck by replacement with the Thompson prosthesis, J. Bone Joint Surg. **58-B:**279, 1976.
22. Sherk, H. H., and others: The treatment of hip fractures in institutionalized patients, Orthop. Clin. North Am. **5:**543, 1974.
23. Albright, J. P., and Weinstein, S. L.: Treatment for fixation complications: femoral neck fractures, Arch. Surg. **110:**30, 1975.
24. Sakuma, J., and others: Rehabilitation of geriatric patients having bilateral lower extremity amputations, Arch. Phys. Med. Rehabil. **55:**101, 1974.
25. Steinberg, F. U., and others: Rehabilitation of the geriatric amputee, J. Am. Geriatr. Soc. **22:**62, 1974.
26. Kerstein, M. D., and others: Rehabilitation after bilateral lower extremity amputation, Arch. Phys. Med. Rehabil. **56:**309, 1975.
27. Stern, P. H., and Skudder, P. A.: Amputee rehabilitation. N.Y. State J. Med. **77:**1436, 1977.
78. Gonzalez, E. G., and others: Energy expenditure in below-knee amputees: correlation with stump length, Arch. Phys. Med. Rehabil. **55:**111, 1974.
29. Fisher, S. V., and Gullickson, G.: Energy cost of ambulation in health and disability: a literature review, Arch. Phys. Med. Rehabil. **59:**124, 1978.
30. Huang, C., and others: Amputation: energy cost of ambulation, Arch. Phys. Med. Rehabil. **60:**18, 1979.
31. Special commentary, Arch. Surg. **110:**760, 1975.
32. American Academy of Physical Medicine and Rehabilitation: Medical knowledge self-assessment program in physical medicine and rehabilitation syllabus, Chicago, 1977, The Academy.
33. Sheldon, J. H.: The effect of age on the control of sway, Gerontol. Clin. **5:**11, 1963.
34. The Parkinson's Disease Foundation: Exercises for the Parkinson patient, New York, 1960, The Foundation.
35. Bliss, M.: The use of ripple beds, Age aging **7:**25, 1975.
36. Brocklehurst, J. C.: Textbook of geriatric medicine and gerontology, Edinburgh, Eng., 1978, Churchill Livingstone.

PROBLEM-SOLVING EXERCISES
Case one

A 76-year-old right-handed man has been admitted to the emergency room after being found lying on the floor of his apartment. He is alert but unable to comprehend instructions or repeat phrases. Physical examination is unremarkable except for a blood pressure of 200/120 and neurological findings.

Questions

1. Which are the most likely neurological findings?
   a. Left foot clonus
   b. Right-sided hemiparesis
   c. Right-sided Babinski's sign
   d. Flaccidity
   e. Spasticity
2. The daughter asks you about her father's prognosis. At present, you can say that it is:
   a. Poor
   b. Good
   c. Unknown
3. As soon as the patient is admitted, your initial rehabilitation prescription includes:
   a. Ambulation training
   b. Passive range of motion to all joints
   c. Hot packs to the right hand
   d. A footboard
   e. Pressure sore prevention by repositioning the patient every 2 hours
4. The next day the patient is able to make an almost complete fist with the right hand. Your prognosis is now:
   a. Unchanged from the initial one
   b. Better than the day before
   c. Not affected by this minor improvement

5. By the end of the first week the patient is able to change his position in bed but has poor sitting balance. He is capable of understanding simple commands but speaks little. Your new prescription should include:
   a. Ambulation training
   b. A short leg brace
   c. Functional activities in occupational therapy to improve motor skills
   d. Speech therapy
   e. Provision of crutches for independent ambulation

6. By the end of the second week the patient has recovered a high level of voluntary muscle control in the affected side and is able to ambulate with minimal assistance. Nonfluent aphasia persists. Your prescription now includes:
   a. Arrangements with social service for prolonged hospitalization to continue speech therapy
   b. Intensive ADL and ambulation training.
   c. Preparation of discharge plans
   d. Active exercises
   e. A wheelchair

7. After another month of physical therapy, complicated by an episode of pneumonia, the patient ambulates with the assistance of a quadripod cane. He plans to return home in 1 week. His aphasia has continued to improve. You should:
   a. Evaluate the home setting prior to discharge so that assistive devices can be provided and any remodeling of the house or apartment completed
   b. Arrange for continued speech therapy at home
   c. Teach the family how to communicate with their aphasic relative
   d. Arrange for at least a year of daily physical therapy at home

Case two

A 76-year-old man had a left AK amputation 2 weeks ago. A corner of the wound shows signs of infection.

Questions

1. Your initial prescription includes:
   a. Flushing of the area with peroxide and the application of Neosporin powder
   b. Wrapping of the stump with an Ace bandage to prevent swelling
   c. Strict bed rest
   d. Active range of motion to prevent contractures

2. Two weeks later the wound is perfectly healed; your prescription now includes:
   a. Discontinuance of the stump wrapping
   b. Strengthening exercises to the stump and remaining limbs
   c. Protective cushioning of the stump
   d. Preparation of a prosthesis

Case three

A 76-year-old woman with coronary artery disease has a unilateral BK amputation due to peripheral vascular disease.

Question

1. During the initial rehabilitation process you should:
   a. Discourage the patient's hopes of ambulation with a prosthesis, since coronary artery disease is always a contraindication
   b. Explain the potential limitations imposed by her coronary artery disease
   c. Monitor her cardiovascular symptoms and signs during training

Case four

A 89-year-old woman has suffered a fracture of the right femoral neck, and an Austin Moore prosthesis has been inserted. She is started on full weight–bearing ambulation a week after surgery. Soon thereafter, she develops pains in the area of the affected hip that are relieved by bed rest.

Question

1. The following can be said about her current problem:
   a. Full weight–bearing ambulation was started too early.
   b. Strict bed rest for 72 hours is indicated.

c. Pain should be regarded as psychologically induced, and the patient encouraged to continue ambulation.

d. Diathermy should be prescribed.

e. An x-ray study of the right hip is indicated to determine whether the endoprosthesis is dislocated.

f. A cane should be provided to relieve weight bearing from the affected limb while the patient continues in ambulation training.

ANSWERS TO PROBLEM-SOLVING EXERCISES

Case one

1. b, c, and d. The patient's lack of ability to communicate suggests aphasia. A left-sided CVA with right-sided hemiparesis and right-sided Babinski's sign is the most likely neurological event. Flaccidity usually accompanies the early stage of a stroke.

2. c. Immediately after a stroke the patient can die from neurological causes, such as herniation from cerebral edema, extension of the infarction, or hemorrhage; or from medical complications, such as aspiration pneumonia or sepsis from urinary retention. Neither a medical nor a rehabilitation prognosis can be given at this early stage.

3. b, d, and e. At this early stage the rehabilitation effort concentrates on prevention of complications. Preventive efforts include range of motion to prevent contractures, a footboard to prevent foot drop, and changing the position of the patient to prevent pressure sores and aspiration pneumonia. It is premature to prescribe ambulation training until the patient is medically stable and has achieved satisfactory sitting balance. Applying hot packs to the right hand has no therapeutic role in the acute phase of rehabilitation of the stroke patient and may cause a burn if there is a sensory deficit.

4. b. Neurological improvement during the acute stage of a stroke is a favorable prognostic sign.

5. c and d. For ambulation training to begin, the stroke patient must first have adequate sitting balance. The need for a short leg brace will be assessed during ambulation training; it is indicated to prevent plantar flexion and inversion of the foot. Crutches are seldom used in the elderly and cannot be used by the hemiparetic or hemiplegic stroke patient, because crutches require two functioning upper extremities. The speech pathologist should assess the degree of the patient's aphasia and begin treatment.

6. b, c, and d. The patient's right-sided hemiparesis has improved markedly, along with some improvement in his aphasia. Improvement in the hemiparesis is an excellent prognostic sign that correlates with an improvement of the aphasia. Speech therapy can be given in the patient's home or in an outpatient setting and is no reason, by itself, for continued hospitalization of the patient. Ambulation, self-care skills, and active exercises should be stressed in an attempt to reach the patient's highest level of functioning. Given this patient's remarkable improvement, it is unlikely that he will require a wheelchair. Prescribing a wheelchair prematurely may be a therapeutic error because it promotes dependence.

7. a, b, and c. An assessment of the home setting is crucial, so that appropriate adaptive equipment can be provided and potential areas for falls (throw rugs, steps, bathtub) can be assessed and altered for the safety of the patient. Speech therapy should continue in an outpatient setting. Involvement and communication with the family should be encouraged for a number of reasons. First, it will be necessary to teach the family members how to communicate with their aphasic relative. Second, the family can provide more intense emotional and physical support during the first few weeks at home. The family should monitor the patient for recurrence of disability or any new problems. There is no need for daily physical therapy for a prolonged period, although it is possible to have the physical therapist come to the pa-

tient's home or apartment if he should need it.

Case two

1. a, b, and d. While local care of the infection is being provided, standard rehabilitation measures aimed at shaping the stump and developing adequate range of motion of the left hip are to be continued. Strict bed rest is contraindicated, since it may lead to pressure sores, thrombophlebitis, contractures, and, possibly, aspiration pneumonia.
2. b and d. Stump wrapping is continued until the prosthesis is fitted. Protective cushioning of the stump is contraindicated, since it would prevent the stump from becoming hard and firmly shaped.

Case three

1. b and c. The patient with coronary artery disease should not necessarily be excluded from a trial of prosthetic ambulation. Continuous cardiac monitoring can be used during ambulation training to detect myocardial ischemia and dysrhythmias. The upper limbs must be strengthened throughout the entire rehabilitation process, since significant amounts of weight will be carried by them, even while the patient is ambulating with a prosthesis.

Case four

1. e. The painful postoperative fractured hip should prompt the clinician to search for a cause. With an Austin Moore prosthesis, the elderly patient can bear weight as soon after the operation as she is able to do so. Strict bed rest for a painful hip is contraindicated because of its adverse side effects. Diathermy is also contraindicated because the hip prosthesis may retain large amounts of heat and injure surrounding tissues. An x-ray study of the hip is the most important diagnostic step after a thorough history and physical examination. The x-ray film will help determine whether there was any dislocation or infection of the hip. Symptomatic treatment by means of bed rest or a cane for weight-bearing relief will,

if not accompanied by a diagnostic effort, be an error.

POSTTEST*

1. Rehabilitation of the elderly differs from that of the young in the following way (s):
   a. The goals are often different.
   b. The rehabilitation process is more likely to be interrupted by a medical problem in the elderly.
   c. The rehabilitation process is often slower in the elderly.
   d. The elderly can only expect relief of pain and discomfort.
   e. The most common rehabilitation problems encountered in the elderly are due to trauma.
2. A physiatrist is a:
   a. Paramedical technician
   b. Nurse certified in physical therapy
   c. Physician
   d. Physical therapist
3. A rehabilitation program for the elderly individual is extremely difficult, perhaps futile, when the patient:
   a. Is a bilateral below-knee (BK) amputee secondary to peripheral vascular disease
   b. Lacks the ability to follow instructions
   c. Lacks the ability to move both his right arm and right leg from a stroke
   d. Lacks the motivation to participate in a rehabilitation program because of depression
4. Occupational therapy:
   a. Provides assessment of, and training for, perceptual disorders resulting from stroke
   b. Provides exercises for the patient us-

---

*Some questions may have more than one correct answer.

ing functional activities for therapeutic purposes

c. Assesses the patient's ability to eat, dress, and toilet by himself

5. An assessment of the elderly stroke patient's ability to perform activities of daily living (ADL) is made during the following stage(s) of stroke rehabilitation:

a. The acute stage, encompassing the first few days following the stroke

b. The intermediate stage, when the patient is medically and neurologically stable

c. The late stage, when the patient stops making progress

6. In the elderly unilateral BK amputee with arteriosclerotic cardiovascular disease manifested by angina and compensated congestive heart failure (CHF), which of the following methods of ambulation would consume the least amount of energy and, therefore, stress the cardiovascular system least?

a. Hopping using crutches

b. Hopping using a standard walker

c. Walking using a BK prosthesis

d. Hopping using a platform walker

7. Phantom pain (a painful sensation perceived by the patient in the nonexistent amputated limb) can be aided by:

a. Helping the patient psychologically adjust to the amputation

b. Deferring the prescription of an artificial limb until the pain subsides or at least improves

c. Expediting the prescription of an artificial limb

d. Giving liberal doses of analgesics

8. Two days ago, an 80-year-old woman had a transmetatarsal amputation of the right foot. The most probable etiological factor is:

a. An automobile accident

b. Osteogenic sarcoma

c. Peripheral vascular disease

d. Embolism

9. A 72-year-old woman sustained a fracture of the left subcapital area of the femoral neck, which was surgically treated with an endoprosthesis of the Austin Moore type. By the end of the third week, her ambulatory status should be:

a. Non-weight bearing (NWB)

b. Partial weight bearing (PWB)

c. Full weight bearing (FWB)

10. The most crucial measure for the prevention of pressure sores is:

a. Adequate nutrition

b. Systemic antibiotics

c. Changing the position of the patient every 2 hours

d. Prevention of urinary and/or fecal incontinence

e. The use of a water bed

ANSWERS TO PRETEST AND POSTTEST

1. a, b, and c. While the goal of rehabilitation of the younger individual is to return to his vocation, the goal for the elderly is often the ability to provide self-care. The elderly, more than the young, are prone to disabling illness and deconditioning. The slower physiological pace of the elderly will often make the rehabilitation process longer. The relief of pain and discomfort should be the least that can be offered at any age. The most common rehabilitation problems encountered in the elderly stem from a cerebrovascular accident, fractured hip, amputation, and arthritis. The younger rehabilitation patient is more likely to have suffered a traumatic injury.

2. c. A physiatrist is a physician with specialty training and certification in physical medicine and rehabilitation. He is an expert in the diagnosis and treatment of disabilities.

3. b and d. To become rehabilitated, the disabled patient must actively participate. If the patient does not follow instructions because of dementia, a communication disorder, or depression, he cannot actively participate in his therapy. Passive therapy is given to the patient who cannot cooperate and should be provided by the nurse or a properly instructed family member. The elderly patient who is mentally clear with a bilateral amputation (a) or a right-sided stroke (c) is definitely a candidate for an agressive rehabilitation program.

4. a, b, and c. The goal of occupational therapy is to improve function.

5. b and c. During the acute stage of the stroke, the patient is medically and neurologically unstable; and an assessment of ADL could not be made at this time. The assessment of the ability to perform ADL occurs after the patient is stable, usually in the intermediate stage or in the late stage.

6. c. Hopping would consume a large amount of energy because the patient would have to overcome the force of gravity with each step. The least amount of energy would be consumed by this elderly patient if he were to ambulate using a BK prosthesis.

7. a and c. Phantom limb sensation is the perception by the patient that the amputated limb is still present. Phantom limb sensation occurs commonly and usually disappears over weeks to months. Phantom pain, a painful feeling coming from the amputated limb, occurs less commonly than phantom limb sensation and usually in patients who have made a poor psychological adjustment to the amputation.

Bombarding the stump with stimuli appears to relieve phantom limb pain. Therefore, the sooner the patient wears a prosthesis, the better. The liberal use of analgesics is usually not helpful in phantom pain and predisposes the patient to the side effects of sedation and confusion, resulting in impaired progress in the rehabilitation program.

8. c. Trauma and malignancy are more frequent in the younger age groups. Although embolism is possible, especially if the patient has atrial fibrillation or a hypercoaguable state, such as hyperosmolar, hyperglycemic, nonketotic coma, arteriosclerotic peripheral vascular disease is the most likely etiological factor.

9. c. One of the reasons for using an endoprosthesis in a fractured hip is to allow early full weight bearing. Most elderly patients can ambulate with full weight bearing on an endoprosthesis as soon as they are medically stable.

10. c. The primary method of pressure sore prevention is the changing of the patient every 2 hours, day and night. Adequate nutrition, the prevention of urinary and/or fecal incontinence, and the use of a water bed are all secondary methods of prevention of pressure sores. Systemic antibiotics should be used when bacterial cellulitis or an abscess complicates a pressure sore.

Chapter 8

Speech and language disorders

FREDRICK T. SHERMAN, SARA MARCHBEIN MEISELLS, EMMANUEL MARGOLIS,
and LESLIE S. LIBOW

EDUCATIONAL OBJECTIVES
Attitudinal

The student should:

1. Recognize and express his feelings of frustration when working with patients with communication problems, particularly elderly patients
2. Become sensitized to the difficulties in communication likely to be encountered by the elderly aphasic patient

Cognitive

The student should:

1. Be aware of some of the current theories regarding the etiology of aphasia, such as neuroanatomic versus holistic theories
2. Know the differential diagnoses of speech disorders in the elderly
3. Know the various types of aphasia, their occurrence in an older population, and their prognosis and therapeutic interventions
4. Understand the role of the speech pathologist in diagnosing and rehabilitating the aphasic or dysarthric patient, know when and how to refer patients to a speech pathologist, and recognize the limitations of speech therapy

Skill

The student should:

1. Develop a general interview approach to the patient who has difficulty communicating
2. Be able to differentiate the aphasic patient from patients with primary hearing, speech, or psychiatric problems
3. Know the differential diagnosis of and proper interview techniques for the patient who speaks little
4. Know the differential diagnosis of and proper interview techniques for the patient who speaks much but makes little sense
5. Be able to explain aphasia to both the patient and the family (spouse, children, attendant) and recommend methods of behavior to optimally integrate the elderly aphasic patient into the social environment

PRETEST*

1. The most common cause of aphasia in the elderly is:
   a. Brain tumor (benign or malignant)
   b. Stroke
   c. Subdural hematoma
   d. Infection
   e. Depression
2. The most likely type of aphasia found in an elderly patient with right-sided hemiparesis is:
   a. Broca's aphasia
   b. Wernicke's aphasia
   c. Conduction aphasia
   d. Anomic aphasia
   e. Global aphasia
3. Match the type of aphasia with its clinical feature:
   Type
   ____ a. Broca's aphasia
   ____ b. Wernicke's aphasia

---

*Some questions may have more than one correct answer.

169

_____ c. Anomic aphasia

_____ d. Global aphasia

Clinical feature

1. Commonly found in patients with metabolic abnormalities or increased intracranial pressure or other diffuse brain involvement
2. Can appear similar to nonfluent aphasia complicated by depression
3. Can be confused with the "word salad" type of speech of a schizophrenic
4. Nonfluent, good comprehension, poor repetition

4. Match the term with the speech pattern that best represents it:

Term

_____ a. Logorrhea

_____ b. Paraphasia

_____ c. Perseveration

_____ d. Jargon

Speech pattern

1. "Do-do-goo-goo-ha-ha"
2. When the patient was asked to say, "The sky is blue," he said, "The sky, sky, sky"
3. When the patient was asked to say, "Knife," he said, "Fork"
4. When the patient was asked why he came to the hospital, his answer was excessively lengthy and contained little information

5. _True or false:_ Most of the spontaneous recovery appears during the first 3 to 6 months after the onset of aphasia in a patient with a stroke.

6. _True or false:_ The elderly patient who has a sudden onset of impaired verbal output is most likely to be having a psychotic episode.

7. _True or false:_ The elderly patient who is aphasic in speech is usually able to write with little difficulty.

Because the elderly patient's ability to live in the community and lead a fulfill-ing existence will often depend on his ability to communicate needs and feelings, the student or clinician should become familiar with the various communication problems that may be encountered by the elderly. In the process, he should become sensitive to his own frustration in communicating with certain elderly patients, develop a rational approach to diagnosis, and become familiar with the methods available to improve communication.

TREATABLE CAUSES OF COMMUNICATION DIFFICULTIES

Treatable causes of communication difficulties in the elderly include:

1. Hearing deficits from a conductive hearing loss from impacted cerumen or otosclerosis; a sensorineural hearing loss from presbycusis; and/or visual deficits resulting from cataracts, glaucoma, senile macular degeneration, a cerebrovascular accident (CVA) — causing hemianopia — and refractive or accommodative deficits, including presbyopia
2. Reversible deficits in mental function (organic brain syndrome) that may be caused, for example, by medication, fever, heart failure, or metabolic abnormalities
3. Other psychiatric disorders, such as depression
4. The inability to articulate speech properly (dysarthria) because of an abnormality in neuromuscular function of the lips, tongue, palate, vocal cords, or muscles of respiration (Primary vocal cord disease, including polyps, tumors, and cricoarytenoid arthritis, can also produce dysarthria.)
5. The loss of previously intact language ability (aphasia) from, for example, a CVA

6. The difficulty of programming motor movements for speech in the face of intact comprehension and motor ability (apraxia of speech)

APPROACH TO THE ELDERLY PATIENT WITH PROBLEMS IN SPEECH: DIFFERENTIAL DIAGNOSIS

In general, if the clinician has problems in interviewing an elderly patient, a number of diagnostic possibilities must be clarified, as noted in the previous list of treatable communication difficulties.

Hearing and/or visual defects

The patient may have a combination of hearing and visual problems impairing communication and creating the erroneous impression of some degree of aphasia or organic brain syndrome. An examination of the external and middle ear may reveal cerumen, chronic suppurative otitis media, or chronic serous otitis media. A simple hearing test and/or hearing aid evaluation (check the battery and tubing) should be performed. The patient's hearing difficulty may be compounded by visual impairment, making compensation by lipreading difficult. The examiner should make sure that the patient is wearing his eyeglasses or contact lenses during the interview to facilitate lipreading. In addition, the following interviewing principles should be followed when communication problems are encountered:

1. Arrange the setting so that light falls on your face, thereby facilitating lipreading by the patient who has difficulty hearing.

2. Eliminate distractions (auditory and visual).

3. Speak clearly and slowly.

4. Do not speak into the patient's ear, thereby eliminating the opportunity for lipreading.

5. Communicate in writing if all of the above do not work. Because the elderly patient may not have learned to write English, it is important to learn what his written language is.

Organic brain syndrome

A patient may have an acute and/or chronic organic brain syndrome and impaired mental function, leading to difficulties with communication. The use of language may suffer as a consequence of loss of drive, inattention, or impaired abstract thinking.

Elderly patients who are acutely confused may display a language problem. They may respond irrelevantly to questions, reflect their disorientation in time and space, or have a reduced perception of their environment. The spoken language such a patient uses, although fluent and grammatically correct, is often abnormal in other ways, with irrelevant comments and inappropriate content. Writing is often especially impaired. A mental status examination should be performed on elderly patients when communication problems appear to stem from organic brain syndrome. Performing a mental status examination on an aphasic patient may be difficult, time consuming, and often impossible. A modified examination seeking "yes" and "no" answers may have to be performed. It is sometimes difficult or impossible to differentiate aphasia from organic brain syndrome.

Psychiatric illness

The patient may be psychotically depressed and display very little verbal output, little physical activity (psychomotor retardation), and affective signs of depression. Consequently, the patient may say little, and the interviewer may confuse him with the aphasic or demented patient. An acute schizophrenic episode, particularly of the catatonic type (admittedly rare in an elderly patient), may be confused with aphasia. A past history of chronic schizophrenia or a premorbid personality aberration frequently precedes overt schizophrenia and helps in differentiating between the two. In general, a sudden onset of a language disorder in an elderly individual results from aphasia rather than a psychiatric problem.

Dysarthria

The patient may be dysarthric and unable to pronounce words correctly. *Dysarthria* is the term given to a group of speech disorders resulting from disturbances in neuromuscular control (weakness, paralysis, lack of coordination) of the speech mechanism due to damage to the central or peripheral nervous system. Neuromuscular impairment of respiration, phonation, accentuation, or articulation from advanced parkinsonism, bulbar paralysis, or a CVA, for example, may cause dysarthria. Mechanical factors, such as vocal cord tumors or cricoarytenoid arthritis, may also cause dysarthria. The most characteristic error made by dysarthric patients is imprecise production of consonants, usually in the form of distortions and omissions. The following types of dysarthria are commonly seen in the elderly:

1. Dysarthria of pseudobulbar palsy results from involvement of upper motor neurons (CVA, multiple or bilateral brain injuries, and amyotrophic lateral sclerosis). Speech is slow, emerges with great effort on the part of the patient, and is produced against certain resistance. In milder cases, speech is often rapid but with very indistinct articulation. Each word is prolonged and hardly intelligible.

2. Ataxic dysarthria results from damage to the cerebellum (degenerative disease, alcohol, multiple sclerosis, or vascular episodes). Typical cerebellar signs are often noted in the extremities and eyes. Speech is impaired and appears slow, staccato, slurred, and jerky.

3. Hypokinetic dysarthria (due to disorders of certain portions of the extrapyramidal system (e.g., parkinsonism), is characterized by hesitation, loss of inflection in the voice, blurring of articulation, stoppages, and bursts of speed. The sentence often ends in a mumble. From a monotonous, soft voice without variation in pitch, there is gradual progression of the dysarthria until the patient's speech becomes hardly audible.

4. Flaccid dysarthria, seen in disorders of the lower motor neurons or neuromuscular transmission (e.g., myasthenia gravis), is characterized by shortness of breath with resulting short phrases, difficulty in producing loud tones, and a harsh voice. The causes are weakness and hypotonia of the respiratory and speech musculature.

Aphasia

See "Aphasia: Neuroanatomic Approach."

Speech apraxia

Speech apraxia is the inability to use the speech musculature in a purposeful manner, despite intact power of movement and complete understanding of what is required. In attempting to speak a word, the apraxic patient grasps for the correct sound and struggles to position his tongue and lips correctly for a consonant or a sequence of sounds. His difficulty is not attributed to slowness, weakness, incoordination, or alteration of muscle tone in any part of the speech apparatus, as in dysarthria; nor is it attributed to his inability to retrieve or comprehend, as in aphasia. He exhibits adequate function in all parts of the speech-generating mechanisms when they are used for reflex, overlearned, or automatic acts (counting; reciting the days of the week, jingles, the Lord's Prayer); but when the patient attempts volitional speech, it is as though he has "forgotten" how to pronounce words. His errors vary and are inconsistent. At times the patient may be free of articulatory errors and display periods of fluency. He is able to express in writing what he cannot say in words. In contrast, the aphasic patient who has difficulty with speech also has difficulty with writing.

The apraxic patient may fail to stick out his tongue on command but may spontaneously protrude it to lick his lips. This ability to perform the movement spontaneously eliminates peripheral neuromuscular dysfunction as a cause of the failure to carry out the command. For example, when the speech apraxic patient is speaking offhand, reciting an overlearned expression, or reacting suddenly to a stimulus, he may produce many words articulately. But when he must concentrate on a verbal target word, he may experience difficulty, grope, and make repeated attempts.

APHASIA: NEUROANATOMIC APPROACH

Aphasia is the loss of previously acquired language facility and results from cerebral dysfunction.[1] In this chapter the neuroanatomic approach to aphasia is stressed, with emphasis on the correlation between the type of aphasia and the cortical lesion, as can be seen in Fig. 8-1.

Two thirds of CVAs occur in people aged 65 and over. By far the most common cause of aphasia in the elderly is a CVA; 94% of all aphasic syndromes are due to thrombosis or hemorrhage,[2] and 40% of major vascular lesions that involve the hemispheres produce language disturbances.[3] Other conditions that may cause aphasia in the elderly are primary or metastatic brain tumor and trauma (subdural hematoma). Viral encephalitis is a rare cause of aphasia.

The cerebral hemispheres differ in language function in accordance with the hand preference of the individual. In the 91% to 95% of the population who are right-handed, the left hemisphere is almost always dominant for speech and language. In people who are left-handed (5% to 9% of the population), language function appears to be more equally divided between the two hemispheres. Of the permanent significant types of aphasia in left-handed people, about 60% have left-sided cerebral lesions and 40% right-sided cerebral lesions. Because of the bilateral representation of language in left-handed individuals, aphasia in them is usually milder.

Since the aphasic patient will have a lesion of the left cerebral hemisphere approximately 98 times out of 100, it is rare to find an aphasic patient with a lesion of the right hemisphere only.[4] Knowing the handedness of the elderly aphasic patient (usually right) may help to localize the lesion to one or the other hemisphere (usually left).

Some elderly individuals who were initially left-handed were compelled to write with their right hands at school because of societal pressure to conform with the right-handed majority. These individuals (crossed laterals) are less likely to suffer a severe language impairment from a stroke and may recover more quickly.[5,6]

History taking

In an investigation of the elderly patient who appears aphasic, the following history must be obtained, either from the patient, the family, or others who know the patient's background:

1. The educational level of the patient
2. His hand preference
3. His native language and learned languages (Has he been known to speak, read, and write in these languages prior to the aphasia? In what order were the languages acquired?)

Since many elderly patients are immigrants and acquired English as a second or third language, the onset of aphasia may have different implications for each of these languages. After the onset of aphasia in a polyglot (a person who knows several languages), there may be more extensive improvement in one language than in another.[7] One cannot be certain whether the language learned first or the language used most commonly prior to the onset of aphasia will be recovered more quickly. The language that is recovered first is often the one used in the treatment modality. In large urban ethnic areas, where the primary language spoken may not be English, assistance from a bilingual speech pathologist is needed.

Functional assessment

In an examination of the aphasic patient, the following six functions should be tested: spontaneous speech, comprehension of spoken language, repetition, word finding ability, reading, and writing. An assessment of these functions will usually lead to a neuro-anatomic localization (Table 8-1 and Fig. 8-2).

Spontaneous speech

Does the patient speak much or little? If he speaks little (less than 50 words per minute) with considerable effort to initiate speech, and if his phrases are short (one- or two-word phrases), the lesion causing the aphasia is likely to be anterior to the central sulcus and the aphasia is called nonfluent. Broca's aphasia is the classic example (area 2 in Figs. 8-1 and 8-2). In the acute stage of a stroke, a lesion posterior to the central sulcus can also cause nonfluency. If the patient speaks effortlessly with normal or high output (100 to 200 words per minute) and easy initiation, but makes little sense and uses incorrect words and grammar, then the patient has fluent aphasia with the lesion located posterior to the central sulcus. Wernicke's aphasia is the classic example (area 1 in Figs. 8-1 and 8-2).

Word-finding difficulty is a salient feature of aphasia and is characterized by failure to find and/or use the correct words. The patient may substitute for the correct word: (1) a circumlocutory phrase (e.g., "what you use to drink water" for a cup); (2) nonspecific words, such as "thing"; or (3) incorrect words (paraphasia). The use of the word "pone" for "phone" is an example of literal paraphasia, and the use of "spoon" for "knife" is an example of verbal paraphasia. The use of "gababyl" for "chair" is an example of jargon.

Table 8-2 presents a clinical evaluation of spontaneous speech.

Comprehension of spoken language

The inability to comprehend instructions (either partially or totally) may seriously affect the elderly patient's living situation and freedom, as well as the rehabilitation outcome, such as after a fractured hip, CVA, or amputation. With poor comprehension, it is likely that many of the activities of daily living (ADL) will have to be performed for the patient by family, friends, and/or health care professionals. Consequently, testing verbal comprehension is extremely important. Assuming the elderly patient can hear, the following methods should be used to test comprehension.

Successful performance of verbal commands. Ask the patient to perform a one-, two-, or three-step command. The failure to perform the command(s) may result from a hearing deficit, aphasia, apraxia, or the inability to retain a sequence. Asking the patient to "remove your eyeglasses, clean them, and place them on the table" is an example of a complex three-step verbal command.

"Yes" or "No" questions. If the patient fails to follow even a one-step command (such as "take off your glasses"), questions requiring a "yes" or "no" answer should be used. Most aphasics can produce "yes" or "no" reliably, and simple or complex questions can be constructed. An example of a simple and concrete question is "Is this a pen?" (The examiner asks this while holding a watch in front of the patient.) A more complex question is "Do you make a cake with an egg beater?"

Object pointing. If the "yes" or "no" form of questioning fails or there is doubt about the answers, the patient can be asked to point to an object (or multiple objects) in the room. "Point to the ceiling" is an example of a simple command, whereas "point to the source of illumination in the room" is an example of a more abstract and difficult command.

Repetition

Both the failure to repeat progressively more complex words, phrases, and sentences and their excessive repetition should be noted. For example, ask the patient to repeat each of the following words or phrases: "comb"; "pencil"; "presidential"; "he was here"; "no ifs, ands, or buts"; or "if he were here, we could go away."

Word-finding ability

In addition to having the patient verbally identify a pencil, an item of clothing (e.g., button, tie), or a watch, ask him to identify the various parts of each, such as the eraser and the stem. The ability to name body parts should also be tested.

Reading (aloud and for comprehension)

One of the pleasures that an elderly aphasic may maintain is his ability to read. The ability of the patient to read aloud should be differentiated from his ability to comprehend written material. One simple test is to present cards with words written in large print describing objects in the room (e.g., chair, desk, window) and to ask the patient to point to the objects. Giving the patient an instructional card that says, "When you have read this, please tear up the card" is a test of comprehension, ability to follow directions, and neuromuscular coordination. Lengthier paragraphs taken from newspapers or magazines can be used to test comprehension.

Writing

Before testing writing ability, one should be sure that the elderly patient has learned how to write. If the patient is aphasic in speaking, he is also likely to demonstrate abnormalities in writing

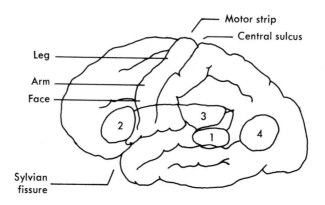

1. Fluent aphasia: Wernicke's area in the posterosuperior temporal gyrus

2. Nonfluent aphasia: Broca's area in the posterior of the third frontal gyrus just anterior to the face region of the motor strip

3. Conduction aphasia: Arcuate fasciculus connecting Wernicke's and Broca's areas

4. Anomic aphasia: Angular gyrus at the tip of the superior temporal sulcus

Fig. 8-1. Localization of common types of aphasia. (From Watson, R. T.: How to examine the patient with aphasia, Geriatrics **30**(12):73, 1975. Reprinted with permission of Geriatrics.)

Table 8-1. Common aphasic disorders*

	Spontaneous speech	Comprehension	Naming	Repetition
Wernicke's aphasia (1)†	Fluent	Poor	Poor	Poor
Broca's aphasia (2)	Nonfluent	Good	Poor	Poor
Conduction (3)	Fluent	Good	Poor	Poor
Global (1,2,3,4)	Nonfluent	Poor	Poor	Poor
Anomic (4)	Fluent	Good	Poor	Good
Isolated speech area (5)	Fluent only in repeating	Poor	Poor	Good
Transcortical motor (6)	Nonfluent	Good	Poor	Good
Transcortical sensory (7)	Fluent	Poor	Poor	Good

*From Watson, R. T.: How to examine the patient with aphasia, Geriatrics **30**(12):73, 1975. Reprinted with permission of Geriatrics.
†Numbers refer to anatomic areas in Fig. 8-2.

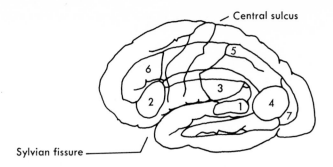

1. Fluent aphasia: Wernicke's area

2. Nonfluent aphasia: Broca's area

3. Conduction aphasia: Arcuate fasciculus

} All are juxtaposed to sylvian fissure, and inability to repeat is common feature.

4. Anomic aphasia: Angular gyrus but more likely to occur with diffuse disease

5. Isolated speech area

6. Transcortical motor aphasia: Nonfluent but with repetition preserved

7. Transcortical sensory aphasia: Fluent without comprehension but with repetition preserved

} All are outside of immediate perisylvian area, and ability to repeat is common feature.

Fig. 8-2. Composite of anatomic localization of aphasia. (From Watson, R. T.: How to examine the patient with aphasia, Geriatrics **30**(12):73, 1975. Reprinted with permission of Geriatrics.)

Table 8-2. Clinical evaluation of spontaneous speech*

	Anterior lesion (Broca's aphasia)	Posterior lesion (Wernicke's aphasia)
Rate of output	Decreased	Normal or increased
Effort	Increased	Normal
Prosody†	Dysprosody	Normal
Content	Use of nouns and action verbs	Use of filler words (e.g., "a," "the,") and circumlocution
Phrase length	Short	Long
Paraphasia	Less often evident	All literal and verbal types may be present

*Modified from Watson, R. T.: How to examine the patient with aphasia, Geriatrics **30**(12):73, 1975.
†All the variations in time, pitch, and loudness that accomplish emphasis, lend interest to speech, and characterize modes of expression.

words. Exceptions are rare, if any. The patient should be asked to write his name. Writing one's name, however, is usually not an adequate indication of writing ability, since the aphasic often writes his name well but fails on other writing tasks, such as monosyllabic words (e.g., cat, dog), multisyllabic words, phrases, and sentences.

Broca's aphasia; Wernicke's aphasia

Broca's (nonfluent) aphasia and Wernicke's (fluent) aphasia are described in detail because they are classic examples of an anterior and posterior lesion. The other, less common types of aphasia are described and localized as shown in Fig. 8-2.

Broca's aphasia

Hemiparesis or hemiplegia almost always accompanies Broca's aphasia. Spontaneous speech is nonfluent, articulation is often awkward, and there is limited vocabulary. Speech is restricted to the simplest, most overlearned grammatical forms. Literal paraphasic errors may also be present. Repetition is usually better than spontaneous speech, but both are abnormal. Oral comprehension may be spared but sometimes is imperfect, whereas reading ability is usually well preserved. Writing is just as involved as speech. An elderly patient with Broca's aphasia may appear to be globally aphasic because of depression. Also, a patient with Broca's aphasia may have initially presented with global aphasia that has subsequently improved.

Wernicke's aphasia

Speech is fluently articulated but marked by verbal and, less often, literal paraphasia and neologisms (meaningless words). Grammatical forms (e.g., sen-

tence types, such as declarative statements or questions; tenses—past, present, and future) are varied but sometimes incorrect. Comprehension is always disturbed, often at the one-word level. Reading and writing are disturbed usually to the same extent as is spoken language. Repetition and word retrieval are impaired. Patients are generally unaware of their speech production and may demonstrate an excessive output of words (logorrhea). Patients with Wernicke's aphasia are often euphoric and occasionally manifest paranoid, bizarre behavior. Consequently, the patient may be misdiagnosed as psychotic.

Systematic examination

1. Observe the patient's conversational speech and describe it in the following terms:
   a. What is the rate of verbal output: "nonfluent" or "fluent"?
   b. Does the patient initiate speech with little effort, or does he strain to talk?
   c. What is the length of each phrase? Are the phrases short (two to three words only), long (four or more words), or logorrheic (excessive and often)?
   d. What is the speech content? Are there more substantive words (nouns, action verbs, significant modifiers) or few substantive words (more cliches, stock phrases, circumlocutions)?
   e. What is the melodic line of speech? Intonational patterns normally encompass the entire sentence. In Broca's aphasia, speech is so stilted that no melodic line exists. In fluent speech, a melodic line is present.
   f. Does the patient perseverate? Per-

severation is the repetition of a response that is no longer appropriate (e.g., "What do you wash with?" [Answer: "Soap"] "What is your name?" [Answer: "Soap"]).

g. What is your general impression? Would you say, for example, that the patient speaks little but conveys more, or that he uses many words but conveys no message?

2. Test the patient's ability to comprehend the spoken word:

a. Ask questions (e.g., "What is your name?" [If no answer] "Is it Mrs. Smith?" "Is it Jane?" "What is your address?" "Are we in New York?" "What time is it?" "Is it Friday?").

b. Give progressively more complex instructions without nonverbal cues. "Raise your left hand," "Touch your nose," "Take off your glasses," and "Grip my hand," are examples of simple commands. "Point to the light in the room" is an example of a more difficult command.

c. Give progressively more complex object identification tasks: (1) ask the patient to identify an object from among a finite number of objects (with an assortment of objects before the patient, ask him to point to one); (2) ask him to identify an object in the room; (3) ask him to identify an object on the basis of a functional description (e.g., "Show me the one you write with" [from a selection of items that includes a pencil]); (4) ask him to identify an object from descriptive cues (e.g., "Show me the long thin object with a point"); and (5) ask him to identify an object on the basis of an abstract concept (e.g., "Point to the source of illumination in the room").

3. Test the patient's ability to name objects:

a. Ask him to name a presented object. Ask, for example, "What is this?" while holding a pen.

b. Ask him to name an object's function (e.g. "What do you do with the pen?").

4. Test the patient's ability to repeat (e.g., "Repeat after me: 'comb,' 'pencil,' 'presidential,' 'The President lives in Washington,' and 'No ifs, ands, or buts' ").

5. Test the patient's ability to read:

a. Test his comprehension of the written word: (1) present written names of objects and ask the patient to point to the objects, (2) ask him to point to a prominent word in a headline, and (3) ask him to read a "yes" or "no" question and respond appropriately.

b. Test his ability to read aloud: (1) ask the patient to read a single word aloud, (2) ask him to read newspaper headlines, and (3) ask him to read a test paragraph.

6. Test the patient's writing ability.

a. Ask him to write his name, since this is the most basic writing skill.

b. Ask him to copy the newspaper headline.

c. Ask him to write a short word and then a phrase. If he succeeds, ask him to write a paragraph.

Factors influencing recovery

There is much controversy in the literature on the factors that influence recovery from aphasia. Prognostic factors include (1) the patient's age, (2) associated defects and poor health, (3) the type of aphasia, (4) speech therapy, (5) the time between the onset of aphasia and speech therapy, (6) the patient's education, (7) the patient's social status, and (8) the patient's personality characteristics and emotional state.

It is commonly accepted that recovery from aphasia is slow (lasting months), with the maximum spontaneous recovery occurring during the first 3 to 6 months.

Acute illness from a superimposed toxic or metabolic state is a factor that can slow the rate of recovery of an older person. Age *per se* is thought by some experts to have no influence on the prognosis. Older patients can make significant gains both spontaneously and with the assistance of a speech pathologist. Therefore, elderly aphasic patients should not be denied the assistance of a speech pathologist, and referral should be made promptly after the loss. Hearing and/or visual defects may interfere with recovery from aphasia. The prognosis is better if there are no coexisting sensory deficits.[8,9] Physical or psychiatric illness may impair or slow recovery. For example, elderly patients with certain illnesses, such as angina pectoris, heart failure, pneumonia, or depression, often have to interrupt their treatment.

The educational level, occupation, and premorbid language abilities may also affect the outcome of therapy. Limited education, which may be present in many elderly persons, however, is not a significant obstacle to language rehabilitation of the aphasic patient. Positive personality characteristics (interest, motivation, aspiration) generally lead to a better outcome of therapy; these personality characteristics are known to affect rehabilitation favorably in all other areas. Although the effect of therapy for aphasia is questioned, and few well-controlled studies exist to confirm its value, there is an impression that improvement in speech is greater when therapy starts early.

The type of aphasia as a predictive factor should be considered with great caution. Presenting symptoms during the period immediately after a CVA are not usually reliable bases for classification[10] or for prognosis, since they change with time. Generally speaking, patients with severe cases of sustained Broca's aphasia do poorly. Conduction aphasia probably has a better prognosis than either Broca's or Wernicke's aphasia. The prognosis of global aphasia is poor. In the case of aphasia from a brain tumor or degenerative disease, much depends on the removal of the tumor and on the course of the underlying disease.

The aphasic patient and the family often ask how much recovery will occur and how soon. Most spontaneous improvement in aphasic patients occurs during the first 3 to 6 months. Thereafter, recovery is usually slow. Any significant improvement in speech during this time brightens the outlook. Some authors have reported a response to speech therapy many months and even years after the onset of aphasia.[11] Periodic reevaluation of the elderly aphasic patient is indicated, especially if communication becomes more difficult.

Role of the environment and the family

The family should be instructed on how to communicate best with their elderly aphasic relative. Specifically, the family should:

1. Not ask open-ended questions, which may lead to frustration in answering
2. Give him time to say what he has on his mind
3. Ask questions that require a "yes" or "no" response, either verbally or with gestures
4. Provide word cues when needed (e.g., a sentence completion cue such

as "you write with a _____?") or provide the first sound of the word (e.g., "pe" for "pen")

5. Not ask several questions at a time

6. Reduce or eliminate competing noises when talking, since the person may also have a hearing defect

The elderly patient with aphasia resulting from a CVA may have other problems affecting his language ability, including depression resulting from loss of physical and verbal ability. Sensory deprivation secondary to isolation from family and friends in a hospital or nursing home environment is another problem. In addition, if all of the needs of the elderly hospitalized patient are met, his motivation to speak may be reduced. Although they are concerned about the patient's needs, family and staff members should make every effort to encourage verbal interaction without frustrating the patient about his inability to communicate.

Elderly patients should not be denied the services of a speech pathologist initially or at a later date for reevaluation. Referral to a speech pathologist should be made as soon as possible after the CVA. Complicating medical and psychiatric problems of late life may make therapy longer and more difficult, but if elderly patients are to return to the community, a maximum effort to improve communication skills must be made.

REFERENCES

1. Darley, F. L.: Treatment of acquired aphasia, Adv. Neurol. **7**:111, 1975.
2. Marks, M., Tailor, M., and Rusk, H. A.: Rehabilitation of the aphasic patient: a survey of three years experience in a rehabilitation setting, Arch. Phys. Med. Rehabil. **38**:219, 1957.
3. Benson, D. F., and Geschwind, N.: The aphasias and related disturbances. In Baker, A. B., and Baker, L. H., editors: Clinical neurology, New York, 1976, Harper & Row, Publishers, Inc., p. 1.
4. Geschwind, N.: Aphasia. N. Engl. J. Med. **284:** 654, 1971.
5. Marquardsen, J.: The natural history of acute cerebrovascular disease: a retrospective study of 769 patients, Acta Neurol. Scand. **45**(suppl. 38): 1, 1969.
6. Isaacs, B.: Stroke. In Brocklehurst, J. D., editor: Textbook of Geriatric medicine and gerontology, ed. 1, Edinburgh, Eng., 1973, Churchill Livingstone, p. 216.
7. Voinescu, I., Vish, E., Sirian, S., and Maretsis, M.: Aphasia in a polyglot, Brain Lang. **4**:165, 1977.
8. Kertesz, A., and McCabe, P.: Recovery patterns and prognosis in aphasia, Brain **100**:1, 1977.
9. Anderson, T. P., Bourestom, N., and Greenberg, F. R.: Rehabilitation predictors in completed stroke: final report, Minneapolis, 1970, American Rehabilitation Foundation.
10. Jenkins, J. J., Jimenez-Pabon, E., Shaw, R., and Sefer, J. W.: Schuell's aphasia in adults, ed. 2, New York, 1975, Harper & Row, Publishers, Inc.
11. Broida, H.: Language therapy effects in long-term aphasia, Arch. Phys. Med. Rehabil. **58**: 248, 1977.

PROBLEM-SOLVING EXERCISES*
Case one

Mr. J. D. is a 75-year-old, right-handed man. He suffered a CVA with right-sided hemiparesis and speech impairment 3 weeks ago. He is an adult-onset diabetic of 20 years, and his diabetes has been complicated by legal blindness from retinopathy and cataracts.

The interview opens with the following questions: "What is your name?" "How are you?" "Where do you live?" "Tell me what happened to bring you to the hospital?" "What is your most serious problem?"

Questions

1. What do these opening questions test?
   a. Spontaneous conversational speech
   b. Word finding
   c. Fluency
   d. Repetition

2. As an answer to the first question the patient utters only his name. Responses to

---

*Some questions may have more than one correct answer.

other questions are: "Da-da," "Chat-to," "Chut-ta," "Da-doo-choo," and "Chee-choo." Such responses exemplify:
a. Jargon
b. Literal paraphasia
c. Verbal paraphasia

3. The patient is unable to recite the days of the week, the months of the year, and numbers from one to ten without initial sound cuing. Melodic line and grammatical form are absent. Phrase length cannot be assessed. Articulation is stiff and labored. Naming is possible only with the introduction of visual (shown a picture or oral posture of the lips), auditory (initial sound production), graphic (shown the written word), and sentence completion ("you write with a . . .") cues. These findings are indicative of:
a. Well-preserved automatic speech
b. Fluent speech
c. Difficulty with word finding

4. Mr. D. is able to move his tongue, lips, mandible, and soft palate; to phonate; to produce; and to sustain his voice. When asked to repeat words in rapid succession (e.g., "tip-top" or "Huckleberry"), he has difficulty in initiating the production of words. When asked to repeat words such as "purple," he says "purkle"; when asked to repeat "what," he says "what"; when asked to repeat "Methodist Episcopal," his answer is completely unintelligible. When asked to say "fifteen," he says "sixteen." These findings suggest:
a. Dysarthria
b. Paraphasia
c. Apraxia
d. Nonfluent aphasia

5. Auditory comprehension is partially functional for single words (body parts, common objects, "yes" or "no" responses). Comprehension of sentences is 60% correct. The following can be said about this patient's language ability:
a. Comprehension is partially impaired.
b. Comprehension is impaired but is superior to expression.
c. Broca's aphasia is the most likely type of aphasia in this patient.

d. Wernicke's aphasia is the most likely type of aphasia in this patient.

Case two

Mrs. S. is a 78-year-old, right-handed woman who has been admitted to a skilled nursing facility for rehabilitation with the following diagnosis taken directly from the transfer note:
1. S/P CVA with moderate right-sided hemiparesis
2. Expressive aphasia
3. Organic brain syndrome
4. History of seizures, etiology undetermined

Past history: Hypertension, arteriosclerotic cardiovascular disease (ASCVD), congestive heart failure (CHF), profound hearing loss, and cataracts.

Mrs. S., who is wearing a hearing aid, answers the opening questions appropriately and produces complete sentences. There are no delays, jargon, or paraphasias. She is able to count and to recite the months of the year.

Questions

1. Which of the following statements can be made?
a. Organic brain syndrome may not be present.
b. Automatic speech is preserved.
c. Spontaneous speech is functional (the patient is able to express thoughts and needs).
d. Comprehension appears to be well preserved.

2. Repetition of single words is functional (i.e., she can repeat seven out of ten words correctly). Repetition of phrases is accurate only up to five words. Normal subjects may retain and repeat as many as 20 to 30 words in a sentence. This reflects an auditory retention deficit in this patient. Examination of the speech musculature reveals adequate verbal and nonverbal movements. This indicates:
a. A severe language deficit
b. That the patient may have conduction aphasia

c. That the patient may have Broca's aphasia

d. Dysarthria

e. Speech apraxia

3. When shown a picture and asked to name what she sees (object naming), Mrs. S. delays her answers and errs about 50% of the time. Responses to solely auditory stimuli are prompt and 85% correct. The patient has difficulty in reading. She is only able to select a given printed word from a group of three. When asked to repeat "the vat leaks," she responds with "the vack leak"; "The spy fled to Greece" becomes "The sky led to Greece." These responses, produced in the face of the ability to name objects and carry on a conversation, could indicate:

a. Poor vision

b. Verbal paraphasia

c. Impaired hearing acuity

d. Conduction aphasia

e. Organic brain syndrome

ANSWERS TO PROBLEM-SOLVING EXERCISES
Case one

1. a, b, and c. By closely observing the verbal responses of the patient to these general questions, the interviewer can make an initial assessment of any speech or language problems. Fluency is the quantity (sparse versus logorrheic verbal output) of the person's speech. Word finding is the person's ability to retrieve appropriate words. Repetition (the ability to repeat) can only be tested by specifically asking the patient to repeat words, phrases, and sentences.

2. a. Mr. D.'s responses are examples of jargon (unintelligible verbal output). Literal and verbal types of paraphasia are more frequently seen in fluent aphasics, but they can also occur in nonfluent types. Verbal paraphasia is the substitution of an inappropriate word during an effort to say a word (e.g., "spoon" for "knife"). Literal paraphasia is the substitution of a similar-sounding word (e.g., "pone" for "phone").

3. c. Automatic speech is the repetition of overlearned sequences, such as counting

from one to ten or reciting the days of the week. The patient does not exhibit fluent speech (effortless speech) with normal or high output. Since visual and verbal cues are necessary for him to name objects, he clearly has difficulty with word finding.

4. b, c, and d. There is no evidence of dysarthria, since Mr. D. is able to move his oral apparatus, phonate, and produce words. He exhibits literal paraphasia ("purkle" for "purple"), as well as apraxia of speech (he has difficulty in initiating speech and in programming motor movements of the speech musculature despite intact speech musculature and complete understanding of what is required). The patient also has nonfluent aphasia.

5. a, b, and c. Comprehension is clearly limited, but appears to be superior to expression. This is typical of Broca's aphasia and is consistent with right-sided hemiparesis.

Case two

1. All of these. Although Mrs. S.'s condition has been diagnosed as organic brain syndrome, her answers to the opening questions are appropriate and without evidence of cognitive dysfunction. Because the initial evaluation does not confirm the diagnosis, a mental status examination should be performed. Automatic speech (e.g., reciting the days of the week), spontaneous speech, and comprehension are intact.

2. b. Mrs. S. appears to be able to communicate but has difficulty in repeating words and phrases. Comprehension is preserved. Her speech is fluent; therefore, Broca's aphasia should not be considered. Conduction aphasia is a fluent aphasia with intact comprehension, impaired object naming, and impaired repetition. This diagnosis must be considered, although there is no comment on the patient's ability to name objects. There is no evidence of dysarthria or speech apraxia. Difficulty with repetition could also be the result of an auditory retention deficit.

3. a and e. Undetected poor visual acuity may be affecting her ability to read and select a specific word from a group of

words. There is no evidence of verbal paraphasia. Impaired hearing acuity could account for the mispronunciation of the phrases, particularly when voiceless speech sounds are involved (e.g., *t, s, p, k*). Finally, conduction aphasia is very unlikely because of Mrs. S.'s preserved ability to name objects, minimal number of paraphasic errors (literal paraphasia is frequent in conduction aphasia), and minimal difficulty with word finding. She is suffering mainly from sensory deprivation (hearing loss and cataracts) and a possible auditory retention deficit, which are affecting her comprehension and therefore her verbal output. Examination of her ear canals for cerumen and an ophthalmological examination will assist in the differential diagnosis.

POSTTEST°

1. The most common cause of aphasia in the elderly is:
   a. Brain tumor (benign or malignant)
   b. Stroke
   c. Subdural hematoma
   d. Infection
   e. Depression
2. The most likely type of aphasia found in an elderly patient with right-sided hemiparesis is:
   a. Broca's aphasia
   b. Wernicke's aphasia
   c. Conduction aphasia
   d. Anomic aphasia
   e. Global aphasia
3. Match the type of aphasia with its clinical feature:
   Type
   _____ a. Broca's aphasia
   _____ b. Wernicke's aphasia
   _____ c. Anomic aphasia
   _____ d. Global aphasia

°Some questions may have more than one correct answer.

Clinical feature

1. Commonly found in patients with metabolic abnormalities, increased intracranial pressure, or other diffuse brain involvement
2. Can appear similar to nonfluent aphasia complicated by depression
3. Can be confused with the "word salad" type of speech of a schizophrenic
4. Nonfluent, good comprehension, poor repetition

4. Match the terms with the speech pattern that best represents it:
   Term
   _____ a. Logorrhea
   _____ b. Paraphasia
   _____ c. Perseveration
   _____ d. Jargon
   Speech pattern
   1. "Do-do-goo-goo-ha-ha"
   2. When the patient was asked to say, "The sky is blue," he said, "The sky, sky, sky"
   3. When the patient was asked to say, "Knife," he said, "Fork"
   4. When the patient was asked why he came to the hospital, his answer was excessively lengthy and contained little information

5. *True or false:* Most of the spontaneous recovery appears during the first 3 to 6 months after the onset of aphasia in a patient with a stroke.
6. *True or false:* The elderly patient who has a sudden onset of impaired verbal output is most likely to be having a psychotic episode.
7. *True or false:* The elderly patient who is aphasic in speech is usually able to write with little difficulty.

ANSWERS TO PRETEST AND POSTTEST

1. b. A stroke, or cerebrovascular accident (CVA), is the most common cause of aphasia in the elderly. The other causes are primarily, but not exclusively, found in younger patients.

2. a. Eighty percent of patients with Broca's aphasia have right-sided hemiplegia or hemiparesis. Wernicke's aphasia, conduction aphasia, and anomic aphasia are all fluent types of aphasia and will result from a posterior lesion of the dominant speech hemisphere. Anomic aphasia may be difficult to localize.

3. a, 4; b, 3; c, 1; d, 2.

4. a, 4; b, 3; c, 2; d, 1.

5. True. Recovery from aphasia occurs less often and more slowly after 3 months have passed. The exceptional aphasic patient will show an improvement years later.

6. False. An acute CVA may manifest itself with only a nonfluent or fluent type of aphasia and no focal neurological findings, such as hemiparesis. A posterior lesion (one behind the central sulcus) can cause a fluent type of aphasia, which can be confused with a psychotic episode.

7. False. There is a rare aphasic patient who is capable of functional writing ability. In general, if the patient is aphasic in the spoken word, he also has difficulty in writing.

Chapter 9

Hearing disorders

EMMANUEL MARGOLIS, BARBARA LEVY, and FREDRICK T. SHERMAN

EDUCATIONAL OBJECTIVES
Attitudinal

The student should:

1. Explore his feelings about elderly people who have difficulty in hearing
2. Experience a conductive hearing loss by plugging his ears with cotton for half a day and describe its effect
3. Become more aware of his reactions to people who wear hearing aides by wearing one himself for a day

Cognitive

The student should:

1. Understand the social, psychological, and medical effects that decreased hearing may have on the elderly patient
2. Be aware of common types of hearing problems in the elderly
3. Be able to define presbycusis and explain how it presents clinically
4. Know the current governmental regulations on hearing aids and know when to refer a patient to an audiologist
5. Be aware of the audiological tests that are commonly used for both screening and comprehensive evaluation of the elderly patient
6. Be aware of the various assistive devices, other than hearing aides, that are available to overcome hearing deficits

Skill

The student should:

1. Be able to discuss and demonstrate the tests used to differentiate conductive (outer and middle ear) from sensorineural (inner ear, cranial

nerve VIII, and central nervous system [CNS] deficits)
2. Know how to evaluate the need for medical, surgical, and/or mechanical (hearing aid) intervention with the elderly patient
3. Be able to instruct the patient on the use of a hearing aid, when it should be worn, and the main problems encountered in using it (battery failure, occluded tubing, inability to handle equipment)
4. Be able to explain to the patient and family simple techniques (lipreading, slower speaking, proper lighting) that will improve communication.

PRETEST°

1. Hearing loss in the elderly may result from:
   a. Paget's disease
   b. Otosclerosis
   c. Senile dementia
   d. Cerumen
   e. Otitis media
2. You are evaluating a patient with supposed global aphasia. You find that the patient has a marked decrease in word discrimination (i.e., decreased ability to understand speech). His condition may be:
   a. Due to presbycusis associated with aging

°Some questions may have more than one correct answer.

186

b. Associated with other pathological conditions of peripheral parts of the auditory system
c. Associated with other pathological conditions of central parts of the auditory system
d. The result of a conductive hearing loss

3. In the patient with presbycusis, which of the following are true?
  a. The onset of hearing loss is gradual.
  b. There is often a family history.
  c. There is often a history of fluctuation (the patient will hear better if not fatigued, e.g., in the early morning).
  d. The patient's hearing is very much disturbed by background noise.
  e. The patient says he watches television but cannot understand it.

4. The elderly individual may purchase a hearing aid:
  a. Only after having the need confirmed by a physician
  b. And receive reimbursement from Medicare
  c. Directly from a hearing aid dealer without prior examination by a physician after signing a waiver

5. The function of the total hearing system (conductive and sensorineural components) is reflected in the:
  a. Air conduction test
  b. Bone conduction test

6. To determine whether a hearing deficit should be classified as conductive, sensorineural, or mixed, the following test(s) should be used:
  a. Air conduction threshold
  b. Bone conduction threshold
  c. Both

7. A patient is referred to you with bone conduction thresholds indicating impaired hearing. He may have:
  a. Otosclerosis
  b. Otitis media

c. A scarred tympanic membrane
d. Impacted cerumen
e. Presbycusis

8. Ototoxic drugs are:
  a. Digoxin
  b. Streptomycin
  c. Gentamicin
  d. Phenylbutazone
  e. Aspirin

9. The elderly individual who is having difficulty in hearing with his new hearing aid:
  a. May not know how to use the aid properly
  b. May not have the appropriate aid
  c. May lack the motivation to use a hearing aid
  d. May have poor speech discrimination

Impaired hearing is common in old age and can result from a combination of age-related physiological changes and superimposed pathological problems. About 30% of the community-residing elderly over the age of 65 have hearing impairments,[1] and at least 90% of the elderly population living in nursing homes have similar deficits.[2] The elderly constitute at least half of the more than 14.5 million people in the United States who have hearing problems.

Because hearing loss can result in psychological problems, such as withdrawal, depression, and paranoia, and in pedestrian accidents resulting from not hearing an oncoming vehicle, it is important to be aware of (1) the common causes of impaired hearing in the elderly, (2) the methods available to the clinician to determine the types of hearing loss, (3) the role of the audiologist, (4) the tests used by the audiologist and the types of test abnormalities seen in the elderly, (5) the benefit of a hearing aid and the difficulties encountered by the elderly in using it, and (6) various communication methods used to overcome decreased hearing.

TYPES OF HEARING LOSS

There are three types of hearing loss: conductive, sensorineural and mixed. Hearing losses caused by abnormalities of the outer and middle ear are called conductive losses, whereas losses caused by abnormalities of the cochlea and cranial nerve VIII or its central connections are called sensorineural losses. Combinations of sensorineural and conductive losses are called mixed losses.

The integrity of the entire auditory system (outer, middle, and inner ear, and the auditory nerve) is measured by testing air conduction. The patient's inability to hear a sound stimulus coming from earphones or a vibrating tuning fork confirms a hearing deficit, but does not tell the site of the lesion. The integrity of the cochlea and cranial nerve VIII or its central connections is measured by testing bone conduction. Placing a bone oscillator or vibrating tuning fork on the mastoid process tests only inner ear and cranial nerve VIII function; outer and middle ear function is bypassed.

When bone conduction thresholds are compared with air conduction thresholds, the lesion can be localized to the outer and/or middle ear (conductive loss), to the cochlea and/or cranial nerve VIII (sensorineural loss), or to both areas (mixed loss). Figs. 9-1 to 9-3 illustrate conductive, sensorineural, and mixed hearing losses with simplified representations of the anatomy of the ear to clarify the type of loss:

1. *Conductive hearing loss* (Fig. 9-1): Air conduction thresholds indicate a 50-decibel (dB) hearing loss. Bone conduc-

tion thresholds reveal normal hearing. The loss is restricted to the outer and/or middle ear.

2. *Sensorineural hearing loss* (Fig. 9-2): Air conduction thresholds indicate a 50-dB hearing loss. Bone conduction thresholds reveal a 50-dB loss equal to air conduction. The pathological condition is restricted to the sense organ (cochlea) and/or cranial nerve VIII.

3. *Mixed hearing loss* (Fig. 9-3): There is a 50-dB hearing loss revealed by air conduction. Bone conduction thresholds indicate a 25-dB hearing loss. The remaining 25-dB loss can be attributed to the outer and/or middle ear; both the conductive and sensorineural areas indicate disease.

Additional tests can differentiate between pathological conditions of the outer and middle ears and between those of the inner ear and cranial nerve VIII. The basic audiological assessment, which measures air and bone conduction and responses to speech stimuli, will determine the need for these additional tests.

Clinically, a patient with a *conductive hearing loss* may manifest the following signs[3]:

1. He usually speaks in a relatively quiet voice, making it difficult to hear him. The conductive blockage is thought to enhance the bone conduction transmission of the sound stimulus, and the individual perceives sound as louder than it would have been without the conductive loss. Thus, the patient speaks in a quiet voice.

2. Speech discrimination (the ability to distinguish and understand sounds) is relatively unimpaired. He will understand what he hears, provided that the speech is made loud enough for him to hear it.

3. He can hear better in the presence

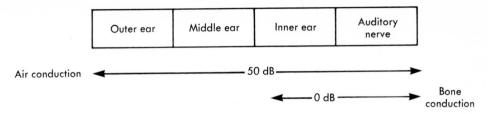

Fig. 9-1. Diagrammatic representation of a pure conductive hearing loss (e.g., cerumen occluding the external canal).

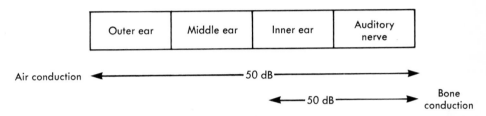

Fig. 9-2. Diagrammatic representation of a pure sensorineural loss (e.g., presbycusis).

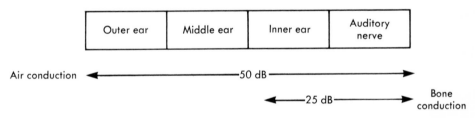

Fig. 9-3. Diagrammatic representation of a mixed hearing loss (e.g., presbycusis and cerumen in the external canal).

of noise than a person with normal hearing.

4. His ear can tolerate loud noises better than other people with normal hearing.

5. He tends to have about the same loss for sounds of all frequency (i.e., the loss is "flat"). This is confirmed by the audiogram.

6. Tinnitus of low frequency is occasionally present.

A patient with a *sensorineural hearing loss* may manifest the following signs:

1. He may speak in an excessively loud voice in many situations where a loud voice is inappropriate, because the cochlea and cranial nerve VIII are impaired and he does not hear his own or other voices normally.

2. Very often, he has difficulty in understanding speech stimuli (impaired speech discrimination), even at levels of loudness that are above threshold. Patients with a sensorineural loss only par-

tially understand what is said to them. They may confuse words like "cake" and "sake," because the frequency of the initial consonant is not easily perceived. Shouting to the patient who has impaired speech discrimination is of no value and actually may hinder understanding.

3. He may be sensitive to loud intensities of sound (recruitment phenomenon). As a rule, patients with a sensorineural loss hear better in a quiet environment, whereas those with a conductive deficit are less disturbed by noise.

4. Tinnitus of a higher pitch than that encountered in the conductive type of deafness is often present. It may be intermittent or constantly occurring during the day as well as at night. Tinnitus may sound like a high-pitched whistle, the sound of escaping steam, or a clicking noise.

Conductive hearing losses
Outer ear conditions

There is little evidence that age-related physiological changes in the outer ear contribute to impaired hearing. Because elderly patients may accept their loss of hearing acuity as part of normal aging, they may not draw attention to their hearing loss. Consequently, it is important to routinely examine the ears for cerumen. The total occlusion of the external canal by cerumen is the most common cause of a conductive deficit in the elderly patient;[4] partial occlusion, however, has little effect on hearing. Cerumen can be removed through the use of a solution that will dissolve the wax, gentle lavage using a specially designed irrigation syringe, curettage under direct visualization, suctioning of the external canal with a specially designed tool, or any combination of these. The cerumen plug may often be dried and hard, making mechanical removal painful. The dried cerumen

can first be softened with a solution of carbamide peroxide or similar agent, 5 to 10 drops two times daily, instilled directly into the ear. Removal of the cerumen can then be accomplished by any of the mechanical means previously mentioned.

Middle ear conditions

Although the tympanic membrane may appear sclerotic and scarred in the elderly, these changes do not usually affect hearing. While middle ear disease is the primary cause of hearing loss in only 3% of the elderly,[5] it may be the clue to more serious illness. For example, acute otitis media may result from impaired immunity caused by leukemia or carcinoma; serous otitis media may occur from blockage of the eustachian tube by benign or malignant nasopharyngeal tumors. Cholesteatomas may also be noticed in late life and can be successfully removed surgically with the patient under local anesthesia.

Other causes

Paget's disease of the bone, which occurs in up to 10% of octogenarians, may involve the outer, middle, and inner ear and cause progressive hearing loss. Hearing loss occurs in 30% to 50% of patients with skull involvement and is usually bilateral.[6] Sensorineural hearing loss is caused by changes around the foramina of the acoustic nerve. Conductive hearing loss may result from stenosis of the external auditory meatus and ossification of the stapedius tendon. Calcitonin therapy may slow the progression of deafness in Paget's disease; middle ear surgery may occasionally correct the conductive deficit.[7]

Otosclerosis, a hereditary disease of unknown cause, usually starts in youth, causing ankylosis (fixation) of the stapes to the oval window. The most frequent cause of progressive conductive deafness in adulthood, it also causes a sensorineural loss when the cochlea is involved. Otosclerosis may not be clinically evident until late life, when presbycusis is superimposed. The patient then presents with a mixed hearing loss. Depending on the type of loss, the elderly patients with otosclerosis can benefit from surgery and/or a hearing aid.

Sensorineural hearing losses

Sensorineural hearing losses can result from age-related changes, environmental influences, or pathological processes that affect the structure of the inner ear, acoustic nerve, and/or its central connections. Medical and surgical treatments of sensorineural hearing loss are generally not effective; aural rehabilitation using hearing aids and lipreading is recommended.

Causes of sensorineural hearing loss in the elderly include presbycusis, noise trauma, ototoxicity from drugs, involvement of the acoustic nerve by benign or malignant tumors, and possible complications of arteriosclerosis.

Presbycusis

Presbycusis is the general term used to denote the gradual, progressive, permanent bilateral loss of hearing for high-frequency (and, eventually, middle and lower) tones due to degenerative changes throughout the entire auditory system. This process, which begins in the third decade and worsens with advancing age, causes a sensorineural deficit that seldom results in total deafness. Presbycusis affects approximately 60% (12 million) of all individuals over the age of 65 in the United States, though only a fraction of this group has functional deficits requiring aural rehabilitation. Eighty percent to 90% of the population of nursing homes and other senior citizens' shelters show hearing impairments attributed to presbycusis.[8]

Presbycusis has been thought to result from the progressive atrophy and degeneration of hair cells of the organ of Corti (sensory presbycusis). More recent investigations[9] have shown that the entire auditory system—including the nerve fibers (neural presbycusis), the stria vascularis leading to changes in the endolymphatic fluid (metabolic presbycusis), the cochlear partition (mechanical presbycusis), the minute blood vessels supplying portions of the inner ear (vascular presbycusis), and the cochlear nucleii and other auditory centers of the brain (central presbycusis)—shows degenerative changes. Although this classification draws attention to the widespread degenerative changes that occur in the auditory system with aging, it is of little practical help, since all processes may occur simultaneously.[10]

While the transmission of auditory information in presbycusis is impaired, the major part of the hearing loss is related to the inability of the central nervous system (CNS) to understand the information that is transmitted by the ear. Normal conversational speech contains a broad range of frequencies. Since consonants are usually of a higher frequency and vowels of a lower frequency, the patient with presbycusis will hear only parts of words and thus be unable to understand what is said (poor speech discrimination). The problem is due primarily to difficulties with clarity rather than the loudness of the stimuli.

When he is initially seen, the patient with presbycusis usually states that he has experienced some or all of the following[11]: (1) gradual and progressive hearing loss during the last 2 to 10 years; (2) loud sounds and noise making him nervous (recruitment); (3) tinnitus that is particularly noticeable in a quiet environment; (4) difficulties in understanding what has been said (poor speech discrimination), particularly if background noise is present; and (5) a history of an experience with a hearing aid that has yielded little benefit.

The patient asks for repetition of statements ("What?" or "I beg your pardon?" is often heard); he often responds to questions with an unrelated answer or no answer at all; he may be inattentive or withdrawn; he may be inconsistent in his responses to sound; and he watches the speaker's face intently.

Although most hearing deficits should be noted during interviewing or specific testing, the clinician may notice a hearing deficit in the patient for the first time when he percusses and auscultates the patient's back from behind. When the clinician asks the patient to "breathe," he may find that the patient does not cooperate, because the patient is unable to see the clinician's lips and face.

Noise trauma

The exposure of the adult to excessive noise can irreversibly damage the hair cells in the organ of Corti and cause a sensorineural hearing loss. Men are affected more often than women because of occupationally related noise trauma. Since the effects of noise leading to presbycusis and acoustic trauma may be cumulative, it is important to ask the elderly individual about previous work history and exposure to loud noise.

Ototoxic drugs

Drugs may be responsible for irreversible damage in cochlear as well as vestibular function. Antibiotics of the aminoglycoside type (gentamicin, streptomycin, kanamycin, and neomycin) should be used with caution in elderly individuals with known hearing deficits. Dosages of these drugs should be altered on the basis of the estimated and measured creatinine clearance.

Gentamicin, a commonly used parenteral aminoglycoside in the elderly, damages the vestibular portion of cranial nerve VIII more frequently than the cochlea portion.[12] Gentamicin ototoxity has been shown to occur in 10% to 20% of a selected group of elderly patients. Gentamicin has a long half-life in the labyrinthine fluids, and its direct application to the inner ear leads to damage of both cochlear and vestibular components.

In two thirds of patients showing ototoxicity from gentamicin, vestibular damage (vertigo, ataxia, nausea, and the inability to walk unaided) is present alone. In the remaining one third of patients with hearing loss, evidence of vestibular toxicity is present in one half. Therefore only 15% of patients with clinically determined gentamicin ototoxicity have auditory dysfunction alone, manifested by high-frequency loss and tinnitus.

Because the ototoxic effects of gentamicin cannot be predicted from the dosage, duration of therapy, or serum levels, it is important to monitor the elderly patient primarily for vestibular toxicity and secondarily for hearing loss.

The elderly person's perception of early hearing deficits and vestibular dysfunction may be poor; and since routine bedside tests are often inadequate in determining other than gross changes, a more rational approach to gentamicin ototoxicity is to determine whether the elderly patient has ataxia or dysequilibrium and assess his ability to ambulate. Repeat audiograms will reveal only one third of cases of ototoxicity. While damage is often reversible if gentamicin therapy is discontinued, permanent cochlear or vestibular damage may result from continued usage. Symptoms may not be present until several weeks after the drug is discontinued.

Bolus doses of furosemide in elderly patients with renal failure may also lead to hearing loss. Aspirin ingestion can lead to decreased hearing and tinnitus when taken in large quantities for arthritis. These symptoms are completely reversible when the aspirin is discontinued.

Tumors

Primary tumors of the acoustic nerve (acoustic neurinomas), metastatic tumors involving the temporal bone, and tumors of the cerebellar pontine angle may result in unilateral sensorineural hearing loss in the elderly. Episodic vertigo or mild dizziness and tinnitus combined with a hearing loss more profound in one ear than in the other may be the presenting complaint. Physical examination may show decreased air and bone conduction, impaired labyrinth function, and an abnormal audiogram. An absent corneal reflex in the ipsilateral eye may be an early sign of acoustic neurinoma. X-ray studies will often reveal an enlarged internal auditory meatus. Computerized axial tomography will show the extent of the lesion.

Arteriosclerosis

The relationship of arteriosclerosis and hypertension to the progressive decrease in hearing associated with aging is controversial, since cause-and-effect evidence is lacking. The cochlear artery is an end-artery; if it is occluded, sudden and total deafness will result.

TINNITUS

Tinnitus is an unpleasant, annoying internal noise, occurring in from 10% to 37% of the elderly population. It may often be quite distressing and occasionally has led to suicide. Tinnitus may be present with or without hearing loss. The sensation is usually high pitched when it is associated with a sensorineural loss and lower pitched when it occurs with a conductive loss. Unfortunately, in most cases a specific cause cannot be found; therefore, no special remedy can be prescribed. In extreme cases, surgical interruption of cranial nerve VIII is necessary in order to relieve the symptom. Occasionally an arteriovenous fistula, glomus tumor, or paraganglioma of the middle ear may cause tinnitus that can be surgically removed.

AUDIOLOGICAL EVALUATION

After a hearing loss has been determined and medical evaluation of the problem completed, an audiologist should be consulted for evaluation and aural rehabilitation. Audiologists may be found in many settings, including hospitals, special speech and hearing centers, some nursing homes, and in the private offices of otolaryngologists. Most communities lack the extensive network to detect elderly patients with hearing deficits, properly test them, and embark on an aural rehabilitation program. Community outreach programs in senior citizens' centers can provide screening for the detection of hearing deficits and subsequent referral to the primary care physician for further assessment. Screening techniques include self-estimates of hearing loss by the individual (often unreliable), pure-tone audiometry, and speech perception tests.

Basic audiometric testing includes the

following types of pure-tone and speech tests: pure-tone air conduction tests, pure-tone bone conduction tests, speech reception threshold tests, and speech discrimination tests.

Pure-tone testing

Pure-tone testing (air and bone) is accomplished by using an audiometer. In the *pure-tone air conduction test,* the signal is presented to both ears independently through the use of earphones, thereby assessing the integrity of the entire auditory system. In the *pure-tone bone conduction test,* the auditory signal is delivered through a bone oscillator placed on the mastoid process behind the auricle; thus, it bypasses the outer and middle ear. The intensity of the sound (tone) used as an auditory stimulus (measured in decibels) and the frequency of the sound (measured in hertz) are both controlled by the audiologist. In the clinical setting, the audiologist will start the test by applying a sound of an intensity (e.g., 50 dB) and frequency (e.g., 1,000 Hz) that he expects (based on impressions from the conversation with the patient preceding the test) the patient to be able to hear. Gradually, the audiologist lowers the intensity. The lowest intensity to which the patient responds correctly 50% of the time is recorded on the audiogram as the patient's tone threshold. Thresholds at 500 Hz, 1,000 Hz and 2,000 Hz (speech frequencies) are averaged, and the result is termed the pure-tone average (PTA).

An audiogram can be presented in graphic or chart form. Fig. 9-4 shows the normal range of hearing as well as degrees of hearing loss. An audiogram typical of the patient with early presbycusis is seen in Fig. 9-5.

The audiometric studies of elderly pa-

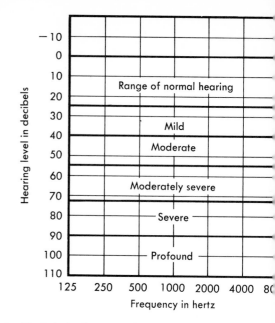

Fig. 9-4. Audiogram showing ranges of hearing loss.

tients show that hearing loss from presbycusis first occurs in the high frequencies (2,500 to 8,000 Hz) and progresses with age to lower frequencies. The thresholds obtained from the air conduction and the bone conduction tests are compared to determine the type and possible site of the lesion in the auditory pathway as described previously.

As presbycusis progresses, there is a loss in all frequencies, as shown by the audiogram in Fig. 9-6. A mixed loss resulting from presbycusis and impacted cerumen in the external canal is shown in Fig. 9-7.

After the type of hearing loss is determined, the degree of hearing loss must be measured. If the patient's threshold (SRT and PTA) is within the range of 0 to 20 dB, he has normal hearing. A threshold between 20 and 40 dB indicates a

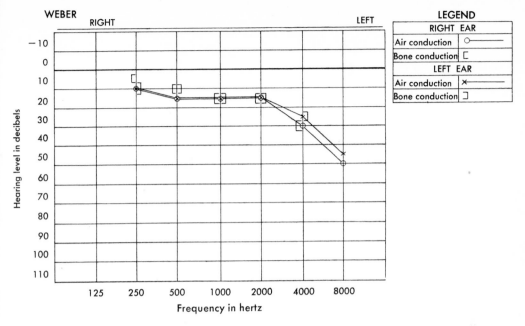

Fig. 9-5. Audiogram showing early presbycusis with loss in the higher frequencies bilaterally and normal hearing in the low and mid frequencies. This loss is typical of early presbycusis. Note that air and bone conduction tests are the same, showing that the loss is purely sensorineural. See Fig. 9-2.

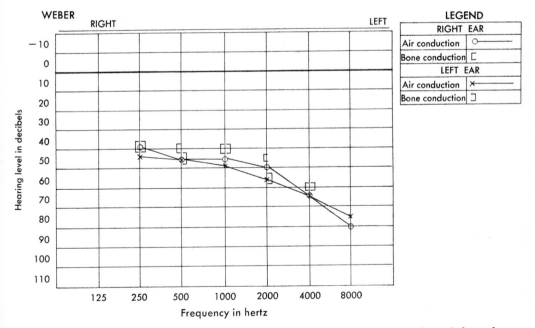

Fig. 9-6. Moderately advanced presbycusis. This pure-tone audiogram shows bilaterally symmetrical moderate sensorineural hearing loss dropping to moderately severe in high frequencies.

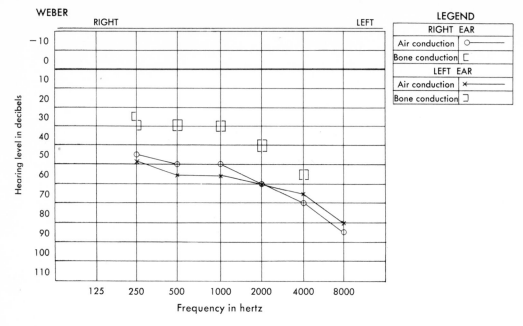

Fig. 9-7. Mixed hearing loss. This audiogram shows a bilateral mixed hearing loss such as would be seen in an elderly individual with presbycusis (the sensorineural component) and impacted cerumen (the conductive component). The brackets are the results of bone conduction testing, and the circle and *x* are the results of air conduction tests. The difference between them is the conductive loss.

mild loss; between 40 and 60 dB, a moderate loss; between 60 and 75 dB, a moderately severe loss; between 75 and 90 dB, a severe loss; and 90 dB and up, a profound loss. (See Fig. 9-4.)

Speech testing

Speech testing takes place after pure-tone results are obtained. These tests are of primary importance, since we communicate using speech, which is a combination of frequencies rather than single tones. The lowest decibel level at which the patient recognizes two-syllable words correctly 50% of the time is called the speech reception threshold (SRT). The SRT and PTA are usually in agreement in geriatric patients (± 5 dB) if allowance is made for the slow reaction time encountered in many elderly patients.

Speech discrimination is then determined through the use of monosyllabic words at a comfortable level (35 dB) above the threshold. At this level, average normal young people will understand 100% of what they hear. The score ranges from 0% to 100%, with many elderly people exhibiting speech discrimination of 50% (i.e., they understand about 50% of what they are hearing at a comfortably loud level). Speech discrimination can be categorized as "excellent" (over 90%), "very good" (over 80%), "good" (over 70%), "fair" (50% to 70%), "poor" (40% to 50%), and "very poor" (less than 40%). For the sake of clarity,

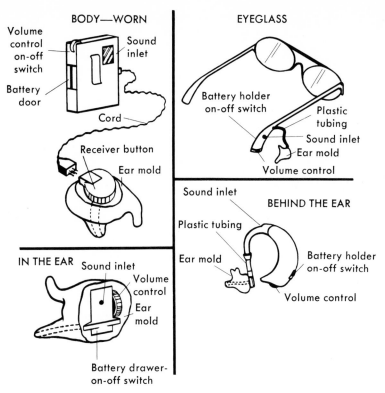

BODY—WORN

Volume
control
on-off
switch

Sound
inlet

Battery
door

Cord

Receiver button

Ear mold

EYEGLASS

Battery holder
on-off switch

Plastic
tubing

Sound inlet

Ear mold

Volume control

Sound inlet

BEHIND THE EAR

Plastic tubing

Ear mold

Battery holder
on-off switch

Volume control

IN THE EAR

Sound inlet

Volume
control

Ear
mold

Battery drawer-
on-off switch

Fig. 9-8. Types of hearing aids. (From Schow, R. L., Christensen, J. M., Hutchinson, J. M., and Nerbonne, M. A.: Communication disorders of the aged: a guide for health professionals, Baltimore, 1978, University Park Press; Courtesy Beltone Electronics Corp., Chicago, Ill.)

the actual percentages should be given in addition to the category.

THE HEARING AID

Despite the high prevalence of hearing loss among the elderly, only about 30% of those who need hearing aids actually have them. This strikingly low percentage may be attributable to (1) the belief that an elderly person may have that his hearing loss is a normal part of aging, (2) the lack of awareness by the physician and/or patient that a hearing loss exists, (3) denial of the hearing impairment by the individual, (4) the often prohibitive cost of a hearing aid (approximately $400 to $500) and the lack of Medicare reimbursement for it, (5) the negative social stigma that is attached to the hearing aid user, and (6) discouraging advice from other hearing aid users who had unrealistic expectations of the device.

Improvements and modifications in design and construction of hearing aids have enabled a greater proportion of the hearing-impaired population to profit from amplification. Many of today's successful hearing aid users would have been regarded as extremely poor risks in the past. Every individual who has communication difficulties due to a permanent hearing loss, no matter how slight or severe the deficit, should have access to an evaluation for amplification and to aural rehabilitation.

Since the majority of elderly people with difficulty in hearing have a sensorineural hearing loss from presbycusis, compensation through the use of a hearing aid should be considered.

Hearing aid components

The electronic hearing aid is similar to a public address system. The three basic components are a microphone for input of the signal, an amplifier to intensify the sound, and a speaker to transmit the louder sound.[13] These components all fit into the body of the ear-level hearing aid. An ear mold, custom fitted to the patient's ear canal, directs the sound into the canal.

Hearing aids come in a variety of styles, including the body aid, the behind-the-ear aid (postauricular), the eyeglass aid, and the in-the-ear aid (Fig. 9-8). Body aids are more powerful, provide a large amount of amplification, and are necessary for those patients with a severe or profound hearing loss. The controls are large, which makes them easier to manipulate — especially for elderly people. Many seriously impaired elderly individuals, however, prefer ear-level hearing aids, although the patient's aural function may be less efficient with this type of aid. The behind-the-ear hearing aid is the most popular type and accounts for 67% of sales; eyeglass aids account for 23% of sales, body aids for 7% of sales, and in-the-ear aids for 3% of sales. In-the-ear aids are very small, which makes them difficult for the aged to manipulate; in addition, they are not suitable for patients with a serious hearing deficit.

There are three basic components to

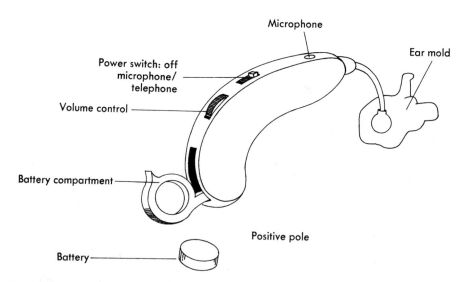

Fig. 9-9. Controls of a behind-the-ear hearing aid. (From Schow, R. L., Christensen, J. M., Hutchinson, J. M., and Nerbonne, M. A.: Communication disorders of the aged: a guide for health professionals, Baltimore, 1978, University Park Press.)

hearing aids: the volume control (to increase or decrease the intensity of the signal), the off/microphone/telephone control, and the battery compartment. These controls, although small and difficult to manipulate for some elderly individuals, can be mastered by most after proper instruction. The controls on the postauricular hearing aid are illustrated in Fig. 9-9.

AURAL REHABILITATION, INCLUDING HEARING AID EVALUATION AND UTILIZATION

The purposes of the hearing aid evaluation are to assess the need for amplification, to estimate the benefit to be derived from a hearing aid, and to determine the aid characteristics needed for effective hearing aid utilization.

The following questions, as modified from Hodgson and Skinner,[14] should be considered during the evaluation:

1. Is there a medical problem that would contraindicate amplification or, if corrected, remove the need for a hearing aid? To ensure that these possibilities are considered, all patients must have medical clearance prior to getting a hearing aid. Examination by a physician prior to the purchase of an aid is required by the Food and Drug Administration.[15]

2. Is the hearing deficit amenable to hearing aid use? The more severe the loss, the greater the need. The patient receives the greatest satisfaction with amplification when the loss is between 55 and 80 dB. When the loss is more than 80 dB, only partial help is obtained from the amplification because of impaired speech discrimination.

3. Is discrimination ability adequate for hearing aid use? How much distortion is present in the hearing mechanism? The poorer the discrimination, the less the satisfaction to be obtained with amplification.

4. Are the patient's expectations from an aid realistic? He must be made aware of the fact that a hearing aid is only one aspect of a comprehensive aural rehabilitation program consisting of speech reading and family counseling, if appropriate. A hearing aid is specifically designed to be useful in face-to-face conversation, and its utility decreases with further distance from the source. Even limited improvement can be beneficial, however, and enhance overall functioning.

5. What are the demands on the patient's hearing?

6. What is the tolerance level for loud sound? Is the patient annoyed or irritated by a loud sound due to recruitment phenomena associated with sensorineural loss, or is the patient just unable to adjust to louder sounds because of psychological reasons?

7. What type of aid is needed? Behind-the-ear or body aid? Monaural (one ear has a hearing aid) or binaural (each ear has a hearing aid)? If a monaural aid is needed, which ear should be fitted, and with what modifications on the aid?

8. What kind of training is needed? A short course in orientation and aid manipulation or full aural rehabilitation including speech reading and counseling?

9. Can the patient handle the aid independently, or is partial or complete assistance required?

10. Does the patient want the hearing aid? Motivation is an extremely important factor in determining success or failure to adjust to amplification.

The answers to these questions should provide information helpful in determining the prognosis regarding the patient's ability to accept and benefit from amplification.

During the evaluation, a decision has to be made regarding whether the aid should be monaural or binaural—and, if monaural, which ear should be fitted. The advantages of a binaural aid, under ideal circumstances, include (1) improved speech reception threshold; (2) improved speech discrimination, especially in a noisy environment, and (3) better localization of sound. Binaural aids, however, are difficult for many elderly to use.

The following guidelines should be considered in the decision of which ear to fit with a hearing aid[16]:

1. In general, choose the ear that results in the maximum functional improvement as measured by formal and informal tests.

2. Fit the ear with the best speech discrimination.

3. If the poorer ear has a moderate loss and the better ear a mild loss, fit the poorer ear to enable the better ear to participate in communication situations.

4. If the loss is more serious and the poorer ear has a profound loss and the better one a severe loss, fit the better ear, since less distortion will be present in that ear.

5. If the ears are similar, the right ear may be chosen if the patient is right-handed.

If the test results indicate that a specific hearing aid will improve functioning and the aid is acceptable to the patient, it should be ordered from the hearing aid vendor for a 2- to 4-week trial. An impression for a custom ear mold is obtained, and within a week's time the ear mold and the hearing aid are dispensed. If the patient cannot adjust to amplification for any reason, the hearing aid is returned to the hearing aid vendor within 4 weeks (allowed by law) of the date it was dispensed. This service may be provided free of charge or for a rental fee.

The relationship between the need for amplification and the need for training and other rehabilitation devices is a function of the magnitude of the hearing loss. Intensive aural rehabilitation, including lipreading, is available if it is suitable to the patient's needs. Poor vision, however, may make lipreading difficult for an elderly patient. The following general guidelines, as recommended by Lundborg and others,[17] should be used to determine the patient's needs:

1. For a 60-dB loss (moderate to moderately severe loss), the patient requires ear-level amplification and an instruction course in the use of the hearing aid and other amplifiers, occasionally along with aural rehabilitation (lipreading, counseling, etc.).

2. For a 60- to 80-dB loss (moderately severe to severe loss), the patient requires a body aid (ear-level, if the patient insists), instruction in the use of amplification and lipreading, and general aural rehabilitation for those able to benefit.

3. For a loss of 80 dB and over (severe to profound loss), the patient requires a body aid and a full aural rehabilitation program. A smaller percentage will benefit in this category.

Some authorities would recommend a hearing aid for those with a hearing loss of 40 to 60 dB.

In addition to hearing aids, there are amplifiers and warning devices using light or vibration that can assist the patient with a hearing loss. These devices can be purchased from hearing aid dealers, the telephone company, and electronic shops, and include light-flashing alarm clocks, vibrating pillows that are connected to an alarm clock, doorbells that activate a flashing light, and various telephone and television amplifiers.

Each patient receiving a hearing aid is scheduled for a course in hearing aid orientation whether or not he is an experienced hearing aid user. This course is designed to familiarize the patient with the controls of the aid, insertion and removal of the ear mold and aid, and battery changing. If a specific task is beyond the capability of the patient, a relative or friend is requested to assist and support the patient so that the hearing aid can be utilized.

After therapy is concluded, regular assessment of the patient's functioning with the aid takes place; if hearing deteriorates, counseling and training are resumed. It is not uncommon after any type of illness, including surgery, for the patient to temporarily regress in his ability to use his hearing aid. Resumption of therapy is then needed if the patient is to readjust to amplification. Monitoring to guard against aid malfunctioning (e.g., dead battery or obstructed plastic tubing) is ongoing in order to ensure continuous utilization of the hearing aid.

Solutions to the problems of rejection of amplification lie in the areas of education, orientation, and a systematic approach to the assessment, fitting, and adjustment of the elderly individual to the effective use of amplification. It is possible to fit any hard-of-hearing patient with a hearing aid, provided that the patient is mentally and physically able to handle it, and thereby enable him to improve his communication ability.

Multidisciplinary cooperation is required to stimulate the desire and the ability of the hard-of-hearing elderly to communicate. There is justification for an optimistic outlook with regard to aural rehabilitation of the elderly patient to ensure effective communication with others.

Patient education material that may facilitate the adjustment to amplification and assist individuals in communicating with the hard of hearing are included here:

Guidelines for hearing aid users

1. Practice inserting and removing the hearing aid until it is done easily. Put the aid on when relaxed. If you are unable to handle the aid, make sure that your relative or friend can help you.
2. Wear the hearing aid 4 to 5 hours at first. Wear it for a longer period of time the next day. After a week, it should be worn all day.
3. Remove the hearing aid before going to bed, bathing, or showering.
4. Make sure the battery is inserted correctly. Follow + sign for placement of + side of battery. If there is no on-off switch, open the battery case at night to shut the aid off; this will conserve battery power. If there is an M-T-O (microphone-telephone-off) switch on the aid, turn to *O* for off at night. Don't forget to turn back to *M* in the morning to turn the aid on.
5. Clean the ear mold daily with a damp cloth. Once a week wipe the mold with a cloth dampened with mild soapy water. If the ear mold gets plugged with wax, clean it out with a toothpick or bent paper clip — carefully!
6. Change the batteries every 10 days to 2 weeks. If a whistle (feedback) is *not* heard when the volume control is fully on, change the battery and the whistle should then be heard. If no whistle is heard despite a new battery, then the problem is in the aid itself.
7. Remember, the aid is a mechanical instrument. Sounds and voices are made louder, not clearer. Expectations should be realistic.
8. Extraneous noises may annoy you at first. Identify the sounds and then forget them.

You will get used to hearing background sounds in a short period of time.
9. If the problem persists, the aid should be tested by the audiologist or hearing aid dealer.

Problems with adjustment faced by patients with a new hearing aid
1. After living in a quiet world, suddenly hearing loud voices and noises can cause the patient to become tense and nervous.
2. Adjusting the hearing aid in public or asking for assistance in caring for it can be traumatic because of embarrassment.
3. Poor memory can lead to problems such as forgetting to turn off the aid or forgetting when and how to change batteries.
4. Poor vision and/or manual dexterity can lead to difficulty in changing the batteries, placing them backward, or problems inserting the mold in the ear.

Communicating with the hard-of-hearing[18]
1. Speak to the patient on his aided side. The head blocks the sound of the voice if you stand on his unaided side. If the patient has a severe hearing loss and needs visual clues to understand speech, stand in front of him so that he can see your face.
2. Do not shout. Speak distinctly and slowly, but do not exaggerate lip movements, which will confuse the listener.
3. Adjust your position so that light from the lamp or window is on your face.
4. Stand close enough to allow easy observation of your face but not so close that the listener is uncomfortable because of your nearness. Stand no closer than 2 feet.
5. Look directly at the patient and encourage him to look at you.
6. Do not cover your mouth with hands or papers.
7. If the patient fails to understand your meaning, rephrase or reword rather than repeat. This method is more effective and less embarrassing.
8. The patient will "hear" better if it is quiet. For example, turn the television or radio down or take him to a quiet area.

9. If the patient indicates that he is not understanding, gesture or write down important words to help him follow the conversation.
10. The individual may not enjoy some activities, because his hearing aid not only makes the speaker's voice louder, but amplifies everyone's speech around him and other noises in the room as well. Activities suitable for him include lectures where he can see the speaker's face and talking with one or two persons rather than a group.
11. Motivation to communicate is essential to satisfactory adjustment to a hearing aid. Your understanding should help to increase this motivation. Speak to the patient whever possible and encourage him to socialize and verbalize. Be considerate and patient. *The attitude of individuals in daily contact with the patient is vitally important to successful adjustment to amplification.*

REFERENCES

1. Prevalence of chronic conditions and impairments, National Health Survey, PHS Pub. No. 10000, Series 12, No. 8, 1967, U.S. Department of Health, Education, and Welfare.
2. Chafee, C. E.: Rehabilitation needs of nursing home patients, Rehabil. Lit. **18**:377, 1967.
3. Newby, H. A.: Audiology, New York, 1966, Appleton-Century-Crofts, pp. 33-34, 46-47.
4. Green, M. F.: Incidence of deafness from wax. In Brocklehurst, J. C., editor: Geriatric medicine and geronotology, ed. 2, Edinburgh, Eng., 1978, Churchill Livingstone, p. 281.
5. Alberti, P. W.: Hearing problems in a geriatric population, J. Otolaryngol. **6**(suppl 4), 1977.
6. Feldman, R. G., Culebras, A., and Schmidek, H. H.: Paget's disease and the nervous system, J. Am. Geriatr. Soc. **27**:1, 1979.
7. Solomon, L. R.: Effect of calcitonin treatment on deafness due to Paget's disease of bone, Br. Med. J. **2**:485, 1977.
8. Hull, R. H., and Trainor, R. M.: Hearing impairment among aging persons in the health care facility: their diagnosis and rehabilitation, Am. Health Care Assoc. J. **3**:14-18, 1977.
9. Schuknecht, H. R.: Further observation on the pathology of presbycusis, Arch. Otolaryngol. **80**:369, 1964.

10. Corso, J. F.: Presbycusis, hearing loss and aging, Audiology **16**:146, 1977.
11. Alpiner, J. G., editor: Handbook of adult rehabilitative audiology, Baltimore, The Williams & Wilkins Co., 1978. pp. 145-146.
12. Appel, G. B., and Neu, H. C.: Gentamicin in 1978, Ann. Intern. Med. **89**:528, 1978.
13. Schow, R. L., Christensen, J. M., Hutchinson, J. M., and Nerbonne, M. A.: Communication disorders of the aged: a guide for health professionals, Baltimore, 1978, University Park Press, pp. 348-349.
14. Hodgson, W. R., and Skinner, P. H., editors: Hearing aid assessment and use in audiologic habilitation, Baltimore, 1977, The Williams & Wilkins Co., pp. 127-128, 215.
15. Federal Register, 1977, pp. 9, 295.
16. Berger, K. W., and Millin, J. P.: Hearing aids. In Rose, D. E., editor: Audiological assessment, ed. 2, Englewood Cliffs, N.J., 1978, Prentice-Hall, Inc., p. 525.
17. Lundborg, T., Linzander, S., Rosenhamer, H., and others: Experience with hearing aids in adults, Scand. Audiol. (Suppl. 3):9, 1973.
18. Haug, O., and Haug, S.: Help for the hard of hearing. Springfield, Ill., 1977, Charles C Thomas, Publisher, p. 17.

PROBLEM-SOLVING EXERCISES*
Case one

Mrs. E. G. is 79 years old and lives with her husband in a retirement community in Arizona. Her medical diagnoses include: congestive heart failure secondary to arteriosclerotic cardiovascular disease, myocardial infarction, a complete recovery from right-sided hemiparesis, and osteoarthritis of the knees. Her prescribed medications include digoxin, furosemide, and potassium supplements. Although not prescribed, she takes five to ten aspirins per day, regularly. On routine audiological screening at a senior citizens' center, Mrs. G. is noted to have impaired hearing manifested by a 38-dB threshold in the right ear and a 50-dB threshold in the left ear. Since these results are poorer than 30-dB bilaterally and 45-dB at 4,000 and 8,000 Hz, she is referred for a complete otolaryngological and audiological evaluation. The otolaryn-

gological evaluation does not reveal any external or middle ear disease. The audiological evaluation shows slightly improved results: 35-dB in the right ear and 38-dB in the left ear, pure-tone average (PTA), indicative of a bilaterally symmetrical mild sensorineural hearing loss. Speech reception tests (SRT) results indicate 40-dB in the right ear and 35 dB in the left ear. (Normal range is 0 to 20-dB.) Speech discrimination is excellent: 96% in the right ear and 92% in the left ear. No further testing is necessary.

Question

1. What could be the cause(s) of this improvement?
   a. Normal variability in testing
   b. Apprehension during screening at the senior citizens' center
   c. Impacted cerumen
   d. All of the above

Three months later, when Mrs. G. is seen by her primary care physician for a routine visit to assess her congestive heart failure, considerable difficulties in communication are noted. Her hearing loss seems to be markedly worse, and tinnitus is present bilaterally. The patient is referred for a second audiological evaluation. The audiogram at this time shows poorer results than previously noted, consistent with a bilateral moderate severe sensorineural hearing loss with an SRT of 70-dB in the right ear and 65-dB in the left ear. Speech discrimination is poorer than before, indicating 72% in the right ear and 52% in the left ear. There is no evidence of vertigo or vomiting. The patient, however, is inattentive and dozes off in the chair.

Questions

2. This dramatic drop in hearing acuity could be attributed to the following:
   a. Normal progression of presbycusis
   b. Impacted cerumen
   c. Meniere's disease
   d. Ototoxicity
3. The most likely drug to be causing this marked loss in hearing is:
   a. Phenylbutazone

---

*Some questions may have more than one correct answer.

b. Aspirin
c. Furosemide
d. Digoxin

Case two

Mr. M. T., an 88-year-old man, has been admitted to a skilled nursing facility for rehabilitation following a fracture of his right hip that occurred when he was hit by a car while crossing the street. During his hospitalization he suffered an uncomplicated myocardial infarction and a catheter-induced urinary tract infection. He is described by the nursing staff as being very deaf.

Question

1. Discuss possible causes of Mr. T.'s hearing loss. What other information would you like?

Otolaryngological examination reveals no corrective outer or middle ear disease. Audiological testing is difficult because the patient is unable to respond to stimuli and dozes in the chair. Depression and hostility are present. Test results indicate a bilateral mixed and moderately severe hearing loss. Speech discrimination is fair in the right ear (48%) and very poor in the left ear (24%). Subsequent hearing aid evaluations are difficult because of the negativism, hostility, and, despair of the patient. Thyroid screening tests performed on admission to the skilled nursing facility reveal a low serum T4 and an elevated TSH level. Thyroxin is started slowly.

Subsequently, the patient has a hearing aid evaluation because the nursing staff report that his attitude has improved.

Question

2. What reversible hearing losses can be detected by audiological evaluation?

Following a period of thyroid replacement and hearing aide usage, the patient appears alert and cooperative, and maintains good eye contact. His physical condition has improved, and he cooperates with audiological testing and with the hearing aid evaluation. The patient's affect improves and he becomes in-

volved in his surroundings and interested in returning home. He is capable of manipulating the hearing aid without assistance and participating in the rehabilitation of his hip fracture.

ANSWERS TO PROBLEM-SOLVING CASE HISTORIES
Case one

1. a and b. Impacted cerumen does not cause a sensorineural loss; rather, it causes a conductive loss.
2. d. Presbycusis progresses more gradually and is bilateral and irreversible. Cerumen causes a conductive hearing loss. The clinical picture is not consistent with Meniere's disease because of the lack of vertigo and nausea. Medication is clearly a possibility for the sensorineural hearing loss. Ototoxic drugs affecting hearing and vestibular function could be a likely cause.
3. b. Aspirin is the nonprescribed drug most commonly used by the elderly. Mrs. G. has been taking it for her arthritis. Tinnitus is often the first indication of aspirin ototoxicity. Discontinuation of the aspirin should result in improved hearing.

Case two

1. Possible causes of Mr. T.'s hearing loss include a sensorineural component caused by presbycusis, noise-induced hearing loss, drug-induced ototoxicity, or Meniere's disease. A conductive loss could be caused by cerumen, external otitis, atresia of the external auditory meatus, or middle ear disease (including otitis media, otosclerosis, chronic serous otitis media, and chronic suppurative otitis media).

   Other information would include any history of hearing loss in the family; medications; associated dizziness; nausea, vomiting, tinnitus, and/or pain; exposure to loud noises; a history of ear infections; and/or trauma.
2. Reversible causes that can be detected by audiological examination include cerumen, any of the otitis medias, and possibly otosclerosis. Presbycusis cannot be re-

versed, but the hearing loss can be improved by amplification. This patient's depression and level of mentation, as well as his hearing, has improved with thyroid replacement and aural rehabilitation.

POSTTEST*

1. Hearing loss in the elderly may result from:
    a. Paget's disease
    b. Otosclerosis
    c. Senile dementia
    d. Cerumen
    e. Otitis media
2. You are evaluating a patient with supposed global aphasia. You find that the patient has a marked decrease in word discrimination (i.e., decreased ability to understand speech). His condition may be:
    a. Due to presbycusis associated with aging
    b. Associated with other pathological conditions of peripheral parts of the auditory system
    c. Associated with other pathological conditions of central parts of the auditory system
    d. The result of a conductive hearing loss
3. In the patient with presbycusis, which of the following are true?
    a. The onset of hearing loss is gradual.
    b. There is often a family history.
    c. There is often a history of fluctuation (the patient will hear better if not fatigued, e.g., in the early morning).
    d. The patient's hearing is very much disturbed by background noise.
    e. The patient says he watches television but cannot understand it.
4. The elderly individual may purchase a hearing aid:
    a. Only after having the need confirmed by a physician

   b. And receive reimbursement from Medicare
   c. Directly from a hearing aid dealer without prior examination by a physician after signing a waiver
5. The function of the total hearing system (conductive and sensorineural components) is reflected in the:
    a. Air conduction test
    b. Bone conduction test
6. To determine whether a hearing deficit should be classified as conductive, sensorineural, or mixed, the following test(s) should be used:
    a. Air conduction threshold
    b. Bone conduction threshold
    c. Both
7. A patient is referred to you with bone conduction thresholds indicating impaired hearing. He may have:
    a. Otosclerosis
    b. Otitis media
    c. A scarred tympanic membrane
    d. Impacted cerumen
    e. Presbycusis
8. Ototoxic drugs are:
    a. Digoxin
    b. Streptomycin
    c. Gentamicin
    d. Phenylbutazone
    e. Aspirin
9. The elderly individual who is having difficulty in hearing with his new hearing aid:
    a. May not know how to use the aid properly
    b. May not have the appropriate aid
    c. May lack the motivation to use a hearing aid
    d. May have poor speech discrimination

ANSWERS TO PRETEST AND POSTTEST

1. a, b, d, and e. These are pathological conditions that cause hearing loss. Senile dementia can cause the patient to be "difficult to test" (i.e., he cannot follow directions or responds inconsistently, leading to unreliable test results). Senile dementia itself does not cause a hearing loss, although it may complicate or invalidate the audiological assessment.

2. a, b, and c. Item a is correct because one of the concomitants of presbycusis is reduced speech discrimination. This is due to deterioration of all components of the auditory system as a result of many years of accumulated insults. Since the auditory nerve and/or the cortex are affected, speech discrimination is poorer than would be expected from the pure-tone test results. Item b is correct because cranial nerve VIII is part of the peripheral auditory system; if a pathological condition is present, reduced speech discrimination results. Item c is correct because speech discrimination is reduced by a pathological condition in the central auditory system. Cortical degeneration is a common finding in many patients with presbycusis. Item d is incorrect because patients with a conductive hearing loss usually have unimpaired speech discrimination if the stimulus is loud enough for them to hear it.

3. All of these.

4. a and c. Item a is correct because the Food and Drug Administration requires an examination by a physician prior to the dispensing of a hearing aid. Item b is incorrect because Medicare does not reimburse the patient for a hearing aid. Item c is correct because if the patient is over 18 years of age and signs a waiver, he may obtain a hearing aid without an examination by a physician.

5. a. In the air conduction test, earphones are placed on the patient's ears, and the air-conducted stimulus passes through and assesses the integrity of the complete auditory system. Bone conduction (item b) does not test the integrity of the total hearing system; rather it tests the cochlea, cranial nerve VIII, and the brain.

6. c. The air conduction test assesses the complete auditory mechanism and determines whether a pathological condition is present (whether the patient has a hearing loss). It does not reveal where the loss is or help to determine the type of hearing loss present. The bone conduction test is the first site-of-lesion test done in the test battery. If air conduction testing reveals a loss of 50 dB (thresholds are averaged across frequencies) and bone conduction testing also indicates an average loss of 50 dB, then the pathological condition exists in the cochlea and/or in the auditory nerve and is a sensorineural hearing loss.

7. e. The other pathological conditions are restricted to the outer and/or middle ear and therefore cause only a conductive loss.

8. b, c, and e. These are ototoxic drugs; the others are not.

9. All of these.

Chapter 10

Visual disorders

CYRUS KAHN

EDUCATIONAL OBJECTIVES
Attitudinal

The student should:

1. Recognize that loss of vision is not necessarily a part of normal aging
2. Recognize that evaluation of vision and of the eye is an integral part of the physical examination.

Cognitive

The student should:

1. Be aware of normal age-related changes in the eye and know their effects on occular function
2. Be aware of common eyelid conditions in the elderly
3. Know the major causes of reversible and irreversible visual loss in the elderly
4. Know the visual symptoms of acute angle-closure and chronic open-angle glaucoma, cataracts, and senile macular degeneration
5. Know how to diagnose primary open-angle glaucoma, cataracts, and senile macular degeneration
6. Know the effects of various topical and systemic drugs used in the treatment of primary open-angle glaucoma
7. Know the visual consequences of cataract extraction and options for correcting them
8. Know the definition of presbyopia

Skill

The student should:

1. Know how to use the tonometer and ophthalmoscope to diagnose glaucoma, cataracts, and macular degeneration
2. Be able to explain to the elderly patient the problems of cataract extraction (aphakic vision)

PRETEST°

1. The leading cause of irreversible blindness in the elderly is:
   a. Cataracts
   b. Diabetic retinopathy
   c. Ischemic optic atrophy
   d. Senile macular degeneration

2. *True or false:* Normal aging is associated with the reduced production of tears.

3. Following cataract surgery, the patient's vision with glasses may not be satisfactory. Explain.

4. *True or false:* Cataract surgery should not be performed until the lens is mature.

5. *True or false:* Open-angle glaucoma results from a buildup of pressure in the posterior chamber.

6. The most common form of glaucoma in the older population is:

a. Primary open-angle glaucoma
b. Secondary open-angle glaucoma
c. Primary angle-closure glaucoma
d. Secondary angle-closure glaucoma

7. What factors must be considered in evaluating the elderly glaucoma patient's need for medication?

8. *True or false:* Senile macular degeneration follows disruption of Bruch's membrane.

°Some questions may have more than one correct answer.

207

9. *True or false:* Topical beta-adrenergic blocking agents have fewer visual side effects than pilocarpine in the treatment of primary open-angle glaucoma in the elderly.

A major consideration in the care of older patients is their visual requirements. As the elderly individual's senses diminish because of normal aging or pathological processes, social withdrawal may occur. It is important to maintain the elderly individuals' visual contact with his environment so that he can actively participate in community life.

HISTORY TAKING AND PHYSICAL EXAMINATION

A brief evaluation of the elderly patient's visual symptoms and status should be performed in the course of the routine history and physical examination. In the course of obtaining a history and systems review, one should ascertain whether the patient has any subjective complaints regarding his eyes.

The examiner should obtain the patient's visual acuity with and without corrective lenses by having the patient read a Snellen chart or a reading card; or, if these are unavailable, the examiner can use any printed material to make a rough approximation of acuity. The visual fields can be grossly determined by the technique of confrontation.

With a penlight, the lids and lashes can be evaluated for any signs of inflammation (loss of lashes, crusting of the lid margins, or discharge) or for malposition or other abnormalities. The symmetry of the pupils and their response to light, both direct and consensual, should also be observed.

With the ophthalmoscope set at about +2 to +3 diopters and the observer positioned approximately 18 inches from the eye, the optical media can be evaluated. Any distortion of the red reflex may be indicative of the presence of a cataract or of vitreous floaters. A simple test to differentiate between the two is to shift the viewing angle slightly from side to side. If the opacities appear in the same position, they are probably located in the lens, whereas if they appear to shift in the same direction as the observer moves, they are probably in the vitreous. The examiner can then move closer to the patient and focus on the retina.

To evaluate ocular motility, the examiner should ask the patient to fixate on a target, such as a finger or penlight, and have him follow the fixation target through the cardinal fields of gaze. While the patient fixates on the target and alternately covers each eye, the examiner can detect a strabismic problem by noting any movement of the covered eye as the cover is removed and shifted to the opposite eye. The inability of the eye to follow the target may be indicative of an extraocular muscle palsy from a cerebrovascular or neoplastic process, or other neuromuscular problem.

The intraocular pressure should be determined. An applanation tonometer is the most accurate way to measure the intraocular pressure. However, this instrument may not always be available. A reliable measurement can be obtained with a Schiötz tonometer. The examiner places a drop of topical anesthetic (proparacaine hydrochloride [Ophthaine, Ophthetic], tetracaine hydrochloride [Pontocaine] into each eye and, with the patient in a reclining position, places the Schiötz tonometer on the cornea. One must be careful not to place any pressure against the globe while holding the lids open, since this will give a falsely elevated pressure reading. It is also necessary that the tonometer be clean, that it be placed perpendicular to the cornea, and that the sleeve of the tonometer arm float freely.

The entire ophthalmic examination can be performed without the addition of more than a few minutes to the time necessary for a complete physical examination of the patient.

CONDITIONS OF THE EYELIDS

In addition to their apparent cosmetic and protective functions, the eyelids are of vital importance to the eye. Indeed, when the functions of the lids are compromised by trauma or disease, the viability of the globe becomes severely jeopardized. By their repeated blinking action, the lids maintain an even distribution of moisture across the surface of the cornea, thereby ensuring the integrity of the corneal epithelium.

Entropion

The normal aging process results in loss of the elasticity of the skin and diminished muscle tone of the lid. With elongation of the lid and loss of lid muscle tone, the lid margin may pull away from its normal approximation to the globe. If the lower lid margin now rotates inward against the globe (a condition called entropion), the lashes, which ordinarily help defend the globe from foreign body intrusion, will now rub against the cornea, causing damage.[1-3] Aside from the annoyance of a constant foreign body sensation, the action of the lashes against the cornea may lead to a breakdown of the corneal epithelium and set the stage for bacterial or viral invasion.

There are many surgical procedures to correct entropion and thereby restore the normal anatomic position of the lid against the globe.[3-5] While awaiting a surgical procedure, the patient with severe entropion can have the lower lid held to its normal position by a small strip of ½- to 1-inch adhesive tape, applied to the lid below the lashes and attached to the skin over the cheekbone.

Ectropion

With laxity and elongation of the lid, a different set of forces may lead to eversion of the lid margin, called ectropion (Fig. 10-1). Although potentially less damaging to the eye, ectropion causes enough symptoms to make the patient uncomfortable.[6-9] In ectropion, the tears overflow and the patient suffers from constant tearing (epiphora). If the degree of ectropion is severe, the exposed palpebral conjunctiva will no longer be bathed in the tear film layer and the resulting chronic dryness will lead to metaplasia and keratinization of the epithelium. The drying effects of ectropion can be partially ameliorated by various lubricating medications in drop and/or ointment form. Ultimately ectropion requires surgical correction, usually in the form of lid shortening.[1-3]

Loss of lid closure

A dramatic example of the importance of the lids is evidenced by the chain of events that follows the loss of normal lid closure. This is most apparent in the comatose patient, but it can also be seen in patients with facial palsies. Without the protective effects of blinking, the corneal epithelium begins to dry and becomes devitalized. The eye quickly reddens as the epithelium sloughs, exposing the corneal stroma. Even without secondary infection, the dried cornea

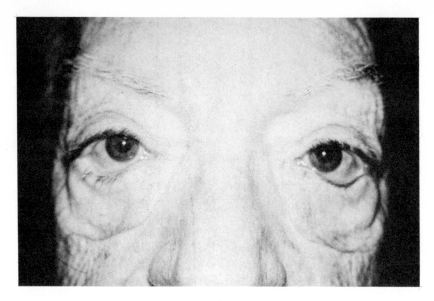

Fig. 10-1. Ectropion revealing exposed conjunctiva.

undergoes thinning and ultimately may result in perforation and loss of the eye.

These sequelae can be prevented if the exposed eye is kept adequately moistened. To tide the patient over the early stages of corneal exposure, a bland ophthalmic ointment or even mineral oil should be instilled into the eyes frequently. The lids can be temporarily closed with strips of adhesive tape. If lid function does not return early and the eye appears compromised, a tarsorrhaphy (surgical fusion of the upper and lower lids) can be performed. At a later date, when the patient's condition improves, the sutures can be taken out.

Chronic blepharitis

One of the most common ophthalmic problems in the older population is chronic blepharitis.[7] This is a form of seborrhea involving the eyelashes. Primarily as a result of poor facial hy-

giene and a lack of stimulation of the lid tissues, secretions accumulate around the roots of the lashes. The secretions lead to chronic irritation and secondary bacterial infection, usually by staphylococci. Blepharitis clinically presents with encrusted lid margins that are inflamed and edematous. In severe cases, there may be a progressive loss of lashes and recurring chalazion. Toxins produced by staphylococci can cause marginal ulcerations of the cornea.

Chronic blepharitis usually responds to topical antibiotics alone (e.g., sodium sulfacetamide) or in combination with low concentrations of a steroid Meticulous attention must be paid to facial hygiene. The lids should be washed frequently with a clean cloth and warm water). In more severe cases the lid margins can be "shampooed" every few days with a dab of nonirritating baby shampoo on a washcloth. The application of a small amount of petroleum jelly or baby oil to the roots of the lashes at bedtime may also be helpful.

Tearing

Tissue laxity of the lids also impairs the drainage of tears from the lacrimal sac. The emptying of the lacrimal sac depends on the contractions of the orbicularis muscle in the closing of the lids: the lacrimal pump mechanism.[1] With loss of tone, the forcefulness of the contractions diminishes and complete emptying of the lacrimal sac does not occur. Consequently, secretions accumulate in the lacrimal drainage system and may lead to infection in the tear sac. Pressure applied over the inner aspect of the lower lid near the nose may cause a mucoid or mucopurulent secretion to be expressed from the lower punctum. Treatment of tear sac infection requires consultation with an ophthalmologist.

As a normal accompaniment of the aging process, there is a reduction in tear production. In some ways this can be viewed as a compensatory reaction: as the lid tissues became more lax and the lacrimal excretory system less efficient the eye would find itself unable to handle the normal rate of tear secretion and epiphora (excessive tearing) would result. The amount of baseline tear production can be readily measured with a small strip of filter paper placed so as to overhang the lid of the anesthetized eye (Schirmer's test). After 5 minutes the paper is removed and the amount of wetting measured. The normal elderly individual will wet 10 to 15 ml of paper within the 5-minute period.[8]

If drying is excessive, the patient will develop a burning sensation in the eyes. Under the biomicroscope, the corneal epithelium will show punctate opacities, which represent devitalized epithelial cells. The problem of the dry eye is frequently seen in the elderly patient with Parkinson's disease, where diminished frequency of blinking makes the patient more vulnerable to the effects of reduced tear production. The dry eye can be treated by frequent instillations of any of the commercially prepared tear substitutes to supplement the patient's own tear production.

GLAUCOMA

The rate at which aqueous humor is produced, and the resistance to its escape from the eye, largely determines the intraocular pressure. When the pressure within the eye becomes elevated, causing damage to the optic nerve and subsequent loss of visual fields, a condition known as glaucoma exists. For purposes of classification, the types of glaucoma are divided into two large groups: primary glaucoma and secondary glaucoma. Each group can then be further divided into subgroups of those with open drainage angles and those with closed drainage angles.

With few exceptions, glaucoma results from an interference with the normal escape of aqueous humor from the anterior chamber of the eye (Fig. 10-2). The ciliary body, which is located behind the root of the iris, produces aqueous humor by an active metabolic process. Aqueous humor is released into the posterior chamber (that part of the eye bounded anteriorly by the posterior surface of the iris and pupil and posteriorly by the zonules of the lens and the anterior surface of the lens) and passes through the pupil into the anterior chamber. The aqueous humor normally leaves the anterior chamber by passing through the trabecular meshwork located at the junction of

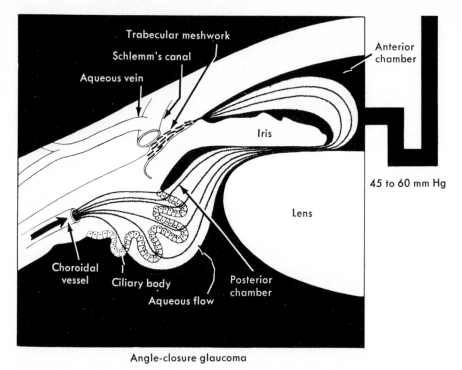

Angle-closure glaucoma

Fig. 10-2. Mechanisms of the rise of intraocular pressure in angle-closure glaucoma and in open-angle glaucoma. In angle-closure glaucoma, the root of the iris is in opposition with the trabecular meshwork.

the iris root and the corneoscleral junction (limbus) into the canal of Schlemm. From the canal of Schlemm, the aqueous humor flows into the systemic venous circulation. In the course of aging, there is a tendency for the trabecular meshwork to work less efficiently and for a gradual rise in intraocular pressure to occur.[9] This is usually offset by a corresponding diminished rate of aqueous production. The net result is that the intraocular pressure will still remain within normal limits in most cases.

Acute angle-closure glaucoma

Because of the apposition of the back of the iris against the anterior surface of the lens, the aqueous humor meets resistance as it works its way through the posterior chamber to the pupil and into the anterior chamber. In individuals with narrow anterior chambers, the slight rise in pressure in the posterior chamber can be sufficient to bow the iris root into apposition with the trabecular meshwork, thus closing off the route of egress of aqueous humor from the eye. Since the ciliary body is still producing aqueous humor, a rather rapid rise in intraocular pressure occurs and a situation known as acute angle-closure glaucoma develops. Because of the elevated pressure, the normal iris circulation becomes compromised and the iris becomes fixed in middilation. This is an ophthalmic emergency and must be dealt with promptly if the eye is to be salvaged.

A diagnosis of acute angle-closure

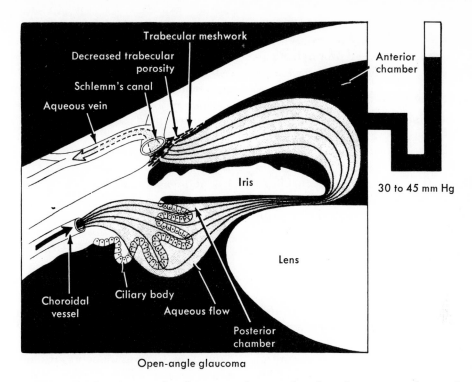

Trabecular meshwork

Decreased trabecular porosity

Schlemm's canal

Aqueous vein

Anterior chamber

Iris

30 to 45 mm Hg

Lens

Choroidal vessel

Ciliary body

Aqueous flow

Posterior chamber

Open-angle glaucoma

Fig. 10-2, cont'd. In open-angle glaucoma, decreased trabecular porosity limits the egress of aqueous humor. (Modified from Kolker, A. E., and Hetherington, J., Jr.: Becker-Shaffer's diagnosis and therapy of the glaucomas, ed. 4, St. Louis, 1976, The C. V. Mosby Co.)

glaucoma can be confirmed only by slit-lamp evaluation of the angle recess with a gonioprism: a contact lens containing an angled mirror that permits observation of the junction of the iris root at the limbus. In any situation, however, in which there is a red, painful eye with elevated pressure and a fixed, mid-dilated pupil, acute angle-closure glaucoma should be suspected; if ophthalmic care is not immediately available, therapy with frequent instillations of 2% pilocarpine should be initiated to pull the iris root out of the angle recess. In some cases it is necessary to supplement this with an oral hyperosmotic agent (glycerin), although the cardiopulmonary risks in the older

population must be weighed. Carbonic anhydrase inhibitors may also be used to reduce the rate of aqueous production.

Once the attack is broken, the patient must be maintained on a regimen of miotics until a peripheral iridectomy can be performed. This procedure equalizes the pressure between the anterior and posterior chambers and prevents the buildup of pressure behind the iris. Approximately one third of these patients are not completely cured by a peripheral iridectomy and still require medical therapy postoperatively in order to maintain their pressure at a normal level (below 20 to 21 mm of mercury). The other eye must also be considered, since the eyes tend to be symmetrical. It can be assumed that the unaffected eye may also be prone to attack and should be treated prophylactically with miotics until proven otherwise.

Chronic primary open-angle glaucoma

Chronic primary open-angle glaucoma, by far the most common type of glaucoma encountered in the elderly, affects approximately 5% of the 70- to 74-year-old age group. It is a complex and insidious problem caused by obstruction to the outflow of aqueous humor from the anterior chamber of the eye because of abnormalities in the trabecular meshwork. In this slowly progressive, usually bilateral type of glaucoma, the elderly patient is generally free of symptoms until relatively late in the disease process, when irreversible disc changes have taken place and the patient has sustained loss of peripheral vision, with perhaps some loss in central acuity. It thus becomes critical to closely monitor the intraocular pressure and the appearance of the optic disc in the older population.

The decision as to when and how to initiate therapy is based on the pattern of the intraocular pressure, the appearance of the optic nerve and visual fields, and experience. In some older patients it is not always possible to obtain accurate visual fields, because the patient is unable to cooperate because of reduced ability to concentrate on the test. Consequently, the decision to treat patients with borderline pressure becomes more dependent on other factors, such as a positive family history and a trend toward elevated intraocular pressure over a period of months. A family history of glaucoma may be helpful in establishing a diagnosis of glaucoma (open or closed), since there have been many reports of an inheritable nature to glaucoma.[10]

An entity that must be differentiated from chronic glaucoma is benign ocular hypertension, which affects 15% of the 70- to 75-year-old age group. While the intraocular pressure is elevated above normal in benign ocular hypertension, the visual fields and optic disc remain unchanged. There is no easy way to differentiate benign ocular hypertension from chronic glaucoma except for frequent measurements of the intraocular tension, the visual fields, and the cup-disc ratio. Benign ocular hypertension does not require therapy.

In recent years there has been an increasing awareness of a condition known as low-tension glaucoma.[11] In this condition, the optic nerve undergoes the characteristic disc changes of glaucoma with associated visual field loss despite normal intraocular pressure and aqueous flow. Low-tension glaucoma can occur in older individuals and affects both eyes similarly. The explanation as to why the optic nerve head is abnormally vulnerable to the intraocular pressure is not completely understood, but it is probably related to poor vascular perfusion of the nerve head.

Before the diagnosis of low-tension glaucoma can be made, it is imperative to rule out other causes. Diurnal measurements are necessary to eliminate the possibility of transient pressure elevations during the course of the day. It is necessary to consider the possibility that the pressure may have been elevated at one time as a result of corticosteroid use or ocular inflammation. Neurological disorders affecting the optic nerve must also be looked into, although disc atrophy from optic neuritis or a tumor characteristically has a different appearance. (Optic atrophy secondary to glaucoma is shown in Fig. 10-3.) The eyes have to be treated

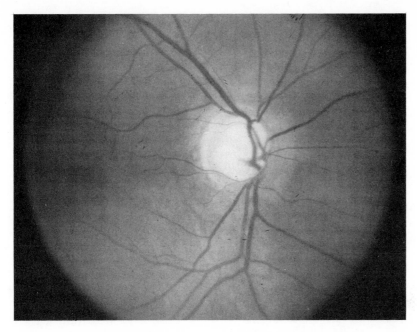

Fig. 10-3. Optic atrophy secondary to glaucoma (right eye). Note nasal displacement of vessels and marked excavation of the nerve head with dropout of fine capillaries on the temporal rim.

in the same manner as for chronic open-angle glaucoma and observed at regular intervals for signs of progression.

Therapy

Once the diagnosis of glaucoma has been established and the decision made to treat it, then a rational approach to therapy becomes imperative. Ideally, a medication should be chosen that will sufficiently lower the patient's intraocular pressure, not significantly alter his life-style, and have a minimum of undesirable side effects.

Miotics, such as pilocarpine and carbachol, are usually effective agents; in the presence of lenticular opacities, however, the narrowing of the entrance to the pupil caused by these parasympathomimetic drugs may have the undesira-

ble effect of reducing the patient's visual acuity.

To minimize the accommodative spasms produced by periodic doses of pilocarpine and to provide a constant level of medication, a delivery system called the Ocusert can be used.[12] This is a thin wafer, impregnated with pilocarpine, that is placed under the patient's lid. The medication escapes from the wafer at a constant rate over the life span of the wafer, which is approximately 1 week. The major drawback to the device is its relatively high cost, compared with a few cents per day for pilocarpine. This cost factor makes it an unreasonable alternative for many older patients. The longer acting cholinesterase inhibitors, such as echothiophate (Phospholine) iodide, have the additional disadvantage of being implicated in the formation of cataracts.

An alternative drug would be the levo form of epinephrine, (Epifrin, Eppy, Epitrate). While usually not affecting the pupil or the accommodative mechanism and thereby not affecting visual acuity, these drugs tend to cause a chronic dilation of the conjunctival vessels and are associated with a high incidence of allergic reaction. In some highly sensitive older patients, cardiac dysrhythmias have been reported due to systemic absorption of the drug. Cystoid macular changes may occur in aphakic eyes from the epinephrine. Therefore, the drugs have limited applicability in patients who have undergone cataract extraction.

A recent addition to the pharmacological armamentarium is a beta-adrenergic blocking agent, timolol.[13] Timolol has proved to be a very safe and effective topical medication, although there have been case reports of bradycardia and bronchospasm in sensitive individuals. The drug, which does not cause miosis, is used in a 0.25% or 0.5% concentration and is instilled twice a day. When topical medications alone or in various combinations are ineffective, systemic carbonic anhydrase inhibitors (acetazolamide [Diamox]) can be used. These act to lower the intraocular pressure by reducing the production of aqueous humor by the ciliary body. They usually cause a lowering of serum potassium. Patients must be monitored closely for hypokalemia, especially if they are taking additional diuretics and digitalis. Anorexia, loss of libido, paresthesia of the limbs, and renal calculi have been associated with the carbonic anhydrase inhibitors.

Once the decision has been made to treat the patient who has glaucoma, the treatment regimen should be individualized for that patient. To ensure compliance, one should start with the weakest drug that produces the desired lowering of pressure with a minimum of side effects and the least disruption of the patient's life-style. Because compliance is a factor in the elderly, pilocarpine, which must be given three to four times a day, may be replaced by drugs that only require twice-daily doses, such as epinephrine, timolol, and/or acetazolamide. These medications do not constrict the pupil, as pilocarpine does, and thus will not interfere with vision if there is any evidence of cataract formation.

CONDITIONS OF THE LENS
Normal changes with aging

The lens is a unique structure in the body in that its entire history is contained within its transparent capsule. As the lens matures, the old lens fibers become compacted toward the center of the lens, thereby increasing its bulk.

The lens and its capsule have elastic properties, which account for the ability of the lens to change shape in order to accommodate for near vision. In the process of accommodating for near vision, there is a contraction of the ciliary muscle, which shifts forward into a circle of lesser radius within the globe. As a result, there is a relaxation of tension on the zonules that suspend the lens and the lens is thus able to contract, becoming more convex. The result is to change the focal point of the eye so that close objects are brought into focus.

With advancing years, the ciliary muscle weakens and the lens, thickened by its increasing density of lens fibers, becomes less elastic. The ability to accommodate diminishes, and the near point becomes increasingly remote until supplementary glasses are required to perform near tasks. This condition is known as presbyopia.

Cataracts

A not infrequent finding in the geriatric population is the presence of opacities within the lens.[14] The term *cataract* is applied to any opacity of the lens whether or not it interferes with vision.[15]

Cataracts can arise from any situation that interferes with the normal metabolism of the lens, such as trauma, diabetes mellitus, inflammation, chemicals, radiation, heat, or cold. The lens, which has no blood supply, is dependent on the surrounding aqueous humor for its nutrition. There are three substances present in large amounts in the normal lens: the sulfur-containing polypeptide glutathione, ascorbic acid, and riboflavin. These substances are found to be greatly reduced, and finally absent, when the lens becomes cataractous.

As the cataract increases in density, the patient becomes increasingly aware of a deterioration in his vision. In some instances, as the lens becomes more dense, its refractive index increases, making the patient increasingly myopic. The patient may complain of a misty vision and may find himself increasingly bothered by glare. Eventually, as the cataract continues to mature, useful vision in the eye is lost.

With modern microsurgical techniques of cataract extraction, there are few medical contraindications to the surgical removal of the opaque lens. The decision to operate should be based on the patient's limitation of vision, not on the "maturity" of the cataract. With the tight wound closure afforded by fine sutures, the patient can ambulate almost immediately following surgery and be discharged from the hospital within a day or two or, in some cases, immediately following the operation.

The management of the patient with cataracts poses many problems because of the difficulties encountered in restoring the binocular vision of these patients. It is a well-known saying among ophthalmic surgeons that aphakia (the absence of the lens) is the greatest complication of cataract surgery. Until recently, the patient with a monocular cataract was faced with a dilemma: because the spectacle lenses used to correct aphakia have a magnifying effect of approximately 25%, the monocular aphake, fitted with an aphakic lens for the eye operated on and with his normal prescription lens for the uninvolved eye, would perceive two vastly different views of an object, so disparate in size as to be unmanageable by the brain.[16,17] By means of a contact lens, the magnification is reduced to about 8%, thereby allowing the brain to fuse the images[18-20] (Fig. 10-4).

Most geriatric patients, however, find they lack the dexterity to handle a contact lens. Until the lens is placed on the eye, their vision is usually impaired, making it difficult to locate the contact lens and prepare it for insertion. Tremor, arthritis, and/or weakening may make the placing of the lens into the eye a monumental task.

If a contact lens could be placed on the eye and left in position for a prolonged period (weeks to months), the problem would be eliminated. A number of soft contact lenses have been approved for extended wear. There are certain risks, however, that must be taken into account. Prolonged wearing of the contact lens may lead to proliferation of blood vessels in the normally avascular cornea. The risk of infection is real and must be taken into account. These complications can usually be controlled by removal of the contact lens.[21]

A controversial area in ophthalmology is the use of the intraocular lens (pseudophakos) (Fig. 10-5). The theoreti-

Aphakic Vision

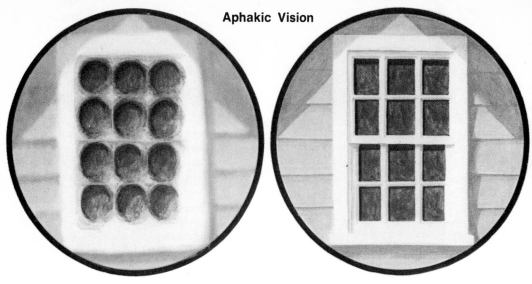

Blurred image of uncorrected
aphakic vision

Aphakic vision corrected with
spectacle or contact lens

Monocular image size

Binocular image
(combination)

E

8% larger than
normal vision

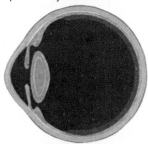

Aphakic eye with contact lens

E

Normal vision

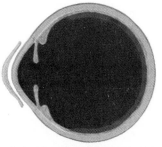

Normal eye

E

Fusion of two
nearly similar
images

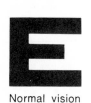

25% larger than
normal vision

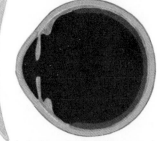

Aphakic eye with spectacle lens

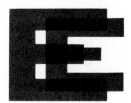

Diplopia because of
inability to fuse
two greatly disparate
images

JOHN A. CRAIG—AD
© CIBA

Fig. 10-4. For legend see opposite page.

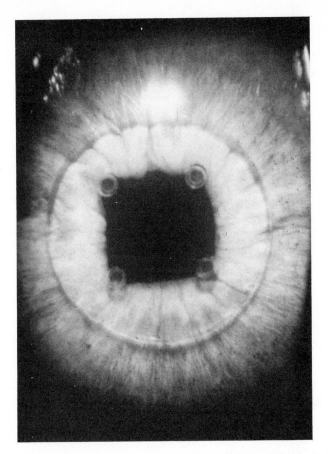

Fig. 10-5. Intraocular lens implant. Note the circular outline of the lens in front of the plane of the iris. The square shape of the pupil is caused by the supports of the implant, which saddle the iris.

Fig. 10-4. Aphakic vision and effect of a contact lens and a spectacle lens on binocular vision. © Copyright 1974 CIBA Pharmaceutical Co., Division of CIBA-GEIGY Corp. Reprinted with permission from Clinical Symposia, illustrated by John A. Craig, M.D. All rights reserved.

cal advantages of the pseudophakos are enormous. The patient is restored to "normal" vision almost immediately following surgery and does not have to contend with the problems of contact lenses or cataract glasses. The artificial lens, sitting near the normal location of the patient's own lens, affords the most "natural" vision.[22]

A large number of lenses have been designed for the purpose of implantation, but there are some serious questions as to the long-range safety of this procedure, the most ideal lens, and the technique of implantation. The procedure is not without risks.

The pseudophakos is not intended for all eyes, and there are a number of contraindications to its use. For example, a pseudophakos should not be implanted in an eye with axial myopia greater than 7 diopters, since the patient would derive little visual benefit. Following removal of the lens, the high myope would be left with little refractive error and therefore not be in need of the implant.

A pseudophakos should not be implanted in a patient who only has vision in one functional eye, or who has already had a poor result with an implant in the fellow eye. The implant is also contraindicated in patients with corneal dystrophy, since there is a likelihood of corneal decompensation following the procedure. Likewise, results have been poor in patients with proliferative diabetic retinopathy and in those suffering from poorly controlled glaucoma.

A history of retinal detachment should also be considered as a contraindication, because the pseudophakos makes visualization of the peripheral retina more difficult. A history of chronic intraocular inflammation would also preclude the use of a pseudophakos.

There are a number of complications that can occur with the implant. At the time of lens implantation and in the postoperative period, contact of the pseudophakos with the corneal endothelium can cause irreparable harm to the cornea. Imperfections in the design or fabrication of the lens or improper handling at the time of implantation can result in inflammation within the eye, which may lead to damage to the iris or trabecular structures. Endophthalmitis resulting from a contaminated lens can be disastrous. A lens can become dislocated within the eye and may require surgical manipulation to reposition or remove it. Nonetheless, in spite of the risks, lens implantation has been gaining steadily in popularity and acceptance.

DISORDERS OF THE MACULA

By far the greatest single cause for visual loss in the elderly results from disorders of the macula.[14] The macula is an area in the retina, approximately 1 disc diameter in size, temporal to the disc and centered around the fovea.

Senile macular degeneration

Much has been learned about the pathogenesis of senile macular degeneration through the use of the technique of fluorescein angiography.[23-25] Deep in the retinal pigmented epithelium and separating it from the choriocapillaris is a structure known as Bruch's membrane.[26,27] Unexplained age-related changes in the underlying choriocapillaris may lead to thickening, hyalinization, and breaks in Bruch's membrane. Choroidal neovascularization resulting from the breaks in Bruch's membrane may lead to the development of new vessels within the subretinal pigment epithelial space. These vessels later may penetrate to the subsensory retinal space, where leakage may cause serous or hemorrhagic detachment of the pigment epithelium and/or sensory retina.

Senile macular degeneration is usually symmetrical, although it is not uncommon for one eye to be more advanced than the other eye.

Patients with senile macular degeneration may maintain adequate central visual acuity for a number of years, but many will suffer rather severe loss as a result of serous or hemorrhagic detachment of the pigment epithelium and/or retina.

At present, there is no effective treatment for senile macular degeneration, although there is some indication that laser photocoagulation of the new vessels may destroy these vessels before they, in turn, destroy the macula. Some patients can be helped with low-vision aids, such as magnifying devices or a telescopic lens, but in the older population, most patients find anything more than the simple magnifying glass difficult to manage.

Diabetic retinopathy

Although senile macular degeneration is the leading cause of blindness in the geriatric population, a significant amount of visual loss can be attributed to diabetic retinopathy. In the adult-onset diabetic with background changes, the visual loss is usually related to vascular changes in and around the macula. Leakage of serous fluid from vessels surrounding the macula lead to macular edema and subsequent deterioration in visual acuity. This can sometimes be remedied by the use of laser photocoagulation. Hemorrhages within the macula may lead to a more permanent visual loss. A dropout of retinal capillaries may lead to macular is-

chemia with an attendant poor prognosis for visual recovery.

SUDDEN VISUAL LOSS

Sudden visual loss in the elderly must always be carefully and thoroughly evaluated. It may be caused by occlusion of one of the major vessels of the eye as the result of hypertension, atheromatous vascular disease, abnormal blood viscosity or hemorrhage in preexisting macular degeneration, vitreous hemorrhage, retinal detachment, or ischemic infarction of the optic disc. Temporal arteritis and glaucoma must also be considered. The visual loss of occlusion of the central retinal artery is usually more severe than that caused by central retinal vein occlusion.

Temporal arteritis is a form of arteritis with segmental areas of destruction of the internal elastic layer accompanied by giant cell formation. The vessel lumen becomes obliterated by the thickened vessel wall. This disorder is frequently marked by low-grade fever, anorexia, and an increased erythrocyte sedimentation rate. There may be pain in the muscles and joints. The pain around the temporal vessels may be so severe that the patient can hardly brush his hair. The optic disc may be slightly edematous with hemorrhage in the area surrounding the optic disc. Optic atrophy follows swiftly. Because this disorder tends to be bilateral, prompt diagnosis and institution of appropriate steriod therapy is necessary to preserve sight.

Ischemic optic neuropathy presents a typical clinical picture of slight edema of the disc, associated with altitudinal field defects. Optic atrophy usually follows resolution of the edema. There is no known relationship with hypertension, carotid atheromatous disease, or diabetes. If the second eye becomes involved, a pseudo–Foster Kennedy syndrome may be observed with optic atrophy in one eye and papilledema in the other. There is no effective treatment of this condition.

• • •

The preservation and restoration of vision is clearly a priority for the elderly person. While multiple pathological processes can affect visual function, many of the deficits are treatable.

REFERENCES

1. Callahan, A.: *Reconstructive surgery of the eyelids and ocular adnexa,* Birmingham, Ala., 1966, Aescolapius Publishing Co., pp. 120-139, 150, 173.
2. Fox, S. A.: *Lid surgery: current concepts,* New York, 1972, Grune & Stratton, Inc., pp. 80, 96-102.
3. Fox, S. A.: *Ophthalmic plastic surgery,* New York, Grune & Stratton Inc., pp. 264, 298-335.
4. Mustarde, J. C., Jones, L. T., and Callahan, A.: *Ophthalmic plastic surgery—up to date,* Aescolapius Publishing Co., Birmingham, Ala., 1970, pp. 85-91.
5. Bodian, M.: A tarsal resection procedure for senile entropion with lid retraction, Ophthalmic surg. **8**(6):34, 1978.
6. Beard, C.: Mechanical, including paralytic, ectropion, *Trans. Am. Acad. Ophthalmol Otolaryngol.* **66**:588, 1962.
7. Smolin, G., and Okumoto, M.: Staphylococcal blepharitis, *Arch. Ophthalmol.***95**:812, 1977.
8. Moses, R.: Adler's *physiology of the eye,* ed. 6, St. Louis, 1975, The C. V. Mosby Co., pp. 25, 27.
9. Kolker, A. E., and Hetherington, J., Jr.: *Becker-Shaffer's diagnosis and therapy of the glaucomas,* ed. 4, St. Louis, 1976, The C. V. Mosby Co., p. 80.
10. Shin, D. H., Becker, B., and Kolker, A. E.: Family history in primary open-angle glaucoma, *Arch. Ophthalmol.* **95**:598, 1977.
11. Chandler, P. A., and Grant, W. N.: *Lectures on glaucoma,* Philadelphia, 1965, Lea & Febiger, pp. 143-146.
12. Hillman, J. S., Walker, A., and Davies, E. M.: Management of chronic glaucoma with pilocar-

pine Ocuserts, *Trans. Ophthalmol. Soc. U.K.* **97**:206, 1977.
13. Zimmerman, T. J., and Kaufman, H. E.: Timolol, a beta-adrenergic blocking agent for the treatment of glaucoma, *Arch. Ophthalmol.* **95**:601, 1977.
14. Kini, M. M., Liebowitz, H. M., Colton T., and others: Prevalence of senile cataract, diabetic retinopathy, senile macular degeneration and open-angle glaucoma in the Framingham Eye Study, *Am. J. Ophthalmol.* **85**:28, 1978.
15. Jaffe, N. S.: The lens-annual review, *Arch. Ophthalmol.* **87**:453, 1972.
16. Woods, A. C.: The adjustment to aphakia, *Am. J. Ophthalmol.* **35**:118, 1952.
17. Christman, E. H.: Correction of anisokonia in monocular aphakia, *Arch. Ophthalmol.* **85**:148, 1971.
18. Ogle, K. N., Burian, H. N., and Bannon, R. E.: On the correction of unilateral aphakia with contact lenses, Arch. Ophthalmol. **59**:639, 1958.
19. Cassady, J. R.: Contact lenses for correction of aphakia—a report of 648 patients, *Contact Intraocular Lens Med. J.* **4**:14, 1978.
20. Kersley, H. J.: Contact lens in aphakia, *Trans. Ophthalmol. Soc. U.K.* **97**:142, 1977.
21. Clements, D. B.: Continuous wear soft lenses in the treatment of aphakis, *Trans. Ophthalmol. Soc. U.K.* **97**:145, 1977.
22. Jaffe, N. S., Galin, M. A., Hirschman, H., and Clayman, H. M.: *Pseudophakos,* St. Louis, 1978, The C. V. Mosby Co., pp. 26-34.
23. Fine, S. L.: Photocoagulation of macular lesions, J. Continuing Educ. Ophthalmol. **41**:17, 1979.
24. Gass, J. D. M.: The pathogenesis of discoform detachment of the neuroepithelium, *Am. J. Ophthalmol.* **63**:573, 1967.
25. Hogan, M. I.: Bruch's membrane and disease of the macula: role of elastic tissue and collagen, *Trans. Ophthalmol. Soc. U.K.* **87**:113, 1967.
26. Sarks, S. H.: Aging and degeneration in the macular region: a clinicopathological study, *Br. J. Ophthalmol.* **60**:573, 1967.
27. Green, W. R., and Key, S. N.: Senile macular degeneration: a histopathologic study, *Trans. Am. Ophthalmol. Soc. U.K.* **75**:180, 1977.

PROBLEM-SOLVING EXERCISES
Case one

A 72-year-old former ballerina who teaches ballet has been complaining of a painless, progressive visual loss in her right eye over a period of a few months. She has also become increasingly bothered by the glare of oncoming headlights when driving at night.

On physical examination, visual acuity is found to be OD 20/200, OS 20/40 best corrected. The ocular adnexae are normal, and the intraocular tensions by applanation are 18 in both eyes. The corneas are clear and the anterior chambers deep. The right lens reveals advanced nuclear sclerotic changes; the left lens reveals early changes. The discs are pink and healthy, and there are some mild arteriosclerotic changes in the fundi. The macular reflexes are normal.

A diagnosis of cataract is established, and the various means of correcting the patient's vision after surgery (implant, contact lens, or spectacles) are discussed. The patient then asks you, "What would you suggest doctor?"

Question

1. What do you reply?

Case two

An elderly man being followed in the general medical clinic comes for his routine appointment complaining of pain and blurred vision in his left eye. His medications include L-dopa and hydrochlorothiazide. Last week, amitriptyline was started for depression. With a penlight, you notice that the conjunctiva is hyperemic and that the cornea appears slightly cloudy. The pupil is about 4 mm in size and reacts very poorly to light stimulation. The eye is very tender and feels hard on palpation, although it is difficult to evaluate because of the hazy cornea and the patient's irritability.

You attempt to locate the consulting ophthalmologist, but he has left his office and his page system is not working. The patient asks you to do something to relieve his discomfort.

Question

1. What is the differential diagnosis and what should you do?

ANSWERS TO PROBLEM-SOLVING EXERCISES
Case one

1. The following should be considered.
   - The pros and cons of doing nothing versus performing a monocular cataract extraction resulting in monocular aphakia
   - The side effects of spectacle correction of aphakia
   - The pros and cons of a contact lens versus a pseudophakos and the risks and contraindications of each

Case two

1. The differential diagnosis of a painful red eye includes acute angle-closure glaucoma, iritis, conjunctivitis, abrasion, and foreign body. Although a definitive diagnosis of acute angle-closure glaucoma can only be confirmed by gonioscopy, a presumptive diagnosis can be made based on the history and physical examination. The anticholinergic effects of the amitriptyline started a few weeks earlier may have caused the attack of acute angle-closure glaucoma. L-dopa also has anticholinergic side effects. The physical examination revealed a reddened eye with a nonreactive and dilated pupil with a cloudy lens. Pilocarpine, 2%, should be instilled directly into the eye to bring the root of the iris away from the Canal of Schlemm. Once the attack has been controlled and the intraocular pressure returned to normal, topical pilocarpine should be used on a daily basis.

POSTTEST*

1. The leading cause of irreversible blindness in the elderly is:
   a. Cataracts
   b. Diabetic retinopathy
   c. Ischemic optic atrophy
   d. Senile macular degeneration

*Some questions may have more than one correct answer.

2. *True or false:* Normal aging is associated with the reduced production of tears.

3. Following cataract surgery, the patient's vision with glasses may not be satisfactory. Explain.

4. *True or false:* Cataract surgery should not be performed until the lens is mature.

5. *True or false:* Open-angle glaucoma results from a buildup of pressure in the posterior chamber.

6. The most common form of glaucoma in the older population is:
   a. Primary open-angle glaucoma
   b. Secondary open-angle glaucoma
   c. Primary angle-closure glaucoma
   d. Secondary angle-closure glaucoma

7. What factors must be considered in evaluating the elderly glaucoma patient's need for medication?

8. *True or false:* Senile macular degeneration follows disruption of Bruch's membrane.

9. *True or false:* Topical Beta-adrenergic blocking agents have fewer visual side effects than pilocarpine in the treatment of primary open-angle glaucoma in the elderly.

ANSWERS TO PRETEST AND POSTTEST

1. d. Senile macular degeneration is the leading cause of irreversible blindness in the elderly. Visual impairment from cataracts is correctable by surgery. Diabetic retinopathy is not a common cause of irreversible blindness in the elderly, because the patient with severe diabetes with proliferative retinopathy usually does not survive into late life.

2. True.

3. Because of the image magnification and distortion produced by the high plus–powered lens needed to correct aphakia (removal of the lens), the patient suffers from a visual disorientation within his environment. This situation is further compounded when only one eye has had surgery and an attempt is made to give the patient binocular spectacle correction. The eye operated on perceives a 25% larger image, and the resulting disparity causes double vision.

4. False. Cataract surgery should be performed when the cataract is dense enough to interfere with the patient's normal life-style and ability to function within his environment.

5. False. Open-angle glaucoma is a condition that results from reduced outflow of aqueous humor from the anterior chamber through the trabecular meshwork and the canal of Schlemm.

6. a.

7. The severity of the pressure elevation and the appearance of the optic nerve and visual fields are of major importance. A family history of glaucoma may be significant in determining therapy.

8. True. It is believed that a disruption in Bruch's membrane leads to proliferation of new blood vessels beneath the pigment epithelium. The incompetency of these vessels results in their leakage, producing a serous or hemorrhagic detachment of the sensory retina.

9. True. Pilocarpine produces miosis with a resultant change in visual acuity. The smaller pupil diminishes the elderly person's ability to function in reduced light. Timolol, a beta-adrenergic blocking agent, does not affect pupil size but can rarely cause systemic side effects, including bradycardia, congestive heart failure, and the exacerbation of a bronchospastic component in chronic obstructive pulmonary disease.

Chapter 11

Hypertension

LESLIE S. LIBOW, FREDRICK T. SHERMAN, and LARRY D. WRIGHT

EDUCATIONAL OBJECTIVES
Attitudinal

The student should:
1. Be cautious in approaching hypertension in the elderly (particularly white women) because of some unclarity as to what levels of pressure should be treated and because of the risks of treatment
2. Recognize that the approach to the elderly hypertensive patient is different from the approach to the "ageless" 70-kg hypertensive patient
3. Consider the quality of life of the patient when deciding on treatment approaches

Cognitive

The student should:
1. Recognize the possible inaccuracy of extrapolating diagnostic categories and treatment regimens from middle age
2. Recognize the significant correlation of diastolic pressure with morbidity and mortality
3. Recognize the similar, perhaps stronger, correlation of systolic pressure with morbidity and mortality
4. Know the differential diagnosis of systolic and diastolic hypertension
5. Know that the diagnostic evaluation of the elderly hypertensive patient should be conservative and simple
6. Know that for black men and women and white men aged 65 to 74 years, the reduction of diastolic pressure initially found in the range of 90 to 104 mm Hg. appears to lead to a reduction in mortality (For white women, there is as yet no evidence of the value of treating diastolic pressure found to be in the range of 90 to 104 mm Hg.)
7. Know that diastolic pressure in the range of 90 to 104 mm Hg may have protective effects in the elderly
8. Recognize the morbidity resulting from treatment of the elderly hypertensive patient
9. Know that orthostatic hypotension in the elderly is common
10. Know that treatment, when indicated, is usually a single medication
11. Know the starting dosages, side effects, and drug interactions of the commonly used antihypertensive medications in the elderly

Skill

The student should:
1. Learn to take the blood pressure in each arm with the patient in supine, sitting, and standing positions
2. Learn the significance of varying types of pulse volume
3. Learn to be cautious in diagnosing hypertension in the elderly
4. Be able to counsel an elderly hypertensive patient in methods of salt restriction, weight loss (when indicated), and medication compliance

PRETEST

1. List five causes of pure systolic hypertension.
2. List four common side effects of antihy-

pertensive medications in elderly patients. Include one example of a drug that can cause each side effect.

3. It has been shown that:
   a. High systolic blood pressure is associated with increased risk of cardiovascular and cerebrovascular morbidity and mortality
   b. High diastolic blood pressure is associated with increased risk of cardiovascular and cerebrovascular morbidity and mortality
   c. Both a and b

4. *True or false:* Elderly white female patients whose diastolic blood pressures are consistently between 90 and 104 mm Hg will clearly benefit in terms of decreased risk of cardiovascular morbidity and mortality by receiving adequate antihypertensive therapy.

5. The most appropriate initial therapeutic trial in treating hypertension in elderly patients is _____.

6. Name a category of antihypertensive drugs that reliably lowers systolic blood pressure without significantly affecting diastolic pressure.

7. The accepted "usual" definition of hypertension:
   a. Sets an upper limit for systolic and diastolic values based on observed end-organ damage, which routinely occurs in patients whose pressures exceed this
   b. Chooses a "normal" blood pressure limit (standard deviation from the mean; e.g., 140/90) that has, as its basis, population statistics that are not usually age relevant
   c. Depends on confirmation of symptoms reported by the patient that can be clearly attributed to the elevated blood pressure
   d. Includes well-established diastolic and systolic blood pressure levels by age for each decade of life

8. Based on cross-sectional population studies, as age increases (going from 20 years of age to 70 years of age):
   a. Systolic blood pressure increases, and diastolic blood pressure is unchanged
   b. Systolic blood pressure is unchanged, and diastolic blood pressure increases
   c. Systolic blood pressure increases, and diastolic blood pressure increases
   d. Neither systolic nor diastolic blood pressure changes significantly

9. Alpha-methyldopa is one of the most commonly used antihypertensive medications. List the adverse effects of this drug in the elderly.

10. For an elderly hypertensive patient with persistently elevated blood pressure despite 100 mg per day of hydrochlorothiazide, the most appropriate additional medication might be:
    a. Propranolol
    b. Guanethidine
    c. Reserpine
    d. Clonidine

The pathogenesis, diagnosis, and treatment of high blood pressure in the latter phase of life (65 years of age and over) is a challenge to the skills of the clinician and to the current state of medical knowledge and research. Since blood pressure, in general, normally increases with age, it is often difficult to clearly establish when the blood pressure is pathologically high in the older patient (Figs. 11-1 and 11-2). Treatment is more difficult than in the young, since side effects occur more often and exert a greater detrimental influence on the daily social, mental, and physical functioning of the older individual. Hence, the clinician and the older patient are frequently faced with the choice of accepting the risks of untreated

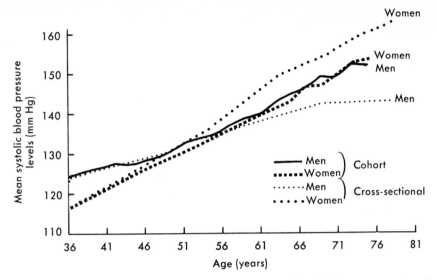

Fig. 11-1. Average age trends in systolic blood pressure levels for cross-sectional and cohort data (Framingham study, Exams 3 to 10). (From Kannel, W. B.: Blood pressure and the development of cardiovascular disease in the aged. In Caird, F. I., Dall, J. L. C., and Kennedy, R. D., editors: Cardiology in old age, New York, 1976, Plenum Publishing Corp.)

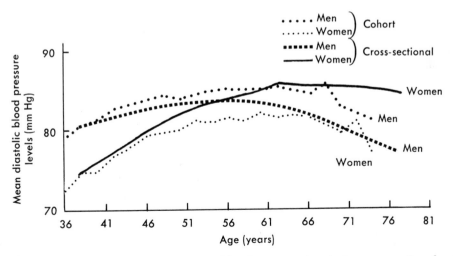

Fig. 11-2. Average age trends in diastolic blood pressure levels for cross-sectional and cohort data (Framingham study, Exams 3 to 10). (From Kannel, W. B.: Blood pressure and the development of cardiovascular disease in the aged. In Caird, F. I., Dall, J. L. C., and Kennedy, R. D., editors: Cardiology in old age, New York, 1976, Plenum Publishing Corp.)

hypertension or coping with the more immediate, often disabling side effects of adequate antihypertensive therapy.

EPIDEMIOLOGY AND RELATIONSHIP TO MORBIDITY AND MORTALITY

Although prevalence data on hypertension among the elderly vary considerably from study to study, hypertension is quite common. The prevalence of hypertension (defined somewhat arbitrarily as systolic pressure above 160 mm Hg and/or diastolic pressure above 95 mm Hg) in those 65 to 74 years of age is in the range of 35% to 50%, with generally greater prevalence in blacks than in whites.[1-3]

In any age group, high blood pressure is a purely statistical concept. Thus, patients who have systolic and particularly diastolic blood pressures greater than two to three standard deviations above the mean for their age are considered hypertensive. There is clearly increased morbidity and mortality in the group of patients who have hypertension on the basis of this definition. The inadequacy of a statistical definition of hypertension

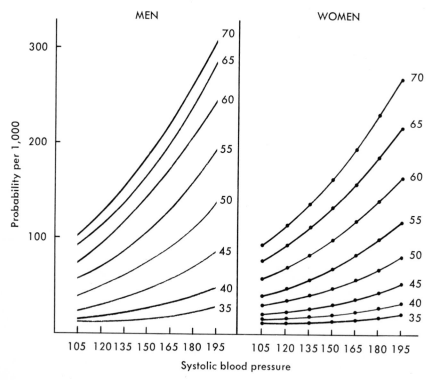

Fig. 11-3. Probability of cardiovascular disease in 8 years according to systolic blood pressure at specified ages in each sex (Framingham study: 18-year follow-up, low-risk subjects). (From Kannel, W. B.: Blood pressure and the development of cardiovascular disease in the aged. In Caird, F. I., Dall, J. L. C., and Kennedy, R. D., editors: Cardiology in old age, New York, 1976, Plenum Publishing Corp.)

becomes apparent, however, when one looks at the longitudinal epidemiological studies of communities such as Framingham, Mass.[3-5] In these studies it has been clearly demonstrated that there is an increased risk of cardiovascular morbidity and mortality associated with each small increment in both systolic and diastolic pressures, even within the so-called normal range. Thus, there is greater risk associated with a systolic pressure of 130 mm Hg than with one of 125 mm Hg and with a diastolic pressure of 85 mm Hg than with one of 80 mm Hg. For any given level of systolic or diastolic pressure, the risk is higher the older the individual (Fig. 11-3 and Table 11-1). Contrary to previous thinking, the correlation of cardiovascular morbidity and mortality with increased systolic blood pressure is equal to or greater than that seen with diastolic pressure.[3-5]

BENEFITS OF TREATMENT

Although these data on the strong correlation of morbidity and mortality with high blood pressure are convincing, clear benefits from correcting hypertension in the elderly have been established only in patients with markedly elevated levels and in black men and women and white men with mild hypertension (90 to 104 mm Hg). There is as yet no clear evidence of benefit in treating older white women who are mildly hypertensive. In managing elderly patients with hypertension, the clinician is confronted with at least two problem areas: borderline diastolic hypertension in white women (arbitrarily defined as 90 to 104 mm Hg) and pure systolic hypertension, in which the current medical literature is not definitive.

The range of diastolic blood pressures between 90 and 104 mm Hg may be termed "borderline" hypertension and is the range for most elderly hypertensive patients. Although the Veterans Administration (VA) study[6-8] showed significant reduction in cardiovascular morbidity in older men (women were not studied) when treating diastolic hypertensives with blood pressures in the range of 105

Table 11-1. Incidence of cardiovascular disease according to hypertensive status by age and sex in men and women 45 to 74 (Framingham study: 18-year follow-up)[*]

| | Five-year incidence per 100 at risk | | | | | |
| | Men | | | Women | | |
Age in years	45 to 54	55 to 64	65 to 74	45 to 54	55 to 64	65 to 74
Blood pressure status						
Normotensive	4.15	7.75	8.20	1.20	3.10	4.15
Borderline	7.33	14.65	15.95	2.50	7.10	12.15
Hypertensive	11.70	22.20	26.15	4.45	11.35	16.60
Regression coefficient	0.534	0.554	0.613	0.662	0.639	0.579
HBP vs. normotensive						
Risk ratio	2.82	2.86	3.19	3.71	3.66	4.00
Difference in risk	7.55	14.45	17.95	3.25	8.25	12.45
Attributable risk (%)	64.50	65.10	68.60	73.00	72.70	75.00

[*]From Kannel, W. B.: Blood pressure and the development of cardiovascular disease in the aged. In Caird, F. J., Dall, J. L. C., and Kennedy, R. D., editors: Cardiology in old age, New York, Plenum Publishing Corp.

to 129 mm Hg, the results in treating diastolic hypertensives with blood pressures in the range of 90 to 104 mm Hg were not nearly as impressive. In this VA study, there is a suggestion that treating patients of all ages with diastolic pressures between 90 and 104 mm Hg is beneficial, but the improvement in cardiovascular morbidity and mortality does not reach statistical significance.

The initial reports of the Hypertension Detection and Follow-Up Program (HDFP)[15,16], which focused only on mortality, suggests that black men and women and white men aged 65 to 74 years do benefit from treatment of diastolic pressure in the range of 90 to 104 mm Hg. There is no evidence that white women benefited from this treatment. No subjects above 74 years of age were included in this study.

Similarly, it is unclear what the clinician should do about treating the older patient with "pure" systolic hypertension (defined as systolic pressure above 160 mm Hg and diastolic pressure below 95 mm Hg). This finding occurs in about 2% of the population in the 30- to 40-year-old age group but in 15% to 43% of the population over the age of 65.[9]

Many clinicians believe that it is important to view systolic hypertension in the elderly as a quantitative pathological entity, distinct from diastolic hypertension,[10-13] and to treat patients for it. Another view is that systolic hypertension results from the process of atherosclerosis of the large vessels, such as the aorta,[14] and that the correlation of high systolic pressure with stroke, heart failure, and coronary artery disease simply reflects the more advanced degrees of atherosclerosis seen in patients with these disorders.

In any case, there are no medications presently available to reduce systolic pressure without also affecting diastolic pressure. Although there is an increased tendency among clinicians to treat patients with systolic blood pressures above 160 mm Hg with medications such as diuretics and/or propranolol, no evidence exists supporting the benefits of lowering the blood pressure in pure systolic hypertension.

PROTECTIVE EFFECTS OF ELEVATED BLOOD PRESSURE

Of further interest are the data from the National Institute of Health's (NIH) longitudinal study of human aging[17,18] and from the longitudinal study of the elderly at Duke University,[19,20] which suggest that minimally increased levels of systolic and diastolic blood pressures within the so-called "normal" and/or "borderline" range may be of protective value in the elderly. The NIH study suggests that in the presence of asymptomatic clinical arteriosclerotic disease, increased blood pressure within a narrow "normal" range protects against slowing of the electroencephalogram (EEG). Furthermore, in the healthy older man without clinically evident arteriosclerosis, there is a positive correlation between fast EEG activity and blood pressure, suggesting a protective effect of increased blood pressure on electrical activity of the brain in late life.

In the study at Duke University, older individuals with diastolic blood pressures in the range of 96 to 105 mm Hg who were followed for 10 years with repeated intelligence quotient (IQ) tests showed improved scores on certain aspects of these tests as compared with a "matched" group of normotensive older individuals whose IQ scores remained unchanged over this period. Patients with definite hypertensive diastolic blood pressures over 105 mm Hg had IQ scores that declined over the 10-year interval. These data suggest that within a limited blood pressure range there is a protective effect of increased pressure on mental function in late life.

Thus both of these studies suggest that the brain is protected by increased blood pressure within a narrow normal to borderline hypertensive range.

Beyond the clinical studies just reviewed, there are many case reports and clinical anecdotes that indicate that treatment of elevated blood pressures in the elderly may produce acute morbidity, such as stroke and myocardial infarction.[21-23] Clinicians have long argued that older persons may require relatively higher pressures in order to maintain normal cerebral, coronary, and renal blood flow through arteries often partially narrowed by atherosclerosis.

Thus, the issue of defining hypertension in the elderly is difficult, and the issue of when to treat the patient is even more difficult. It would be wrong, however, to conclude from this discussion that elevated blood pressure in the elderly does not require treatment. There is no doubt that lowering diastolic pressure that exceeds 104 mm Hg decreases morbidity. Less certainty exists as to the benefits derived from treating patients (especially older white women) with borderline diastolic hypertension (90 to 104 mm Hg) and/or patients with pure systolic hypertension. Our specific recommendations for treating patients with borderline diastolic hypertension (90 to 104 mm Hg) and pure systolic hypertension above 160 mm Hg are presented later in this chapter under "Treatment."

DEFINITION

Normally, hypertension has been defined in statistical terms. Traditionally, systolic/diastolic pressures of 140/90 mm Hg in the 70-kg "younger or ageless man" have been held as the upper limits of normal for blood pressure. Of course, there is no specific basis for applying this arbitrary definition to all age groups, as can be appreciated from the foregoing discussion. It fails to recognize the very important differences in patterns of blood pressure among individuals of different age groups, especially the elderly.

There is considerable debate about the definition of systolic hypertension. Many clinicians use the definition of systolic pressure over 160 or 180 mm Hg. Others use "a person's age plus 100." Complicating this definition is the observation that as the radial arteries harden with age, there appears to be an increasing gap between the pressure recorded via a cuff applied externally and simultaneous measurement of intra-arterial blood pressure.[24] Data from the Framingham Study[3-5] show that as systolic pressure increases, particularly to levels above 160 mm Hg in the elderly, even when diastolic pressure is below 90 mm Hg, there is still a significant correlation with morbidity and mortality.

There is also controversy about patients with "labile" hypertension and whether they should be treated. These controversies can be put aside fairly readily with the realization that the correlations of blood pressure levels with morbidity and mortality come from two major sources: the Build and Blood Pressure studies,[25] which correlate blood pressure readings with later events, as recorded in thousands of applicants who were accepted for life insurance, and the Framingham study (mentioned above) and other community studies. In all of these studies, blood pressures were recorded once or twice externally and these recordings were then correlated with ensuing events over several years.

Thus, we cannot make light of the prognostic meaning of the traditionally recorded, single external blood pressure measurement.

PATHOPHYSIOLOGY

Most hypertension in the elderly is "essential" (i.e., of unknown etiology). A very modest percentage, certainly less than 5%, are related to primary demonstrable pathological conditions in the kidneys (nephrities), renal arteries, or endocrine system (Cushing's syndrome, aldosteronism, pheochromocytoma). Occasionally medications may cause hypertension (ergot derivatives, estrogens, or other steroids).

Sodium, aldosterone and other mineral corticoids, renin, and angiotension are all believed to have some role in the pathophysiology of essential hypertension.[26] In contrast to the situation with the young, studies of renin and aldosterone in the elderly[27] show a decline in serum levels and/or decreased responsiveness to stimuli. There is no clear linkage of the renin-aldosterone mechanism to essential hypertension in the elderly.

HISTORY TAKING

Hypertension at any age is usually a symptomless problem. However, questions focusing on symptoms such as headaches, dizziness, angina, intermittent claudication, and renal problems are appropriate. Knowing the medication history and dietary habits will also be of value in evaluating the patient. Medications such as salt-retaining steroids, including estrogens and cortisone (as well as excessive licorice ingestion), are examples of drugs that may induce hypertension. At times, an older person will report a history of hypertension and the clinician will find an absence of hypertensive levels on repeated measurement. This may reflect lability of the blood pressure, effects of treatment, or a recent myocardial infarction.

Careful evaluation of the mental status, including the use of brief mental status questionnaires, such as FROMAJE (see Chapter 4), is indicated.[28-31] The patient's mental status has implications for both decision making in the choice of treatment and compliance with the treatment prescribed. The history should also focus on cardiac symptoms, including episodes of chest pain consistent with angina or infarction, with the recognition that ischemic chest pain in the elderly may present with atypical manifestations. A history of dyspnea, orthopnea, or ankle edema could suggest congestive heart failure (CHF), giving indications of further end-organ involvement. Focal neurological symptoms, such as speech, visual, sensory, and/or motor changes, may reflect cerebrovascular symptoms.

Secondary types of hypertension, although rare, should be explored via the history. Thus, in Cushing's syndrome, weight gain, carbohydrate intolerance, and hirsutism are characteristics. Of course, these three symptoms are very common in the elderly and are usually unrelated to Cushing's syndrome. Weight gain may occur from excess caloric intake or from CHF. Carbohydrate intolerance may be due to primary, adult-onset diabetes mellitus. Hirsutism is quite prevalent in normal elderly women. Pheochromocytoma and its accompanying tachycardia, hyperglycemia, and sweating should also be excluded. These symptoms are usually due to anxiety and primary diabetes mellitus.

The history should also focus on the

differential diagnosis of pure systolic hypertension. It includes, in addition to age, high–cardiac output states, such as hyperthyroidism, arteriovenous fistula, Paget's disease of the bone, hyperkinetic heart syndrome, anemia, aortic insufficiency, and fever.

PHYSICAL EXAMINATION
Blood pressure

The blood pressure should be taken with the patient in the supine, sitting, and standing positions and in both arms. As a practical matter, the blood pressure should be taken in both arms while the patient is sitting. An occasional patient will have obstruction of blood flow to one arm, reflecting a potential subclavian steal syndrome. The standing blood pressure should be taken after the patient has been standing 30 to 60 seconds to provide an opportunity for orthostatic abnormalities to occur.

The pulse

A full large-volume pulse usually accompanies systolic and/or diastolic hypertension. An even sharper upswing of the pulse accompanied by an abrupt downswing is considered a collapsing pulse (or Corrigan's pulse) and accompanies the high-output states mentioned earlier, such as aortic insufficiency, hyperthyroidism, arteriovenous fistula, high fevers, complete heart block, and anxiety states (such as at the time of the physical exam). A collapsing pulse is often associated with marked bilateral pulsations in the neck and is best seen with the patient sitting. A small pulse volume occurs with aortic stenosis or with hypotension secondary to hypovolemia or infarction. It is of interest to note that aortic stenosis is not uncommon in the elderly and, somewhat contrary to the situation with the young, may be accompanied by systolic and/or diastolic hypertension.

Fundi

Characteristically, minimal hypertension of the diastolic type is accompanied by modest, if any, changes in the funduscopic picture. There may be narrowing of the arteries with some nicking of the arteriovenous crossings. This is difficult to differentiate from the similar findings of arteriosclerosis unrelated to hypertension. In an occasional elderly person with more advanced hypertension, there will be hemorrhages or exudates. Hypertension rarely will be accompanied by papilledema. Hypertensive encephalopathy is distinctly uncommon in late life.

Aneurysms and bruits

Abdominal examination should seek out aneurysms via gentle palpation and auscultation. Although a bruit heard in the midepigastrium and in the loin may suggest renovascular stenosis, it is more-likely to come from an arteriosclerotic aorta.

Systolic hypertension and various physical findings

Systolic hypertension syndromes may be accompanied by physical findings such as a palpable goiter (with or without eye signs) and/or tremor, indicative of hyperthyroidism. Aortic insufficiency produces a diastolic murmur as well as peripheral signs, such as femoral artery "pistol shots," and Quincke's pulse in the nail bed.

LABORATORY INVESTIGATION

The laboratory investigation of the elderly hypertensive patient should include the following (clinical implications are in parentheses).

1. Hemoglobin, hematocrit, and white blood cell count (erythremia, anemia, vascular inflammatory states)
2. Urinalysis (albuminuria, casts, hematuria)
3. Blood tests
   a. Serum electrolyte levels: sodium, potassium, chloride, carbon dioxide (Cushing's syndrome; aldosteronism)
   b. Serum glucose, blood urea nitrogen, creatinine values (diabetes mellitus, renal diseases)
   c. Cholesterol, calcium, phosphorus, and alkaline phosphatase values (atherosclerosis, renal stones)
   d. Triglycerides (high-density lipoproteins)

4. Electrocardiogram (left ventricular hypertrophy as well as ischemic heart disease)

With regard to the laboratory value for cholesterol, the effect of cholesterol as a risk factor of cardiovascular disease is diminished in late life, while that of hypertension persists and/or increases[3] (Fig. 11-4).

More extensive laboratory investigations are unwarranted except under the following conditions, most of which are quite rare:

1. Diastolic pressure above 115 or 120 mm Hg
2. Advanced retinopathy, such as grade III or IV
3. Recent onset of significant diastolic hypertension or marked further ele-

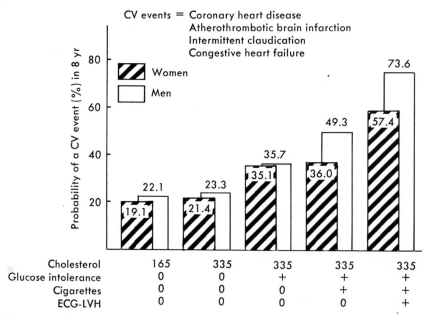

Fig. 11-4. Probability in men and women 70 years of age of cardiovascular disease at systolic blood pressure of 165 mm Hg according to risk factors (Framingham study: 18-year follow-up). (From Kannel, W. B.: Blood pressure and the development of cardiovascular disease in the aged. In Caird, F. I., Dall, J. L. C., and Kennedy, R. D., editors: Cardiology in old age, New York, 1976, Plenum Publishing Corp.)

vation of blood pressure in a known elderly hypertensive patient

4. Persistent low serum potassium level without kaliuretic medication (diuretics, L-dopa) or licorice ingestion

5. Signs or symptoms suggestive of pheochromocytoma

6. A diastolic pressure in the range of 105 to 115 mm Hg in a patient who does not respond to standard treatment

Steps in the more extensive workup for the above-listed indications include:

1. Rapid-sequence intravenous pyelogram (IVP)

2. Urine vanillylmandelic acid (VMA) – "catechol pathway")

3. Renal angiography

The major question regarding the last procedure listed (renal angiography) is whether the patient should be subjected to the morbidity and mortality associated with this procedure? The answer rests with whether an operative procedure is anticipated should a renovascular lesion be confirmed. Renal angiography should usually not be done in the elderly, because most elderly patients with renovascular hypertension respond well to medical approaches (medications), and also because the elderly often have impairment of the other kidney and significant other illnesses, making the risks of surgery even higher. There are, however, occasional instances where operative intervention is appropriate; in such instances, renal angiography should be performed. The angiogram, when abnormal, shows a stenosis or obstruction quite close to the aorta, in contrast to the obstructions in the renal artery that are closer to the kidney and characteristic of fibromuscular hyperplasia in younger women. Contrary to the high cure rate following corrective surgery for fibro-

muscular hyperplasia in younger women, the clinical improvement in blood pressure following correction in renal artery stenosis due to atheromata in the elderly is approximately 35%.

TREATMENT

The evidence is clear that elderly male patients with elevated diastolic pressures above 104 mm Hg benefit from antihypertensive treatment with a reduction in morbidity from stroke, heart failure, and renal impairment (though not a reduction in coronary artery disease).[6-8] Although there are no comparable data to serve as guidelines for treatment of diseases in older women, we believe that until we know otherwise, older women, too, should be treated if their diastolic levels are above 104 mm Hg.

For diastolic pressures between 90 and 104 mm Hg, the benefits of antihypertensive treatment in reducing morbidity in elderly male patients are not statistically significant, although they are suggestive.[7,8] Little data exist regarding reduction of hypertensive morbidity in older women.

The HDFP[15,16] study, focusing only on mortality and hypertension, reported decreased mortality resulting from treatment of black men and women and white men aged 60 to 74 years whose diastolic pressures were in the range of 90 to 104 mm Hg prior to treatment. There was no decrease in mortality in white women.

For patients with diastolic pressures within the 90 to 104 mm Hg range, the so-called "mild" range, we recommend cautious treatment with weight loss, salt restriction, and the safest of medications. The "safest" medications would be, in general, the thiazide diuretics. The risks of hypotension include end-organ ischemia[19-21] and/or possible subtle changes in certain aspects of cerebral electrical activity and/or mental function, as noted previously.[17,18]

Weight loss

Overweight hypertensive middle-aged adults have shown a significant decrease in their blood pressures with weight loss.[32,33] Weight loss may have a similar effect in the elderly hypertensive patient (data to substantiate this are not available). Weight loss diets at any age, however, are unlikely to be successful as a long-term approach because of poor compliance.

Salt restriction

There is suggestive, though not definite, evidence that simple moderate dietary salt restriction will produce a modest reduction in blood pressure. The study cited[34] was not age specific, however, and the reduction was not as great as with medications. It is well known that sodium is closely linked to hypertension, and there are cultures where salt is not part of the diet and there is no known hypertension. Animals studies, too, suggest a relationship between hypertension and salt.[35] Thus, the recommendation of salt restriction, commonly given to middle-aged and young hypertensive patients, is applicable to the elderly. However, compliance will be even more of a problem in the elderly, since salt restriction is not well tolerated.

Physical activity

Most studies showing the benefit of increased physical activity in lowering blood pressure refer to younger patients; there is some suggestion that this benefit would have to be gradual and well monitored in the elderly. This, too, would not be easily applied to the elderly, particularly those who are chronically ill.[36]

Medications
Diuretics

Thiazide diuretics should be prescribed in the form of hydrochlorothiazide at probably one half the usual adult dosage (or 25 mg PO once or twice per day). Alternatively, chlorthalidone, 12.5 mg PO in the morning, can be prescribed and increased to 25 to 100 mg once a day, if necessary.[36] Diuretics are the primary approach to treatment of elderly hypertensive patients who are in need of a medication approach. Most elderly patients who need medication will respond to a single medication, and this medication should be a diuretic except where there are appropriate contraindications. The side effects of diuretics are not pleasant, although they impair the quality of life less than most other antihypertensive medications. They cause frequent urination, which is bothersome—particularly to men with prostatic obstruction—and they produce nocturia, which interferes with sleep. Other side effects include glucose intolerance, worsening of previously existing diabetes mellitus, and hyperuricemia. Diuretics can also impair renal function, particularly in late life, when the renal blood flow and glomerular filtration rate are already decreased by about 50%. Diuretics may induce hypokalemia.[37] Elderly patients being treated with L-dopa for Parkinson's disease may develop hypokalemia because of the kaliuretic effect of the compound.[38] Consequently, elderly hypertensive patients taking thiazide diuretics and L-dopa (but not L-dopa with a decarboxylase inhibitor) are at a high risk for developing hypokalemia. When symptoms of hypokalemia occur, such as weakness and difficulty in walking, and are clearly related to a low serum potassium level, the diuretic should be supplemented with an oral potassium liquid or tablet. A wax material tablet containing potassium chloride may be too large for some elderly patients to swallow. An alternative approach to diuretic-induced hypokalemia in patients without renal insufficiency is to add triamterene, a potassium-retaining medication, or spironolactone, an antagonist of aldosterone. Each of these potassium-sparing diuretics is also available commercially in combination with a thiazide diuretic. Giving the elderly patient these combined medications may decrease compliance problems. When significant renal failure exists, a loop diuretic (furosemide) is indicated, rather than a thiazide diuretic, for the control of hypertension.

Antiadrenergics

Alpha-methyldopa. The occasional older hypertensive patient who will not respond to diuretic treatment will need an additional or substitute medication. One of the theoretical advantages of alpha-methyldopa is its lack of effect on the renal blood flow. Dosage should begin at 250 mg per day and be increased to 3,000 mg per day, as necessary. Problems include mental confusion, hepatitis, sedation, impotence, orthostatic hypertension, a positive direct Coombs' test in up to one fifth of patients, and hemolytic anemia in only a few.

Beta-adrenergic blocking agents: propranolol. An excellent alternative to alpha-methyldopa is a beta-adrenergic blocking agent, such as propranolol. The beta-adrenergic blocking agent lowers pressure via a reduction in cardiac output as well as suppression of renin and some central nervous system (CNS) effects. Significant side effects include exacerbation of CHF; bronchial asthma; chronic obstructive pulmonary disease; and occasional instances of confusion, nightmares, or sleep disturbance. The typical antihypertensive dosage for propranolol would be in the range of 20 to 80 mg, two to three times per day (40 to 240 mg/day). Of benefit is the absence of orthostatic hypotensive effects.

The Rauwolfia alkaloids: reserpine

These are excellent mild hypotensive agents but should not be used frequently with the elderly because of induction of depression, mental confusion, impotence, and peptic ulcer syndromes. The dosage range is 0.1 mg per day to about 0.25 mg per day in divided doses. Fluid retention, orthostatic hypotension and Parkinson's disease are other complications.

Vasodilators

Peripheral vasodilatation via hydralazine is, to some clinicians, a worrisome approach with the elderly because of induction of tachycardia and/or worsening or induction of myocardial ischemia. Other experts[39] prefer hydralazine to alpha-methyldopa, since hydralazine does not induce mental symptoms and may produce less tachycardia in the elderly than in the young. Prazosin, a new peripheral vasodilator, produces less tachycardia and more orthostatic hypotension than hydralazine.[40]

Ganglionic blocking agent

Guanethidine should not be used in the elderly, because of its many side effects and interactions with both prescribed and nonprescribed drugs and with tyrosine in food. Orthostatic hypotension, diarrhea, sodium retention, and inhibition of ejaculation are its most troublesome side effects.

Other problems with many antihypertensive medications

Postural hypotension. Postural hypotension is not a significant problem with propranolol. It is a significant problem with methyldopa, guanethidine, prazosin, and occasionally with the diuretics.

Mental confusion. Mental confusion or drowziness is a rare significant complication of the thiazide diuretics but a more common complication of propranolol, alpha-methyldopa, reserpine, and clonidine.

Costs. Guanethidine and the spironolactone-thiazide combination are expensive drugs. The theoretical benefits of the spironolactone-thiazide combination have already been mentioned.

Sexual impotence. Sexual impotence may accompany the use of any of the antihypertensive medications other than the thiazide diuretics. Sexual impotence is much more likely to occur with medication such as alpha-methyldopa, guanethidine, and reserpine. It is an infrequent accompaniment of treatment with propranolol.

Blocking effects of tricyclic antidepressants and phenothiazines on guanethidine or clonidine

Of interest is the blocking effects of tricyclic antidepressants and phenothiazines on the effects of guanethidine or clonidine. Since neither clonidine nor guanethidine is frequently used with the elderly, this is not a likely problem.

Effects of nonprescribed medications

Nonprescribed medications for respiratory infections include sympathomimetic amines and may produce rapid increases in blood pressure.

CONCLUSION

The likelihood of an older person with hypertension (systolic and/or diastolic) having simultaneous and perhaps related problems in either the brain, kidney,

heart, or peripheral vasculature is much greater than would occur in a young or middle-aged person. Adverse symptoms of the side effects of treatment and/or of lowering the blood pressure are more likely with the elderly than with middle-aged hypertensive patients. Some elderly patients appear more likely to develop hypokalemia when given diuretics, Also, orthostatic hypotension appears to be a greater problem in the elderly than in the middle-aged. Therefore, therapeutic decision making is difficult and requires extensive knowledge of the side effects and interactions of the medication.

Deciding on the appropriate diagnostic investigations and treatment of hypertension in the elderly requires a considerable command of the body of knowledge of geriatric cardiovascular disease. This includes an understanding of the available facts in the literature relating to age-specific morbidity factors, reversibility, and drug side effects. It is because hypertension remains a strong morbidity factor in late life that the decision about treatment is so important. Other factors, such as cholesterol, tend to become less significant in late life. Elderly hypertensive patients with diastolic pressures between 90 and 104 mm Hg should be treated with relatively "safe" medications (thiazide diuretics and/or anti-adrenergics) when simpler treatments, such as weight reduction, salt restriction, and increased activity fail. Although mortality of black men and women and white men is reduced, it is uncertain whether lowering of diastolic pressure in this range will reduce morbidity. On the other hand, those with diastolic pressures above 104 mm Hg appear to definitely benefit from antihypertensive treatment. There is no evidence at this time to support treatment of pure systolic hypertension. The issue in the treatment of hypertension is the risk of end-organ damage (the brain, in particular). In the elderly, the risk-benefit balance seems even more tenuous than in the younger adult hypertensive patient and thus requires greater skill from the clinician and further research.

REFERENCES

1. Dyer, A. R., Stemler, J., Shekelle, R. B., and others: Hypertension in the elderly, Med. Clin. North Am. **61**:513, 1977.
2. Ostfeld, A. H.: Elderly hypertensive patient, N.Y. State J. Med. **78**:1125, 1978.
3. Kannel, W. B.: Blood pressure and the development of cardiovascular disease in the aged. In Caird, F. I., Dall, J. L. C., and Kennedy, R. D., editors: Cardiology in old age, New York, 1976, Plenum Publishing Corp., p. 142.
4. Kannel, W. B.: Role of blood pressure in cardiovascular morbidity and mortality, Prog. Cardiovasc. Dis. **17**:5, 1973/1974.
5. Kannel, W. B., Castelli, W. P., McNamara, P. M., and Sorlie, P.: Some factors affecting morbidity and mortality in hypertension, Millbank Mem. Fund Q. **27**:116, 1969.
6. Veterans Administration Cooperative Study Group on Antihypertensive Agents: Effects of treatment on morbidity in hypertension. 1. Results in patients with diastolic hypertension averaging 115-129 mm Hg, J.A.M.A. **202**:116, 1967.
7. Veterans Administration Cooperative Study Group on Antihypertensive Agents: Effects of treatment on morbidity in hypertension. 2. Results in patients with diastolic blood pressure averaging 90 through 114 mm Hg, J.A.M.A. **213**:1143, 1970.
8. Veterans Administration Cooperative Study Group on Antihypertensive Agents: Effects of treatment on morbidity in hypertension. 3. Influence of age, diastolic pressure and prior cardiovascular disease, Circulation **54**:991, 1972.
9. Colandrea, M. H., Friedman, D. G., Nachman, M. Z., and Lynd, C. M.: Systolic hypertension in the elderly, Circulation **41**:239, 1970.
10. Koch-Weser, J.: The therapeutic challenge of systolic hypertension, N. Engl. J. Med. **289**:481, 1973.
11. Tarazi, R. C.: Should you treat systolic hypertension in elderly patients? Geriatrics **33**:25, 1978.
12. Brest, A. M., and Haddad, M.: Should systolic hypertension be treated: controversies in cardiology **8**(1):217, 1977.
13. Gubner, R. S.: Systolic hypertension: a pathogenetic entity, Am. J. Cardiol. **9**:773, 1962.
14. Halloch, P., and Benson, L. C.: Studies on the elastic properties of human isolated aorta, J. Clin. Invest. **16**:595, 1937.
15. Hypertension Detection and Follow-up Program Co-operative Group: Five-year findings of the hypertension detection and follow-up program. 1. Reduction in mortality in persons with high blood pressure, including mild hypertension, J.A.M.A. **242**:2562, 1979.
16. Hypertension Detection and Follow-up Program Co-operative Group: Five-year findings of the hypertension detection and follow-up program. 2. Mortality by race, sex, and age, J.A.M.A. **242**:2572, 1979.
17. Obrist, W., and Sokoloff, L.: Physiological-medical-EEG comparisons. In Birren, J. E., Butler, R. N., Greenhouse, S. W., and others, editors: Human aging. 1. A biological and behavioral study, DHEW Pub. No. (ADM77-122), 1971, U.S. Department of Health, Education, and Welfare, Public Health Service, p. 285.
18. Libow, L. S.: Interaction of medical, biologic, and behavioral factors on aging, adaptation and survival: an 11-year longitudinal study, Geriatrics **29**:75, 1974.
19. Wilkie, F., and Eisdorfer, C.: Intelligence and blood pressure. In Palmore, E., editor: Normal aging, vol. 2, Durham, N.C., 1974, Duke University Press.
20. Wilkie, F., and Eisdorfer, C.: Intelligence and blood pressure in the aged, Science **172**:959, 1971.
21. Jones, J. V.: Hypertension and the cerebral circulation—its relevance to the elderly, Am. Heart J. **96**:270, 1978.
22. Hypertension in the elderly, Lancet **1**:684, 1977.
23. Jackson, G., Piercianowski, T. A., Mahon, W., and Condon, J.: Inappropriate antihypertensive therapy in the elderly, Lancet **2**:1317, 1976.
24. Spence, J. D., Sibbald, W. J., and Cape, R. D.: Pseudohypertension in the elderly, Clin. Sci. Mol. Med. **55**:399s, 1978.
25. Society of Actuaries: Build and Blood Pressure Studies, Chicago, 1959, The Society.
26. Essential hypertension: new concepts about mechanisms: UCLA Conference, Ann. Int. Med. **79**:411, 1973.

27. Weidmann, P., Myttenaere-Bursztein, S., Maxwell, M. H., and Lima, J.: Effect of aging on plasma rennin and aldosterone in normal man, Kidney Int. **8**:325, 1975.

28. Libow, L. S.: Senile dementia and pseudo-senility: clinical investigation by appropriate laboratory tests and a new mental status technique. In Friedel, R., editor: Cognitive and emotional disturbances in the elderly, Seattle, 1977, University of Washington Press.

29. Jacobs, J. W.: Screening for organic mental syndromes in the medically ill, Ann. Intern. Med. **80**:40, 1971.

30. Kahn, R. L., Goldfarb, A. I., and others: Brief objective measures for the determination of mental status in the aged, Am. J. Psychiatry **3**:326, 1960.

31. Perlin, S., and Butler, R. M.: Psychiatric aspects of adaptation to the aging experience. In Birren, J. E., Butler, R. M., Greenhouse, S., and others, editors: Human aging. 1. A biological and behavioral study, DHEW Pub No. (ADM77-122), 1971, U.S. Department of Health, Education and Welfare, Public Health Service, p. 159.

32. Reisin, R., Abel, R., Modan, M., and others: Effect of weight loss without salt restriction on the reduction of blood pressure in overweight hypertensive patients, N. Engl. J. Med. **298**:1, 1978.

33. Tobian, L.: Hypertension and obesity, N. Engl. J. Med. **298**:46, 1978.

34. Morgan, T., Gillies, A., Morgan, G., and others: Hypertension treated by salt restriction, Lancet **1**:227, 1978.

35. Tobian, L.: Salt and hypertension, Ann. N.Y. Acad. Sci. **304**:178, 1978.

36. Report of the Joint National Committee on Detection, Evaluation and Treatment of High Blood Pressure, DHEW Pub. No. 77-1088, U.S. Department of Health, Education, and Welfare, Public Health Service.

37. Dall, J. L. C., Paulose, S., and Fergusson, J. H.: Potassium intake of elderly patients in hospital, Gerontol. Clin. **13**:114, 1971.

38. Granerus, A. K., and others: Kaliiuretic effect of L-dopa treatment in Parkinson patients, Acta Med. Scand. **201**:291, 1977.

39. Finnerty, F. A.: Hypertension in the elderly: special considerations in treatment, Postgrad. Med. **65**:119, 1979.

40. Kincaid, Smith, P.: Prazosin in the treatment of hypertension, Med. J. Aust. (spec. suppl.), August 1977, p. 27.

PROBLEM-SOLVING EXERCISES°
Case one

A 72-year-old, obese, black woman has a long-standing history of adult-onset diabetes mellitus and a history of angina pectoris brought on by exertion and promptly relieved by sublingual nitroglycerin, gr 1/150. During her annual physical examination you discover that the patient has a blood pressure of 180/110 mm Hg. Funduscopic examination reveals arteriovenous (AV) nicking and microaneurysms.

Questions

1. Would you treat this patient for hypertension on the basis of this single blood pressure reading?

2. On repeated exams over the next week the patient's blood pressure remains 180/110. Further investigations convince you that this is essential hypertension. Renal function appears normal for the patient's age. Is diet therapy advisable?

3. The patient will not accept diet restrictions. Which one of the following medications would you use as a drug of first choice?
   a. Hydralazine
   b. Hydrochlorothiazide
   c. Prazosin
   d. Guanethidine

4. Having chosen hydrochlorothiazide, what would be your starting dosage?
   a. 25 mg once per day
   b. 100 mg bid
   c. 100 mg qAM

5. Two weeks later the patient returns with a blood pressure of 170/110. Your next step would be to:
   a. Increase hydrochlorothiazide to 25 mg bid and then by further increments of 25 mg to a maximum of 100 mg/day
   b. Add hydralazine
   c. Add propranolol

6. After adequate efforts with the diuretic,

°Some questions may have more than one correct answer.

there is only a modest change in blood pressure; the level now is 160/108. You decide to add a second medication. You could choose:

a. Hydralazine
b. Propranolol
c. Guanethidine

7. The addition of propranolol brings the patient's pressure down to 150/90. Physical exam is unremarkable except the heart rate is now 55/min and regular (previously 80/min and regular). An ECG shows regular sinus rhythm and left ventricular hypertrophy (LVH), but no other abnormalities. The patient exhibits no symptoms. You would:

a. Discontinue propranolol
b. Not alter the present medication regimen
c. Change to hydralazine

Case two

A 75-year-old, white man with a history of CHF treated with digoxin and adult-onset diabetes mellitus treated with 40 units of NPH insulin is found to have a blood pressure in the range of 200/105. Reserpine is added to his regimen. One month later the patient is seen by you. His blood pressure is 150/80, and he complains of feeling depressed, not eating, and at times not being able to find things about the house.

Questions

1. Which medication is most likely contributing to the mental depression (choose only one):

a. Reserpine
b. Digoxin
c. Thiazide diuretic

2. Reserpine is discontinued, and propranolol is started; the blood pressure is still 150/80. The depression, however, continues; 5 days later the patient is admitted to the emergency room in a coma with a blood glucose determination of 30 mg and no other signs or symptoms of hypoglycemia. Significant factors in producing the

coma in the absence of signs or symptoms of hypoglycemia are:

a. Anorexia related to depression
b. Propranolol
c. Insulin
d. All of the above

3. The patient is treated with glucose, and propranolol is discontinued. His blood pressure increases to 180/100. What treatment for hypertension would you institute at this time?

a. Clonidine
b. Guanethidine
c. Thiazide diuretic

Case three

A 78-year-old white man, recently admitted to a skilled nursing facility is noted to have a blood pressure of 180/100. He has no prior history of hypertension. An ECG reveals LVH, and a chest x-ray film is unremarkable. Fundi reveal AV nicking. No hemorrhages or exudates are noted. Renal function is normal for this patient's age. His mental state is clear.

Questions

1. You decide to:

a. Tell the patient that his blood pressure is normal
b. Consider the patient's blood pressure as "borderline" elevated – you would like to reevaluate him in a few weeks

2. The patient is seen again in 1 month, and this blood pressure at this time is 180/106. Physical examination is unchanged, and the patient offers no symptoms. You would:

a. Do nothing, because 180/106 is not a pathological level
b. Start antihypertensive therapy
c. Do nothing because the patient is old, ill, and in a nursing home

3. Prior to starting antihypertensive therapy, you want to rule out secondary causes for hypertension. You would order as a first line of investigation:

a. T_4
b. Hematocrit
c. BUN

d. Serum sodium
e. Serum potassium
f. Blood glucose
g. Uric acid
h. Urine analysis
i. Urine VMA
j. IVP

Case four

A 75-year-old white woman had persistent blood pressure readings of 160/110. After ruling out secondary causes for hypertension, her prior physician found it necessary to combine a thiazide diuretic with guanethidine. Her blood pressure is now controlled at 140/90. The patient complains of severe depression because her husband has recently been hospitalized for CHF. You reassure her and start her on a tricyclic antidepressant.

Questions

1. Two weeks later the patient returns to your office, less depressed but with a blood pressure of 160/110. You suspect:
   a. The patient is not taking her antihypertensive medications because of depression
   b. A drug interaction
   c. The patient has become refractory to diuretics
2. After suspecting a drug interaction between the tricyclic antidepressant and guanethidine you would:
   a. Add alpha-methyldopa
   b. Abruptly discontinue the tricyclic antidepressant
   c. Continue the tricyclic antidepressant and increase the dosage of guanethidine to overcome the interference from the tricyclic antidepressant

Case five

A 72-year-old white woman has a history of hypertension and transient cerebral ischemic attacks. On physical examination the patient's blood pressure is 170/108. You record her blood pressure on three separate visits, and it

remains at 170/110. You start the patient on an appropriate dosage of diuretics and alpha-methyldopa.

Questions

1. One month later the patient returns to you with complaints of feeling dizzy after arising from a sitting position. Her blood pressure is 140/80. You would:
   a. Caution her to get up slowly from a resting position and evaluate her for orthostatic hypotension
   b. Dismiss her symptoms and tell her that her blood pressure is well controlled and not to worry
2. The patient returns to your office in 2 weeks with the same complaints of dizziness on arising. She also states that when she doesn't take the alpha-methyldopa, she feels better. Her blood pressure in the sitting position is 160/105; on standing it is 110/80. You would:
   a. Continue alpha-methyldopa and add a tricyclic antidepressant
   b. Continue alpha-methyldopa and add hydralazine
   c. Discontinue alpha-methyldopa and if the blood pressure remains significantly elevated, continue treatment with either a diuretic or propranolol

ANSWERS TO PROBLEM-SOLVING EXERCISES
Case one

1. No. Although a single blood pressure reading meaningfully correlates with morbidity, it is common clinical practice to classify someone as hypertensive only after repeated measurements.
2. Yes. When an obese, hypertensive middle-aged person loses weight, his blood pressure decreases. Although not tested in the elderly, weight reduction appears to be a sensible, early step in treatment of the obese, elderly hypertensive patient.
3. b. A thiazide diuretic is generally chosen as the first medication to be used, because of its reasonably well-tolerated and easily

measured chemical and clinical side effects.

4. a. "Start slow": thus, 25 mg PO once per day.

5. a. "Go slow": increase dosage gradually.

6. b. Propranolol is generally chosen rather than hydralazine or guanethidine because of its lesser side effects. (Alpha-methyldopa is probably more commonly used than propranolol.)

7. b. The propranolol (beta-adrenergic blocking agent)–induced bradycardia is not clinically troublesome in this patient; thus, do not alter the medications.

Case two

1. a. Reserpine is well-known to produce depression, sometimes quite serious in nature.

2. d. Anorexia coupled with insulin may lead to hypoglycemia. Propranolol may obscure the tachycardia and other signs of hypoglycemia.

3. c. A diuretic appears to be the best first step. Obviously the diuretics, too, have troublesome side effects.

Case three

1. b. A blood pressure of 180/100 mm Hg is abnormal at any age. However, solid evidence is lacking that lowering this pressure will reduce morbidity and/or mortality in the elderly (or in any age group for that matter). This pressure should be re-evaluated.

2. b. The patient should be treated, probably starting with a diuretic. The patient's being in a nursing home should not stop him from receiving proper care for this problem.

3. a to h. Simple, inexpensive, and noninvasive tests are appropriate.

Case four

1. a and b. Depressed patients may not be taking medications as prescribed. The interaction of guanethidine and a tricyclic antidepressant produces an inhibition of the effect of the guanethidine.

2. c. It may be necessary to increase the dosage of guanethidine to overcome the inhibition.

Case five

1. a. Orthostatic hypotension is a frequent side effect of many antihypertensive medications, including alpha-methyldopa.

2. c. When the orthostatic symptoms are troublesome, it is necessary to reduce dosage and, at times, discontinue the medication.

POSTTEST

1. List five causes of pure systolic hypertension.

2. List four common side effects of antihypertensive medications in elderly patients. Include one example of a drug that can cause each side effect.

3. It has been shown that:
   a. High systolic blood pressure is associated with increased risk of cardiovascular and cerebrovascular morbidity and mortality
   b. High diastolic blood pressure is associated with increased risk of cardiovascular and cerebrovascular morbidity and mortality
   c. Both a and b

4. *True or false:* Elderly white female patients whose diastolic blood pressures are consistently between 90 and 104 mm Hg will clearly benefit in terms of decreased risk of cardiovascular morbidity and mortality by receiving adequate antihypertensive therapy.

5. The most appropriate initial therapeutic trial in treating hypertension in elderly patients is _____.

6. Name a category of antihypertensive drugs that reliably lowers systolic blood

pressure without significantly affecting diastolic pressure.

7. The accepted "usual" definition of hypertension:

a. Sets an upper limit for systolic and diastolic values based on observed end-organ damage, which routinely occurs in patients whose pressures exceed this

b. Chooses a "normal" blood pressure limit (standard deviation from the mean; e.g., 140/90) that has, as its basis, population statistics that are not usually age relevant

c. Depends on confirmation of symptoms reported by the patient that can be clearly attributed to the elevated blood pressure

d. Includes well-established diastolic and systolic blood pressure levels by age for each decade of life

8. Based on cross-sectional population studies, as age increases (going from 20 years of age to 70 years of age):

a. Systolic blood pressure increases, and diastolic blood pressure is unchanged

b. Systolic blood pressure is unchanged, and diastolic blood pressure increases

c. Systolic blood pressure increases, and diastolic blood pressure increases

d. Neither systolic nor diastolic blood pressure changes significantly

9. Alpha-methyldopa is one of the most commonly used antihypertensive medications. List the adverse effects of this drug in the elderly.

10. For an elderly hypertensive patient with persistently elevated blood pressure despite 100 mg per day of hydrochlorothiazide, the most appropriate additional medication might be:

a. Propranolol

b. Guanethidine

c. Reserpine

d. Clonidine

ANSWERS TO PRETEST AND POSTTEST

1. Five of the following:
   - Atherosclerosis of the aorta and large arteries
   - Hyperthryroidism
   - Aortic insufficiency
   - Arteriovenous fistula
   - Hyperkinetic heart disease
   - Fever

2. Four of the following:
   - Postural hypotension: guanethidine, prazosin
   - Impotence: alpha-methyldopa
   - Depression: reserpine, alpha-methyldopa
   - Hypokalemia: thiazide diuretics
   - Hyperglycemia: thiazide diuretics
   - Hyperuricemia: thiazide diuretics
   - Exacerbation of congestive heart failure: propranolol
   - Bronchospasm: propranolol
   - Confusion, lethargy: alpha-methyldopa, reserpine, clonidine, propranolol

3. c. Elevated systolic and/or diastolic blood pressures correlate with increased cardiovascular and cerebrovascular morbidity and mortality in late life, although a decrease in pressure may not be reverse this morbidity and/or mortality.

4. False. Reports of studies vary on this point. The VA study (see references 6 to 8 in text) showed a decline in morbidity at all ages for men with diastolic blood pressures in the range of 90 to 105 mm Hg. This decline, however, was not statistically significant. The HDFP study (see references 15 and 16 in text) revealed a decline in mortality for black men and women and white men, but not for white women.

5. Weight reduction (where applicable) and moderate salt restriction.

6. None exist at this time.

7. b. Although this is the correct answer, it is not the correct approach.

8. c. The diastolic blood pressure reaches a plateau at the 50- to 60-year-old range and does not further increase.

9. Depression of the central nervous system (lethargy, confusion); postural hypotension; hepatitis; and Coombs' positive hemolytic anemia.

10. a. A single medication (thiazide diuretic) usually suffices for control of most elderly hypertensive patients who need a medication. When a second has to be added, an antiadrenergic is a good choice. Alpha-methyldopa has been used extensively, although it causes orthostatic hypotension and lethargy. It is an alternative to propranolol. Either propranolol or alpha-methyldopa is preferred by many clinicians for the elderly in contrast to a vasodilator (hydralazine, prazosin) or ganglionic blocking agent (guanethidine). However, some clinicians would choose hydralazine as a second drug. There is neither enough experience nor any clear role for clonidine in the elderly. It may cause mental confusion and a "rebound" cardiovascular problem on abrupt cessation of the medication. Reserpine has a beneficial effect on blood pressure, but its side effects, especially mental depression, make it less useful in the elderly.

Chapter 12

Thyroid function and disease

PAUL D. GILBERT

EDUCATIONAL OBJECTIVES
Attitudinal

The student should:
1. Recognize that thyroid disorders are the second most common endocrinopathic disorder in the elderly
2. Recognize that thyroid disorders in the elderly are easily misdiagnosed and/or mistreated
3. Realize that there are serious dangers in simply extrapolating treatment and/or diagnostic approaches from the young or middle aged

Cognitive

The student should:
1. Recognize the altered thyroid physiology accompanying normal aging (e.g., changes in thyroid hormone metabolism and thyrotropin-releasing hormone [TRH] responsiveness)
2. Recognize that hyperphagia, diarrhea, and hyperalertness may not be present as accompaniments of hyperthyroidism
3. Recognize that interpretation of a screening T_4 test requires the concomitant testing of the T_3 resin uptake or the thyroxine-binding globulin (TBG)
4. Recognize that the T_3 suppression test is dangerous in the elderly
5. Recognize that hypothyroidism is an easily missed diagnosis in the elderly

Skill

The student should:
1. Learn to examine the neck and thyroid gland
2. Learn to look for key symptoms and signs in the elderly with thyroid dysfunction
3. Learn to interpret the often conflicting laboratory results reflecting thyroid disorders
4. Learn to treat thyroid disease cautiously and safely in the elderly, especially those with cardiovascular disease

---

PRETEST

True or false
1. The T_3 suppression test generally should not be used in the older patient.
2. The response of thyroid-stimulating hormone (TSH) to thyrotropin-releasing hormone (TRH) is blunted in healthy older men.
3. The T_3 resin uptake measures serum T_3.
4. The T_3 resin uptake and the calculable free thyroxine index (FT_4I) can be very helpful in gaining insight into the meaning of serum T_4 by radioimmunoassay (RIA).
5. The major body source of T_3 in the elderly is direct synthesis of T_3 by the thyroid gland.
6. Low serum T_3 levels are common in older persons and/or persons with a variety of acute and/or chronic illnesses.
7. Weight loss, anorexia, and/or constipation are common in the history of older hyperthyroid patients.
8. Nodular hyperthyroidism is the most common type of hyperthyroidism in the elderly.
9. ^{131}I is the usual treatment of choice in older patients with hyperthyroidism.

10. In most elderly hyperthyroid patients, especially those with cardiac disorders, ^{131}I should be preceded by 4 to 6 weeks of antithyroid drugs, followed by 48 to 72 hours of withdrawal of such drugs. The antithyroid drugs should then be started again 3 to 4 days after ^{131}I is given.

11. Hypothyroidism is easily missed, because the slowing of physical and mental activity may be incorrectly attributed to "old age."

12. The best screening laboratory tests for the diagnosis of hyperthyroidism are T_4 by RIA, coupled with T_3 resin uptake test or thyroid-binding globulin (TBG) level.

13. TSH and creatine phosphokinase (CPK) are both elevated in hyperthyroidism.

14. Thyroxine is the best replacement therapy in hypothyroidism and should generally be given in lower doses than in the young and slowly increased.

Thyroid dysfunction is common in the elderly. Many of the symptoms, signs, and laboratory tests are altered by normal age-related changes. Furthermore, the clinical presentation is often different from that in younger patients (e.g., the prevalence of constipation and/or anorexia as part of the history of hyperthyroidism in the elderly, or the decrease in serum triiodothyronine [T_3] with age).

This chapter focuses on the body of knowledge of thyroid function and dysfunction as specifically applied to the older person.

THYROID FUNCTION AND THYROID FUNCTION TESTS
Normal changes with aging
Anatomy

Although there is some question raised by a few studies, it is generally accepted that the size and weight of the thyroid gland diminish with advancing age. There is an increase in lymphocytic infiltration with dense collagenous replacement of the fine perifollicular reticulum fibers, fibrosis, decreased mitotic activity, quantitative changes in the colloid, distention and obliteration of follicles, and increased nodularity.[1-4] By the eighth decade there is an almost 100% incidence of microscopic nodularity.[5] However, the functional reserve of the thyroid gland appears to be little affected by these anatomic changes.

Basal metabolic rate

It has long been recognized that the basal metabolic rate (BMR) decreases with advancing age. This appears to be a consequence of a normal decrease in lean body mass rather than of decreased thyroid function. If the BMR is expressed as a function of oxygen consumption per unit of functioning tissue mass (as reflected by body water or total potassium content), it does not change with age.[6]

Radioactive iodine uptake studies

There is decreased renal clearance of iodide with advancing age, which parallels the decline in glomerular filtration rate. This is reflected in increased plasma iodide levels, and finally in increased intrathyroidal iodide levels. The latter, via intrathyroidal autoregulatory mechanisms (not involving thyroid-stimulating hormone [TSH]), result in decreased trapping of iodide by the gland.[7,8] The overall effect is for a decrease in the absolute iodine uptake and a minor decrease in the 24-hour ^{131}I uptake.[9-12] These decreases are compensatory to increased plasma iodide levels and, as we shall see, to decreased peripheral turnover of T_3 and T_4.

TSH levels

TSH is present in the serum in concentrations of $0.5\mu U$ to $6.0\mu U/ml$. Levels are invariably high in primary hypothyroidism and usually low in secondary and tertiary hypothyroidism. Patients with decreased thyroidal reserve may have slightly elevated TSH levels. The adequacy of replacement in the hypothyroid patient can be assessed by the return of TSH levels to normal.

Most studies indicate no alteration in TSH levels in the elderly.[12-14] A few studies suggest that basal TSH levels may be higher than in a younger population but still within the range of normal.[15-17] Since the elderly can have strikingly raised TSH levels in hypothyroidism, it appears that the anterior pituitary gland is capable of producing TSH normally and that the pituitary does not sense any difference in thyroid hormone levels in older patients. There is no change in the fractional turnover rate of TSH.

Response of the thyroid gland to TSH

The thyroid glands of patients with secondary (pituitary) and tertiary (hypothalamic) hypothyroidism are atrophic but are capable of responding if sufficiently stimulated by TSH. The glands of primary hypothyroid patients are not capable of responding. This is the basis of a test. The vast majority of secondary and tertiary hypothyroid patients will show an increase in their 24-hour ^{131}I uptake to 20% with a doubling of the baseline value and an accompanying rise in the T_4 of $1.5\mu g/dl$ to $2\mu g/dl$ when 10 U of TSH is injected daily for 3 days.

Most studies indicate a normal thyroidal response to exogenous TSH in the elderly, although a few suggest some blunting.[18-20] This is unresolved, but a real question exists as to what extent the doses of TSH used in testing reflect a realistic physiological challenge. Secondary and tertiary hypothyroidism are rare in the elderly, and better tests for their diagnosis exist; thus, the TSH test is rarely used.

T_3 suppression test

In the hyperthyroid patient, the gland functions autonomously (not under TSH control). The administration of T_4 in doses sufficient to suppress pituitary secretion of TSH will not affect the ^{131}I uptake or T_4 as it will in a normal patient whose thyroid gland is functioning in response to TSH. The administration of $75\mu g$ to $100\mu g$ of T_3 a day for 10 days will suppress the 24-hour ^{131}I uptake of a normal (nonautonomous) gland to less than half the baseline value and usually to less than 15% in 24 hours.

There is a concomitant decrease in T_4, since thyroidal production of this hormone is turned off by the T_3. Hyperthyroid patients will rarely if ever suppress the 24-hour uptake. In as much as most patients with exophthalmic Graves' disease are nonsuppressible, the test has value in the diagnosis of endocrine exophthalmos as well. Finally, one can use this test to demonstrate autonomous nodules on scan. Thyroid glands of older patients are normally suppressible; therefore, the T_3 suppression test is normal. The T_3 suppression test is hazardous in the elderly, because one is apt to perform it on a patient with an autonomous gland—and the effects of the administered T_3 and endogenous hormone will then be cumulative. Cardiovascular complications of hyperthyroxinemia may result.

TSH response to TRH

The pituitary response to thyrotropin-releasing hormone (TRH) is modulated by the primary effect of thyroid hormone on the pituitary gland; an excess of thyroid hormone inhibits and a lack of hormone enhances the pituitary secretion of TSH in response to TRH. The administration of $400\mu g$ of TRH intravenously results in a prompt twofold to threefold increase in TSH levels, which peak at 30 minutes and return to baseline values in 2 hours. In addition, there is a significant increase in T_3 levels (40 to 60 ng/dl) 4 hours later. The effects on T_4 and ^{131}I uptake with this dosage are not impressive or predictable. The administration of this dosage of TRH to patients with primary hypothyroidism or decreased thyroidal reserve results in a larger increment in TSH levels, which takes a longer period of time to return to baseline and is not associated with a rise in T_3. Secondary hypothyroid patients usually start with low or unmeasurable levels of TSH and do not respond to TRH. Tertiary or hypothalamic hypothyroid patients have pituitary and thyroid glands capable of responding; although they may start out with low levels of TSH, they do increase these levels in response to TRH, albeit the response may be somewhat delayed and blunted. A few patients with pituitary hypothyroidism may have measurable levels of TSH or may respond to TRH in the same manner as tertiary hypothyroid patients. It is believed that in the first instance there may not be complete atrophy of the thyrotrophs, and in the second that either there is some interruption in the hypothalamic-pituitary portal circulation, so that TRH does not normally reach the pituitary gland, or that there is an abnormality of the thyrotrophs such that the basal secretion is impaired but that pharmacological doses of TRH can elicit a response.

A variety of chronic and acute illnesses (including coma) have been associated with a damping of the TSH response to TRH for varying periods of time in patients without demonstrable thyroid or central nervous system (CNS) disease.[21]

Thyrotoxic patients start off with low or unmeasurable TSH levels that do not increase in response to TRH. This is as expected, since the effects of thyroid hormone predominate at the pituitary level and block any response to TRH. Decreased pituitary responsiveness to TRH may be the most sensitive index of thyroid hormone excess.

Whereas TRH testing in thyrotoxic patients reflects either increased intrapituitary levels of thyroid hormone or slight serum elevations (which might be in the range of normal but are elevated for that patient at that time), the T_3 suppression test reflects the presence or absence of autonomy of the thyroid gland. These two tests frequently, but not always, parallel each other. The relationship of these tests to the persistence of active Graves' disease and the presence and titers of thyroid-stimulating antibodies has not yet been determined.

In patients who are receiving suppressive doses of L-thyroxine (Synthroid), it takes about 6 weeks after discontinuation of therapy for the hypothalamic-pituitary-thyroid axis to return to baseline responsiveness.[22]

Although the data are confusing, it appears that the response of TSH to TRH is often blunted in normal men over the age of 50 and may be suggestive of a hyperthyroid or secondary hypothyroid pattern.[12,16,21,23,24] This seems to be less so in elderly women, who often have relatively normal responses.[25] However, in elderly people of both sexes, the secondary rise in T_3 is blunted. The explanation for these phenomona is unknown. A good rise in TSH levels after the administration of TRH excludes hyperthyroidism in the elderly patient, but a blunted response (unless flat) does not necessarily mean that hyperthyroidism is present (especially in a male patient).

Serum levels of T_3, T_4, and thyroid-binding proteins

On release from the thyroid gland, T_3 and T_4 are immediately and almost completely bound to specific plasma proteins in a firm and reversible bond. Thyroid-binding globulin (TBG), an inter-alpha globulin, is the most important of three proteins, binding about 60% to 70% of the thyroid hormones. Although it has a limited number of binding sites, which are normally one third saturated with hormone, it has the greatest affinity (binding coefficient) for thyroid hormone. Thyroid-binding prealbumin (TBPA) binds 20% of the bound hormone, and the number and affinity of its binding sites are intermediate between TBG and thyroid-binding albumen (TBA), which is the least important of these proteins, binding less than 10% of thyroid hormone in an almost nonspecific bond. Only minute amounts of hormone exist in the free and metabolically active state: 0.02% to 0.04% (1.2 to 4 ng/dl) of the total T_4 (4.5μg/dl to 12μg/dl) and 0.2% to 0.4% (0.2 to 0.8 ng/dl) of the total T_3 (90 to 190 ng/dl) exist free; the remaining 99+% is bound. The binding coefficient of T_3 is significantly less than that of T_4, so that less of its binds and that which does so is less tightly bound. Free T_4 (FT_4) and free T_3 (FT_3) exist in a dynamic equilibrium, with T_3 and T_4 bound to the thyroid-binding proteins ($T_4 \cdot$ TBP, $T_3 \cdot$ TBP). From the equation below, describing the relationship between FT_4, thyroid-binding protein (TBP), and $T_4 \cdot$ TBP, it can be seen that the level of free hormone is directly related to the amount bound and inversely proportional to the number of free binding sites on the binding proteins.

$$(FT_4) \ (TBP) \rightleftharpoons T_4 \cdot TBP$$

or

$$(FT_4) \rightleftharpoons \frac{(T_4 \cdot TBP)}{(TBP)}$$

or

$$FT_4 \rightleftharpoons T_4 \cdot TBP \times \frac{1}{(TBP)}$$

It is the serum level of free and metabolically active thyroid hormones in which we are interested, but these measurements are not yet routine. Our determination of thyroid hormone levels in the blood measures hormone bound to the binding proteins (T_4 by radioimmunoassay [RIA], T_3 by RIA) and the number of unoccupied binding sites on these proteins (T_3 resin uptake or T_3 binding ratio). As long as the levels of TBP remain normal, these tests accurately reflect the level of free hormone and the metabolic state of the patient. As the level of TBP rises (or falls), the number of binding sites rises (or falls) and the amount of bound T_3 and T_4 rises (or falls) — the T_4 and T_3 by RIA rise (or fall). In the presence of a normal hypothalamic-pituitary-thyroid axis and normal cellular metabolism, the absolute levels of free and metabolically active T_3 and T_4 remain constant and normal despite alterations in TBP levels and the patients remain eumetabolic.

The maintenance of normal levels of free hormone in these circumstances is explained by several mechanisms. As TBP levels rise, free hormone is bound to these proteins and the resultant transient decrease in free hormone levels is immediately sensed by the pituitary gland, which increases its TSH secretion with resultant increased thyroidal production and release of T_3 and T_4 with maintenance of normal levels of FT_3 and FT_4 and the eumetabolic state. The reverse is true with decreased levels of TBP.

It is the intracellular levels of free thyroid hormone that determine its rate of degradation. In the above example, an increase in TBP levels would be reflected by decreased levels of free hormone in the serum and at the cellular level. The resultant decreased turnover rate of thyroid hormone would quickly be reflected by a rise to normal of free hormone in the blood without the interposition of altered TSH secretion. The converse would be true with decreased levels of TBP.

The measurement of T_3 and T_4 by RIA are now routine tests in almost all thyroid laboratories. They reflect not only the sum production and disposal rates of thyroid hormone, but also the levels of TBP. Conditions and drugs raising the levels of TBP raise the levels of T_3 and T_4 by RIA. Conversely, the situations lowering the levels of TBP also lower the levels of T_3 and T_4 by RIA.

Chief among the states in which there are increased levels of TBP in the elderly are the administration of estrogenic substances during menopause, the acute stage of viral hepatitis, chronic hepatitis, and occasionally cirrhosis. Decreased levels of TBP are commonly seen with prolonged and major illness, with the administration of androgens and anabolic steroids, after surgical stress, and in hypoproteinemic states such as nephrosis and chronic liver disease. Dilantin (in addition to altering the hepatic metabolism of TBG), penicillin, and aspirin in large doses occupy binding sites on the binding proteins and thus behave as if they decreased the levels of TBP. Up to 20% of patients admitted to geriatric units show disturbances reflecting low TBG levels, often associated with decreased serum albumin concentration.[26] There are, of course, genetic increases and decreases of these proteins.

The T_3 resin uptake, or *binding ratio*, reflects the number of unoccupied binding sites on the binding proteins. *It does not measure T_3 levels.* If the serum of the normal patient is incubated with radioactive T_3 (T_3^*), the T_3^* will bind to unoccupied binding sites on the binding proteins in proportion to their number. The amount of T_3^* that does not bind and is removed by a secondary binder (usually a resin) is then inversely proportional to the number of free binding sites available. The serum of the thyrotoxic patient has a normal number of binding sites, most of which are occupied by thyroid hormone, leaving fewer free binding sites. If this serum is incubated with T_3^*, less of the T_3^* will bind (since there are fewer free binding sites available) and more will be picked up by the secondary binder. Conversely, the hypothyroid patient has fewer binding sites occupied by T_4 and more free sites available. When the serum of this patient is incubated with T_3^*, more of the T_3^* will bind and less will be accumulated by the secondary binder. In patients with elevated levels of TBP, the increased number of binding sites available results in more T_4 binding to them (T_4 by RIA would be elevated, often to hyperthyroid levels). The increase in the number of binding sites is greater than the increased T_4 binding, so that more free binding sites remain. As a result, when this serum is incubated with T_3^*, more of the T_3^* will bind to these available binding sites and less will be available to be picked by the secondary binder. The T_3 resin uptake will look like that of hypothyroidism. The level of free hormone and the metabolic state of the patient remain normal. In patients with decreased levels of TBP there are fewer total binding sites available, less T_4 binds to them (T_4 by RIA would be decreased, often to hypothyroid levels), and fewer free binding sites available. When this serum is incubated with T_3^*, little of the T_3^* binds (since there are so few free binding sites) and larger amounts are left over for the secondary binder to accumulate. The T_3 resin uptake then looks like that of hyperthyroidism and the T_4 by RIA looks like that of hypothyroidism; the levels of free hormone and the metabolic state of the patient remain normal.

When the T_3 and T_4 by RIA go in one direction and the T_3 resin uptake goes in the other, suspect an alteration in levels of TBP, not an alteration in metabolic status.

From the preceeding, it is obvious that one can accurately estimate the levels of free hormone by examining the T_3 and T_4 by RIA and the T_3 resin uptake. The free thyroxine index (FT_4I) is obtained by multiplying the T_4 by RIA by the T_3 resin uptake (when this is obtained by counting the radioactive T_3 bound to the secondary binder). It comes very close to the actual FT_3 and FT_4 as measured by equilibrium dialysis. The mathematical justification of this can be appreciated from the formula on p. 250. T_4 by RIA measures T_4 bound to TBG. The T_3 resin uptake, measuring the T_3^* picked up by the secondary binder, actually measures the inverse of the number of free binding sites. A free T_3 index (FT_3I) may be similarly measured.[27]

In clinical settings where there are marked alterations in the level of TBG,

the T_3 resin uptake does not accurately reflect the magnitude of these changes; thus, the calculated FT_4 and FT_3 indices may vary significantly from the level of free hormone as determined by equilibrium dialysis. This is particularly true in cases in which there are marked reductions in TBG levels in acutely ill patients. Here, the levels of FT_4 measured by equilibrium dialysis are usually elevated (albeit transiently), and the calculated FT_4I may be falsely low. The explanation for this phenomonon is not clear.[28,29] The magnitude of change in free hormone levels exceeds that which is explicable by decreased TBPA levels. This damping effect may be fairly well overcome by relating the amount of T_3^* picked up by the secondary binder to the amount of T_3^* that is unbound (rather than to the total amount of T_3^* used in the test). Likewise, performance of the T_3 resin uptake at a physiological pH rather than at a pH of 5.4 (as is usually done) tends to correct much of this error. Chopra[30] postulates and has some evidence suggesting the presence of a heat-labile substance in the sera of such patients that interferes with the binding of thyroid hormones to their binding proteins at physiological pHs. It may be that the measurement of reverse T_3 (normal values are 20 to 60 ng/dl — see later) in these circumstances would be a more rewarding index of thyroid function.

Basic information: T_3 and T_4 metabolism

Under normal circumstances the thyroid gland produces and secretes about $90\mu g$ of T_4 and $5\mu g$ of T_3 daily. The major route of T_4 disposal (85%) is via deiodination. Of the $30\mu g$ of T_3 generated and turned over daily, $25\mu g$ (80%) arises not from the thyroid gland but from the 5'-

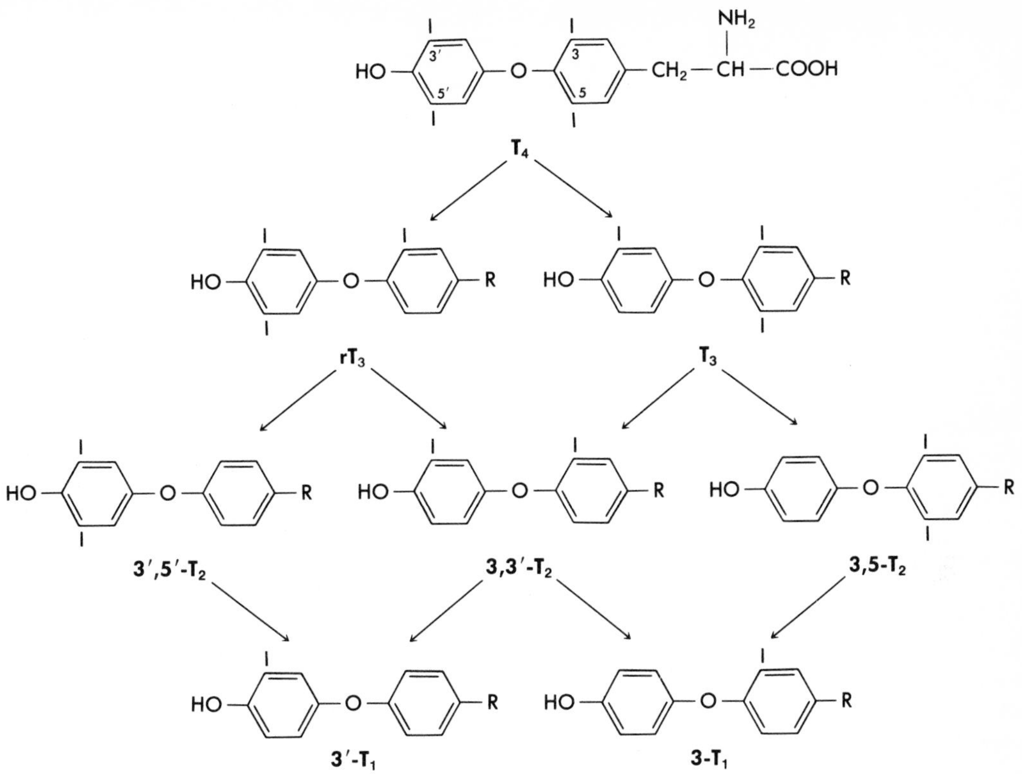

Fig. 12-1. Metabolic pathway demonstrating T_4 deiodination.

deiodination of T_4 by those peripheral tissues that have nuclear binding sites for T_3 and that are capable of utilizing it. This accounts for 40% of the T_4 deiodinated daily. The remaining 60% is deiodinated at the 5 position to the metabolically inert reverse T_3. Less than 2% of the reverse T_3 generated each day originates from the thyroid gland (Fig. 12-1). That these deiodinations are not random but are under tight metabolic control, most likely involving separate 5'- and 5-deiodinases, is evidenced by the following: (1) levels of T_3 and reverse T_3 rise proportionately in response to the administration of increasing amounts of T_4 (suggest-

ing that both routes of deiodination are high capacity and neither substrate, enzyme, nor product limited); and (2) in a variety of clinical situations the levels of T_3 and reverse T_3 move in opposite directions.[31,32] See Table 12-1.

It is important to recall that the peripheral rate of turnover of thyroid hormones is directly related to the levels of hormone at the cellular level (i.e., the half-life [$T_{1/2}$] of T_4 may decrease to as little as 2 days in hyperthyroidism or increase to as much as 10 days in hypothyroidism).

Before one can properly interpret T_3 values, one must understand the T_3 syndromes.

Table 12-1. Summary of the metabolic characteristics of T_3 and T_4

	T_4	T_3
Total	$4\mu g/dl$ to $12\mu g/dl$	90 to 190 ng/dl
Metabolically active		
Percent free	0.03% to 0.04%	0.2% to 0.4% ($10 \times T_4$)
Amount free	1.2 to 4 ng/dl	0.2 to 0.8 ng/dl ($5 \times T_4$)
Volume of distribution	12L	40L
Total extrathyroidal pool	$900\mu g$	$60\mu g$
$T_{1/2}$	7 days	1 day
Daily production	$90\mu g$	$30\mu g$ ($25\mu g$ from T_4)

Eumetabolic low T_3 syndromes

Patients with a wide variety of nonthyroidal illnesses (acute disease; starvation and fasting; chronic liver, cardiac, renal, and neoplastic disease; postoperatively; after epidural anesthesia; patients receiving steroids or antithyroid drugs; and diabetic ketoacidosis) have very low T_3 levels (reduced significantly beyond what could be explained by decreased TBP levels) in the presence of eumetabolism. These patients may have normal or low-normal T_4 levels, often with decreased TBP levels, so that their FT_4 levels are either normal or slightly increased. They have normal levels of TSH and normal TSH responsiveness to TRH. Many of them have increased reverse T_3 levels but do not always parallel the fall in T_3.[13,20,31-34] That this is tightly controlled metabolically is quite clear, but the mechanism is not known. It may be a simple shunting of T_4 deiodination to reverse T_3. However, one need not postulate increased reverse T_3 production; if there were an inhibition of the 5'-deiodinase, there would be a decreased production of T_3 and continued production of reverse T_3. The lack of a 5'-deiodinase would result in a decreased turnover of reverse T_3 with a resultant rise in its serum concentration due to a decreased removal rate rather than to an increased production rate. If this were true, one would expect decreased levels of 3,3'-diiodothyronine, since this compound results from the 5'-deiodination of reverse T_3; indeed, this has been observed in a number of these states (Fig. 12-1).

T_3 toxicosis

In the majority of patients with hyperthyroidism, the thyroid gland produces an excess of T_3 and T_4. The thyroidal production of T_4 may rise two to three times (to $270\mu g$ per day) and that of T_3 seven to eight times (to over $200\mu g$ per day), most of it coming from the thyroid gland and not from the 5'-deiodination of T_4. For reasons that are not well understood, a small group of thyrotoxic patients produce an excess amount of T_3 and normal or reduced amounts of T_4. These patients with T_3 toxicosis have all of the manifestations of hyperthyroidism and the basic disease causing it.[35] The ^{131}I uptake may be high, low, or normal; TBP levels are normal. Thyroid function is nonsuppressible, and there is no TSH response to TRH. We recognize that in intrathyroidal iodide deficiency and in those patients with a decreased iodide pool, preferential formation of monoiodotyrosine (MIT) and T_3 results. T_3 toxicosis is much more common in areas of endemic iodide deficiency[6] and in recurrence of hyperthyroidism after ^{131}I therapy.[37] Some cases of T_3 toxicosis may occur on this basis; however, this does not explain all cases. T_3 toxicosis is more commonly seen in nodular goiter (especially uninodular).

Eumetabolism in the presence of high-normal, elevated, or occasionally normal T_3 levels and low-normal T_4 levels

Iodide deficient glands, prior to the development of frank hypothyroidism, may maintain a eumetabolic state for months in the presence of increased levels of T_3, often elevated TSH concentrations, and low T_4 concentrations. This phenomenon, so-called T_3 euthyroidism, results from the preferential intrathyroidal formation of MIT and T_3 over DIT and T_4 in iodide-depleted glands. Such severe iodide deficiency may result from dietary lack,[38,39] antithyroid medication,[40] and failing thyroid glands (after ^{131}I therapy[41-44] or burnt-out Hashimoto's thyroiditis). This attempt at compensation may continue after clinical hypothyroidism develops, as evidenced by the fact that a significant number of hypothyroid patients have normal levels of T_3.[46]

T_4, TBP, T_3 levels, and age

T_4 and TBP levels do not change significantly as a part of the aging process in otherwise healthy patients.[47-49] It must be borne in mind that many elderly patients (especially a hospital population) are chronically ill with nonthyroidal disease. In the study by Davis and Davis,[49] 83 of 85 elderly hyperthyroid patients had significant nonthyroidal illnesses with an average of three other diseases. Acute and chronic illnesses often decrease the level of TBP[21,26,28,33,34,49-51] with resultant lowering of the T_4 and the moving of the T_3 resin uptake into the hyperthyroid range. Calculation of the free hormone values may then give a more accurate reflection of the patient's thyroid status.

T_4 metabolism

There is a progressive decrease in the rate of disposal (turnover) of T_4 with advancing age to the ninth decade, when it is 50% of that in the third decade.[52,53] Since T_4 and TBP levels and the thyroid-pituitary relationship are unaltered with age, a proportionate decrease in thyroidal synthesis and release of T_4 results.[54] *The primary event is a peripheral one due to retardation of cellular processes and decreased functioning tissue mass, not to thyroidal failure.* This is attested to by the facts that (1) no fall in T_4 levels occurs, as it should if this were thyroidal failure; (2) the thyroid gland responds relatively normally to exogenous TSH; (3) TSH levels are normal, and the TSH response to TRH is certainly not a hypothyroid type of curve; (4) the ability to increase peripheral turnover rate and thyroidal production and release is preserved, as evidenced by the fact that it does so in acute infections and other stress situations; and (5) the ability to generate large increases in TSH is present in elderly patients when they become hypothyroid.

T_3 levels and T_3 metabolism

There is a concomitant decrease in T_3 disposal in the elderly that parallels that of T_4. However, most studies have indicated decreasing T_3 levels in the blood to the age of 90, at which time they are about 60% of that seen in 30-year-old patients.[13,17,21,23,31,48,54-56] This cannot merely reflect decreased turnover of T_4, since most of the T_3 generated is via peripheral monodeiodination of T_4, and T_3 levels fall and T_4 levels do not. This all suggests a shift in T_4 metabolism away from T_3, and a few studies have indeed demonstrated increased levels of reverse T_3[57] and decreased levels of 3,3'-diiodothyronine, strongly suggesting an inhibition of the 5'-deiodinase, as is seen in a variety of nonthyroidal illnesses. In caloric and carbohydrate deprivation states, wherein T_3 values fall and reverse T_3 levels rise, some investigators have demonstrated a decrease in nuclear binding of T_3 (decreased number of binding sites). If this should turn out to be so in the aged, perhaps the decreased nuclear binding might explain the altered peripheral T_3 (and T_4) metabolism. However, Oppenheimer recently demonstrated no change in the number of hepatic nuclear binding sites in older rats (albeit they did not have decreased T_3 or T_4 levels either) but did show a decreased response of two T_3 responsive hepatic enzymes (alpha-glucophosphate and malic enzyme) to administered T_3 in older rats, suggesting a modulation of receptor interaction by unidentified factors distal to the receptor.

Recall that a variety of acute and chronic nonthyroidal illnesses can reduce T_3 levels and that these conditions are more common in the elderly. A study of elderly and otherwise healthy outpatients in Scandinavia (not yet confirmed by others) found no significant decrease in T_3 levels with aging and ascribed the low T_3 in this group of patients to unrecognized chronic disease.[58]

It is generally stated that every case of hyperthyroidism is associated with elevations in serum levels of T_3. Recently, a number of case reports of T_4 hyperthyroidism (i.e., hyperthyroidism with elevated T_4 and normal T_3 levels) have been published.[59] The most likely explanation for most of these cases is a reduction in T_3

levels because of associated nonthyroidal illness or aging.[60]

T_3 binds less well than T_4 to the binding proteins, so that proportionately ten times more T_3 exists in the free state; and it is the free hormone that is metabolically active. On a gram molecular basis, T_3 is five times more potent than T_4, and it does bind specifically to nuclear binding sites in target cells, whereas T_4 does not. Its volume of distribution is greater than T_4 and its turnover rate is more rapid than that of T_4. Most of the T_3 generated daily originates from the 5'-deiodination of T_4 by those peripheral tissues that have binding sites for T_3 and are capable of utilizing it. For these reasons, it is thought that T_3 is the active hormone and that, except under the most unusual circumstances, T_4 serves as a prohormone, having no metabolic effect without prior conversion to T_3. If T_3 is the active hormone and if T_3 levels are low in the aged, if T_3 and T_4 disposal rates and secondary thyroidal hormonal production rates are decreased as a consequence of peripheral cellular mechanisms, if cholesterol and serum lipid values are elevated, and if there is a blunted T_3 secretory response to administered TRH in the elderly, *are these patients eumetabolic or is there tissue hypothyroidism?* They appear eumetabolic clinically, have normal TSH levels, and certainly are not hyperresponders to TRH; they maintain normal T_4 levels, and they are able to generate significant increases of endogenous TSH in response to hypothyroidism when it develops. Peripheral disposal rates and secondary hormonal production rates increase appropriately under stress. Cardiac systolic ejection and deep tendon reflex relaxation times are normal, as are the acute phase enzymes (including creatine phosphokinase [CPK] levels).

If these patients are eumetabolic with

low T_3 and normal FT_4 levels, we must consider whether T_4 may not have a metabolic effect of its own without prior conversion to T_3. Certainly the elderly, the acutely and chronically ill, and calorically deprived groups of patients with low T_3 levels and normal T_4 and TSH levels would appear to be so maintained. Normal or elevated T_3 levels are not always sufficient to maintain the eumetabolic state, as evidenced by a group of clinically hypothyroid patients with such T_3 levels, low T_4 levels, and elevated TSH levels. It is argued that the demonstration of specific nuclear binding sites for T_3 (but not T_4) indicate the primary and sole role of T_3 in tissue metabolism, but recently Sterling has presented convincing work suggesting specific microsomal binding sites for both thyroid hormones. It would appear that T_4 may have a metabolic effect of its own. However, it need not be the explanation for these low T_3 states. Both logic and Larsen's recent work suggest that the ambient levels of T_3 do not necessarily reflect its concentration at the receptor site, but that the intracellular monodeiodination of T_4 could be accelerated and that the T_3 thus generated could be utilized at the receptor site on the spot, without its getting back into the circulation, where it could be measured. Alternatively, there might be an actual decrease in receptor concentration of T_3; but, under certain circumstances, an intracellular multiplier might operate to magnify the hormonal signal, thus maintaining eumetabolism.

Does the decreased TRH responsiveness of the pituitary gland in aged men reflect and parallel altered responsiveness to T_3 and/or T_3 elsewhere? Or is it an isolated phenomenon? A question exists as to whether the set point of the pituitary may be altered in low T_3 states, either via TRH or by the disease processes (or ag-

ing) themselves. It is possible that the pituitary responsiveness to T_3 differs from that of the periphery and that what constitutes eumetabolism for the pituitary gland reflects tissue hypothyroidism elsewhere in these low T_3 states.

Presently, we believe that these elderly persons are eumetabolic, but we cannot exclude the possibility of tissue hypothyroidism in these low T_3 states (which generally occur during periods when tissue oxygen and substrate conservation are important for the survival of the organism).

THYROTOXICOSIS

In 1926 only 3% of all cases of thyrotoxicosis were seen in patients over the age of 65; in 1940 reviews of the subject reported 12%; and today we estimate that 25% to 35% of all cases of thyrotoxicosis occur in patients over the age of 65. As patients liver longer, our understanding of pathophysiology increases, our methods of testing improve, and our clinical awareness increases; we recognize the presence of the disease with greater frequency. Ordinarily we do not associate hyperfunction with aging. Weakness, weight loss, and tremor tend to be associated in our minds with the aging process and not with hyperthyroidism. The vast majority of the elderly with thyrotoxicosis present with significant diseases of other organ systems that distract our attention from the thyroid gland. The results of thyroid testing may be influenced by these nonthyroidal diseases; indeed, these diseases may trigger the onset of hyperthyroidism or cause the flare-up of underlying smoldering thyrotoxicosis. Thyrotoxicosis seems to have a more insidious onset in the elderly; this may be due in part to the fact that the majority of cases are secondary to nodular goiter, which characteristically has episodic periods of hypersecretion. However, the elderly may have altered adrenergic responses. They also tend to complain less, inappropriately accepting many symptoms as a part of growing older. Finally, thyrotoxicosis in the elderly often presents atypically.

As in younger patients, the disease is more common in women than in men. Although we speak of hyperthyroidism in the elderly as being atypical and often masked or apathetic, the majority of cases (perhaps 75%) present rather typically and only a fourth may give real difficulty in diagnosis. The terms "masked" and "apathetic" hyperthyroidism are often used synonymously, but I use the term "masked" to indicate (1) that the hyperthyroidism is masked by another condition that overshadows the thyroid disease or (2) that the thyrotoxicosis is so monosystemic in its presentation that it presents looking like a disease of that organ system. The term "apathetic" I reserve for those patients who present with few or none of the sympathomimetic manifestations of the disease and appear apathetic, depressed, wasted, and lethargic on examination.

The disease tends to be more monosystemic in symptomatology in the elderly, with the cardiovascular system predominating, although gastrointestinal or neuromuscular complaints may be primary.[49,54,61] Weight loss (often greater than 20 pounds) is a typical symptom in the elderly. Up to two thirds present with symptoms of CHF, and most of these with palpitations as well. Anorexia is a more common complaint than hyperphagia, and constipation is seen as often as hyperdefecation.[49,62] Insomnia is a rather uncommon complaint, and heat intolerance is more common than in the young. Almost a third of older patients present with lassitude and asthenia, rather than nervousness or hyperkinesis.[49] Angina pectoris, either new or increased in intensity, is a common presenting complaint of elderly hyperthyroid patients.[54]

Gland size and configuration

As the size of the thyroid gland decreases and the incidence of nodularity increases with advancing age, it is not surprising to find that the overall incidence of goiter in elderly hyperthyroid patients is less than that seen in younger patients and the incidence of nodular goiter is greater. Davis and Davis, and Iverson[49,63] state that in 12% of their elderly hyperthyroid group, no thyroid tissue was palpable. My own experience and that of others[54,64-66] suggests that perhaps 10% to 20% of elderly hyperthyroid patients do not have thyromegaly and that almost three fourths of the goiters in elderly hyperthyroid patients are nodular. Graves' disease is more than the simple hypersecretion of thyroid hormones; it is now considered an autoimmune disease and is associated with a multiplicity of thyroid-stimulating immunoglobulins, which play an important role in the genesis of the disease, and with infiltrative exophthalmos and pretibial myxedema, which are peculiar to Graves' disease. Indeed, Graves' disease may exist without hyperthyroidism. Toxic nodular goiter is a more common cause of thyrotoxicosis in the elderly than is Graves' disease. A few patients with hyperthyroidism and nodular goiters may have Graves' disease of the internodular areas and not hypersecreting nodules; of course, the symptoms of these patients are similar to those of patients with Graves' disease.

Cardiovascular effects

Thyroid hormones have direct chronotropic and ionotropic effects on the heart appear to act synergistically with catecholamines (perhaps by increasing the number of cardiac catecholamine receptor sites), cause peripheral vasodilitation, and increase the peripheral demands of the body on the heart. It is not surprising to find an increased incidence of cardiac arrythmias, angina pectoris, and CHF (in up to two thirds of cases) in the thyrotoxic older age group,[49,54,61-63,67,68] in whom there is a high incidence of underlying cardiovascular disease. As the hyperthyroidism increases, the peripheral demands of the body exceed the capacity of the heart to supply them and these complications ensue. Myocardial infarction is very rare in or as a result of hyperthyroidism. The question as to whether a specific thyrotoxic myocardiopathy of hyperthyroidism exists is a moot one.

It is generally accepted that tachycardia is an almost universal finding in hyperthyroidism at all ages, although it is not as marked in the elderly as in younger patients. When absent, it casts some doubt on the diagnosis and the patient should be checked by an electrocardiogram (ECG) to exclude heart block. Contrary to this, Davis and Davis[49] found 42% of their patients to have pulse rates less than 100 and one fourth of these patients to have heart rates less than 80 (the percent of patients taking negative chronotropic medication, such as digitalis, was not noted); only 15% of the elderly patients studied had pulse rates greater than 120. In this series 10% of the elderly thyrotoxic population had tachycardia as the only cardiovascular abnormality.

Atrial fibrillation is the most common dysrhythmia and is seen in 20% to 40% of thyrotoxic elderly patients. Only 30%

to 40% of these patients revert to normal sinus rhythm (NSR) with control of their disease.[49,54,61,69] This no doubt reflects underlying heart disease, since almost 100% of young patients revert to normal rhythms with control of the hyperthyroidism. Heart block and premature atrial and ventricular contractions are seen less commonly, wheras paroxysmal atrial tachycardia, paroxysmal atrial flutter, and ventricular arrhythmias are rare. *Any unexplained tachyarrhythmia with or without CHF, especially if poorly responsive to digitalis, requires a thorough thyroid evaluation.* The explanation for so-called "digitalis resistance" in atrial fibrillation secondary to hyperthyroidism is most likely a shorter half-life of the drug in the system resulting in lower serum levels.

Lack of eye signs

Exophthalmos is less common and much less severe in elderly hyperthyroid populations.[49,54,61,70] Severe or malignant exophthalmos is almost never seen, and the extraocular muscles are rarely involved clinically. Mild, measurable exophthalmos is seen in up to 40% of patients. However, enophthalmos and blepharoptosis may also be seen in this group of patients. Since exophthalmos is believed to be part of the autoimmune process of Graves' disease, and since toxic nodular goiter does not have any autoimmune pathogenesis, it may be the predominance of toxic nodular goiter in the elderly that explains the lower incidence of eye problems. There may also be damped adrenergic responses in this age group, which would explain the lower incidence of spastic eye findings as well. Despite the above, I have found that "bright eyes" are often a helpful finding in thyrotoxicosis in the elderly, once parkinsonism and ectropion have been excluded.

The acute onset of psychosis may be the presenting finding in elderly thyrotoxic patients. Similarly, such a patient may be inappropriately labeled as senile, depressed, or psychotic when apathetic hyperthyroidism is present. As the metabolic abnormality is corrected, so is the psychiatric problem.

Hyperthyroxinemia is often associated with increased carbohydrate intake, is thought to be associated with increased carbohydrate absorption from the intestine, and is associated with accelerated glycogenolysis and with a shortened half-life of insulin in the blood. It is not surprising that the sudden development of hyperglycemia or loss of control in a previously well-maintained diabetic may be the first clue to thyrotoxicosis in an elderly patient, and such a finding should stimulate an investigation for this condition.[49,54,61,66]

Although 25% of elderly thyrotoxic patients present with the expected hyperkinetic picture, an equal number present with an apathetic one.[49,54,68] This is most unusual in younger populations.

Neuromuscular signs

Refined neuromuscular testing will usually demonstrate myopathy in almost every patient with hyperthyroidism.[71,72] Elderly hyperthyroid patients very often present with significant clinical findings of myopathy with marked proximal muscle wasting. Although muscle strength decreases slightly with normal aging, profound weakness is an abnormal finding and should trigger an investigation. Specifically, the functions of the quadriceps and deltoid muscles should be included in the history and examination (ability to get up steps, squat, and comb hair), since these muscle groups are usually involved earliest and to the greatest extent.

Fine skin and tremor are common enough in old age as to be of little help in making a diagnosis of thyrotoxicosis. The same may be said of a widened pulse pressure, which may result from increased cardiac output and decreased peripheral resistance in hyperthyroidism and from decreased elasticity of the aorta in old age. Osteoporosis is a common finding in the elderly and may result from accelerated bone turnover in hyperthyroidism. There is no increase in pathological fractures in hyperthyroidism. The finding of mild asymptomatic hypercalcemia in the presence of osteoporosis in an elderly patient should suggest the possibility of hyperthyroidism as well as hyperparathyroidism; serum parathormone levels are low, and phosphorus levels are normal or elevated in the hypercalcemia of hyperthyroidism. It is worth noting that the incidence of hyperthyroidism is higher in patients with hyperparathyroidism (1%) than in the general population.

Toxic nodular goiter is more common in the elderly, and T_3 toxicosis is more common in toxic nodular goiter. It is my impression that T_3 toxicosis is more common in the aged.[54]

Screening tests

Every series indicates that a significant number of cases of hyperthyroidism will be missed if only one screening test of thyroid function is performed.[49,54,61,73] The T_4 by RIA should be the basic thyroid function test made, and a T_3 resin uptake should also be done to pick up any alterations in binding proteins from drugs or disease. From these two values an FT_4I may be calculated. If T_3 toxicosis is suspected, a T_3 by RIA should be performed with the knowledge that a multiplicity of acute and chronic nonthyroidal diseases, and perhaps old age itself, may decrease the circulating levels of T_3. One can calculate an FT_3I in the same manner as for T_4.

It is conceivable, then, to see an elderly thyrotoxic patient who has weight loss, anorexia, and constipation; who has enophthalmos and blepharoptosis; who has a small innocent-feeling nodular goiter (or none at all); who appears depressed and apathetic; who may have atrial fibrillation at a slow rate with or without mild CHF; and who has few other historical or physical findings of thyrotoxicosis. Indeed, in some series up to 15% of elderly hyperthyroid patients present in such a manner. With such a clinical picture, a diagnosis of gastrointestinal malignancy, depression, or even hypothyroidism may be entertained. If, in addition, the patient has significant nonthyroidal disease, depression of his TBP level may result in a normal T_4 by RIA; and his T_3 by RIA may be normal for reasons already mentioned. The T_3 resin uptake must be performed and an FT_4I (and FT_3I) calculated. A normal TSH response to administered TRH will exclude hyperthyroidism, but one that is blunted is not necessarily diagnostic of the disease, as it is in younger patients. Elderly men often have blunted responses to TRH for unknown reasons, and the administration of thyroid hormone, corticosteroids, and L-dopa affect this test similarly. A 4- and 24-hour ^{131}I uptake may be helpful in establishing the diagnosis, and a scintiscan of the thyroid gland will certainly be helpful in assessing the nature of the goiter. The demonstration of nonsuppressibility of the gland, as by a T_3 suppression test might be helpful; but non-suppressibility does not always parallel hypersecretion, and the administration of such doses of thyroactive materials to elderly patients is hazardous. In this regard, the demonstration of thyroid-stimulating antibodies by in vitro techniques may be helpful when they become more generally available. In such a situation as described above, a high index of suspicion and a thorough understanding of the pathophysiology of thyroid disease is essential.

Therapy for hyperthyroidism

The treatment of choice is ^{131}I except in the very rare large goiters that obstruct or in the even rarer situation where a question of malignancy exists.[49,54,61]

The administration of a therapeutic dose of radioactive iodine results in 7 to 10 days in radiation thyroiditis with breakdown of cell and basement membranes and extrusion of hormone-rich colloid into the interstices of the gland and then into the circulation. This acute outpouring of thyroactive material can result in a significant, albeit transient, exacerbation of the disease, which in an elderly patient with underlying cardiovascular disease can be catastrophic. Since this discharge of hormone is not physiological, it is not inhibited by the administration of iodides. Although I have seen serious problems in only two or three occasions, in Davis and Davis's series,[49] 3 of 29 patients so treated died within 10 days of ^{131}I administration, suggesting this mechanism. This catastrophe can be avoided by depleting the gland of stored hormone prior to treating with ^{131}I (see below).[49,54,61]

Antithyroid drugs (propylthiouracil and methimazole [Tapazole]) act by inhibiting thyroidal organification of iodides and thus blocking the further production of hormone by the gland. They have no effect on that hormone previously formed and present in the thyroid; this hormone must be released from the gland and metabolized peripherally before a clinical effect from these drugs becomes manifest. Propylthiouracil may also inhibit the peripheral monodeiodination of T_4 to T_3. As therapy with these drugs is continued, the gland depletes itself of stored hormone. When the patient is then given radioactive iodine, he may develop a radiation thyroiditis, but one unaccompanied by an extravasation of thyroactive materials into the circulation and its consequences. Further, when these drugs are discontinued, the iodide-depleted gland (via intrathyroidal autoregulatory mechanisms) transiently traps more iodide without a concomitant increase in hormone production. This "rebound phenomenon" is utilized clinically to deliver a greater percentage of an administered dose of ^{131}I to the thyroid gland and thus cut down total body radiation. One never administers ^{131}I to a patient who is taking antithyroid drugs. These antithyroid drugs block organification; ^{131}I trapped by such a gland remains in equilibrium with plasma iodide – it is rapidly discharged from the gland and thus cannot exert its effect on the gland. These patients must be monitored for the rare hematological complication of agranulocytosis and the more common dermatological and gastrointestinal (cholestatic hepatitis) side effects of these drugs.

Iodides do block release of hormone from the thyroid within 12 hours of administration and are a very useful adjuvant to therapy in acutely ill patients. However, they have many other effects on the thyroid gland and should be used only when the clinical situation dictates and never as the sole therapy. In the acute situation, when they are needed, the patient should first be given a loading dose of antithyroid drug and then be maintained on it during the period of iodide administration. This prevents organification of the iodide and hormonal enrichment of the gland and yet does not interfere with the ability of the iodides to block hormonal release.

Propranolol (Inderal) is an excellent adjuvant to therapy and is effective in blocking most of the peripheral catecholaminelike effects of thyroid hormone. It does not alter thyroid function, but may inhibit peripheral monodeiodination of T_4 to T_3. It is contraindicated in patients with asthma or non–rate-related CHF.

Our routine in most elderly thyrotoxic patients is to treat them with an antithyroid drug for 4 to 6 weeks, until they are euthyroid and their thyroid glands are depleted of stored hormone. If indicated, propranolol is given during this period to slow the heart and relieve the adrenergic symptoms. The antithyroid drug is then discontinued; 48 to 72 hours later, a repeat uptake is performed and the patient is treated with radioactive iodine "on the rebound." Since ^{131}I does not manifest any clinical effect for a month and may not have a peak effect for 2 to 3 months, the antithyroid drug may be started again 3 to 4 days after therapy for a period of 4 to 6 weeks; or propranolol may be given during this period. In the acutely ill patient, we may use iodides along with the antithyroid drugs in the first weeks of therapy but not for a month or so prior to ^{131}I treatment, since exogenous iodides do decrease trapping and do increase the iodide pool, so that less radioactive iodine gets into the gland. *Our aim in treating thyrotoxicosis in the elderly is to attain and maintain the eumetabolic state as quickly as possible in view of the high incidence of underlying cardiovascular disease. We use larger doses of* ^{131}I *and concern ourselves less with resultant hypothyroidism.* In this age group the theoretical concerns regarding genetic damage, thyroidal malignancy, and/or leukemogenesis consequent to ^{131}I are not applicable. The theoretical possibility of radiation-induced neoplasms is 10 to 20 years down the line.

Multinodular goiters require even larger doses of radioactive iodine, since the amount of radioactivity accumulated by the nodules varies and as the more active nodules are destroyed by the ^{131}I, the less active ones (which got little or none of the ^{131}I) become active and the disease reactivates. Single nodules suppressing the remainder of the gland often require extremely large doses of ^{131}I. It is more difficult to render a nodular goiter hypothyroid for the same reason that it is more difficult to cure it with ^{131}I.

Repeated doses of ^{131}I may be required to render the patient permanently eumetabolic, especially in toxic nodular goiter. As a rule, we try not to treat more frequently than every 2 to 3 months, since this is the period required for the maximal effect of the beta emissions of ^{131}I to become manifest. Such adjuvant therapy as is indicated is used in the intervals between ^{131}I therapy. As helpful as thyroid testing is, we treat patients, not numbers. Careful clinical evaluation at 2-month intervals (minimally) is most important.

Radiation destroys some cells in a period of several months and injures others, so that their ability to reproduce themselves is interfered with. In Graves' disease, continuation of the basic autoimmune processes results in the ongoing destruction of thyroid cells long after the effects of radiation are dissipated. These factors give rise to a continuing incidence of hypothyroidism following ^{131}I therapy of 3% per year, so that at the end of 15 years almost half of the patients with Graves' disease treated with ^{131}I are hypothyroid. *The incidence is only a fraction of this in patients with toxic nodular goiter.* Since hypothyroidism may begin particularly insidiously in the elderly, they must be warned of this possibility and carefully followed periodically for many years after ^{131}I therapy.

There is a significant incidence of hypothyroidism following surgical therapy of hyperthyroidism and a lesser recurrence rate. The recurrence rate of the disease in the first year after therapy with antithyroid drugs alone is close to 50%.

All elderly patients treated for hyperthyroidism require lifelong follow-up. In the first year after therapy they should be seen at least every 3 months, examined carefully, and screened with T_3 and T_4 by RIA, T_3 resin uptake, and TSH levels, with an awareness of the limitations of these tests and how they may be altered in thyroidal and nonthyroidal illness. Testing does not replace careful clinical appraisal; tests must be interpreted in terms of what is going on clinically. For example: rising T_3 levels in the presence of low or unmeasurable TSH levels mean recurring thyrotoxicosis, whereas rising or high T_3 levels found in the presence of elevated TSH levels indicate impending thyroidal failure; low levels of T_3 may represent eumetabolism in the presence of nonthyroidal illness or may be seen in hypothyroidism; and up to 20% of hypothyroid patients have normal T_3 levels. Elevated or borderline TSH levels require frequent monitoring for hypothyroidism despite the clinical state or normal levels of T_4. In the period following testing, those patients who apparently are normal may be seen once or twice a year and those in whom hypothyroidism is present or suspected, more often.

Any acute stress or illness (infection, surgery, diabetic acidosis, fracture, myocardial infarction, cerebrovascular accident, gastrointestinal bleeding) in a partially treated or untreated thyrotoxic patient may precipitate an acute exacerbation of the hyperthyroidism and result in *thyroid storm*, an acute medical emergency.[74] Significant hyperpyrexia is present in true storm but may be absent in impending storm. In the elderly, tachyarrhythmias and CHF are almost invariably present and predominant findings. Therapy consists of a large loading. dose of methimazole or propylthiouracil, followed shortly by the infusion of potassium iodide intravenously by drip infusion; large doses of corticosteroids intravenously (the turnover of cortisol is rapid in hyperthyroid states and the hypothalamic-pituitary-adrenal axis, which may have been working close to maximal capacity to maintain normal cortisol levels, may not be able to further increase cortisol production to meet the needs of the body in response to this additional stress), and the administraion of propranolol to block the peripheral effects of thyroid hormone (if there is no heart failure or if that failure which is present is felt to be mostly rate-related). The precipitating factors are treated vigorously; fever is brought down by appropriate measures; heart failure, if present, is treated with diuretics and cardiotonics; and necessary supportive measures are utilized (intravenous fluids, vasopressors, oxygen, etc.). As the acute state is brought under control, the iodides and steroids are discontinued and the antithyroid drugs and propranolol continued. Once the patient has been rendered eumetabolic and his

gland depleted of stored hormone, therapy with ^{131}I is undertaken.

HYPOTHYROIDISM

Old age does not represent a hypothyroid state. Despite the anatomic changes in the thyroid gland, the decrease in absolute iodine uptake, the decreased rate of turnover of T_3 and T_4 in the periphery with resultant decreased hormonal production, and the significant lowering of T_3 levels with advancing age, T_4 levels are normal, the thyroid gland maintains its ability to respond to exogenous TSH, TSH levels are normal and rise markedly and appropriately in hypothyroidism, and the peripheral turnover of thyroid hormones increases markedly in response to stress states. Elderly patients generally appear eumetabolic. Their reflex relaxation time, left ventricular ejection time, and acute-phase enzymes (including CPK) are all normal.

Hypothyroidism is a disease primarily of the aged; after diabetes mellitus, it is the most common endocrine abnormality of older persons, occurring in about 4% of a hospitalized population over the age of 65.[26,75] As with all other thyroid disease, hypothyroidism is most common in women, affecting women five times as frequently as men.

Etiology

Primary hypothyroidism may result from surgical or ^{131}I ablation of the thyroid gland; burned-out Hashimoto's thyroiditis, Graves' disease, or colloid goiter; from high doses of radiation to the neck or thorax for nonthyroidal malignancies (e.g., laryngeal carcinoma or lymphoma); from the rare very late manifestation of congenital lesions of intrathyroidal iodide metabolism, and from the administration of drugs that interfere with intrathyroidal iodide metabolism. In addition, patients may present with hypothyroidism on the basis of having discontinued thyroid replacement started by another physician or of having continued large doses of antithyroid medication without proper monitoring.

Pituitary and hypothalamic hypothyroidism are not dealt with here; differentiation of these states is discussed in the section on testing.

In a genetically susceptible population the autoimmune system may break down; and as clones of cells directed against self (in this case thyroid) arise, they are not destroyed by the immune system. Occasionally they may stimulate the tissue against which they are directed (as with thyroid-stimulating immunoglobulins in Graves' disease or as with Hashimoto's thyroiditis); and late in the course of Graves' disease they may gradually destroy the gland, resulting in hypothyroidism. There is an almost linear temporal incidence of hypothyroidism after radioactive iodine and surgical therapy of Graves' disease of about 3% a year, which is in large part believed to be related to continued autoimmune destruction of the thyroid cells. These patients almost uniformly have small, fibrosed glands. In addition, a number of patients with nontoxic nodular goiter eventually burn out and present as hypothyroid patients. There is a high incidence of antithyroglobulin and antimicrosomal antibodies in low titer found in the normal elderly population, so that the presence of such antibodies in this group is difficult to evaluate with regard to the genesis of hypothyroidism. In a large group of normal euthyroid patients over the age of 50, 5% of the men and 30% of the women had low titers of these antibodies.[76] Of the elderly hypothyroid

population, 64% have positive antimicrosomal antibodies by hemagglutinic testing and almost 85% have one or both antibodies in low titers. These antibodies are not seen in secondary and tertiary hypothyroidism. The above is not to suggest that this large percentage of elderly patients have hypothyroidism on an autoimmune basis; rather, it is to emphasize the difficulty in establishing a cause.[77]

Lithium, which has come into wide use for manic-depressive states, interferes with the thyroidal organification process and hormonal release and occasionally results in goitrous hypothyroidism.[78] The sulfonylureas (oral hypoglycemic agents), para-aminosalicylic acid (PAS), and rarely phenylbutazone may result in goitrous hypothyroidism by interfering with the organification process. On occasion, the administration of iodides may result in goitrous hypothyroidism.[79,80] Normally, the administration of iodides in milligram doses results in very high intrathyroidal iodide levels, which in turn cause a block in organification via unexplained mechanisms (the Wolff-Chaikoff effect). High levels of intrathyroidal iodide are required for the maintenance of this phenomenon. After 24 to 48 hours, via unexplained intrathyroidal autoregulatory mechanisms, trapping of iodide is inhibited, intrathyroidal iodide levels fall, the block in organification disappears, and organification proceeds normally (escape from the Wolff-Chaikoff effect occurs). However, in glands with underlying organification defects (such as in Hashimoto's thyroiditis, and after ^{131}I therapy for Graves' disease) escape from the Wolff-Chaikoff effect does not occur, organification remains blocked, decreased levels of thyroid hormone are present in the blood, TSH is turned on, and the gland enlarges. Iodide-induced goitrous hypothyroidism results.

Clinical picture

Sluggishness, lethargy, withdrawal, atrophic skin, hair loss, constipation, and impaired memory and hearing may be common accompaniments of old age. They are also the most common presenting complaints in hypothyroidism.[54,61,67,76,81] The diagnosis will be delayed or missed if one requires the classic appearance of myxedema. This is especially true since the onset of this disease is typically gradual and insidious in this age group and many patients do not have goiters. The clinical picture is a nonspecific one, often with impaired general health, psychomotor retardation, apathy, and depression predominating. A high index of suspicion is required with particular attention to recent deterioration of the mental state, proximal muscle weakness, and recurrent falls.[82,83] Weight loss is more common than weight gain. When present, bradycardia, a croaky voice, and macroglossia are helpful findings. "Hung" deep tendon reflexes[84] (slow relaxation time) are a very important physical finding when present, although they may be seen in other conditions, including hypothermia, where there is an equal prolongation of both contraction and relaxation times. The ankle jerk may be absent in up to 40% of elderly patients; however, these "hung" reflexes are as easily demonstrable elsewhere, especially in the triceps and biceps muscles. Weakness and myopathy are invariable, but these are usually interpreted as part of other diseases or advancing age. The resulting myalgias, weakness, stiffness, and cramps are likely to be overlooked. Similarly, the arthralgias of hypothyroidism are apt to be attributed to arthritis associated with aging.[85-87] Percussion myxedema and carotenemia (best seen when examining the creases of the palmar surfaces) are helpful findings. Baggy eyelids, even in the absence of typical myxedematous facies, may be a sign of hypothyroidism. Deposition of mucopolysaccharide under the flexor retinaculum may lead to a carpal tunnel syndrome that completely resolves with replacement of thyroid hormone. Constipation is so common in the elderly as to be of little diagnostic value, and hypothermia is a useful but often overlooked finding.

Laboratory findings

The T_4 by RIA is the best screening test for hypothyroidism and should be performed along with the T_3 resin uptake to exclude the possibility of decreased TBP levels causing a low T_4 or elevated TBP levels moving a hypothyroid T_4 into the normal range. TSH levels are invariably elevated in primary hypothyroidism. The expected exaggerated response of TSH levels to the administration of TRH with a delayed return of the TSH levels to baseline is seen in elderly hypothyroid individuals. There is always a myopathy in hypothyroidism, which may be detected by rises in CPK, lactic dehydrogenase (LDH), aldolase, and serum glutamic-oxaloacetic transaminase (SGOT) levels with appropriate rises in the skeletal muscle isoenzymes in the former tests. Unexplained elevations of CPK levels should suggest the possibility of hypothyroidism.[88] Anemia (usually macrocytic, often refractory) may be present. Ascites and pleural and pericardial effusions (low-voltage ECGs) are common and occasionally are unexplained presenting findings. The T_3 by RIA is of little help in making the diagnosis of hypothyroidism and may even be misleading.

Therapy

The disease is treated by the administration of thyroid hormones. Guidelines to therapy are:

1. Replacement is rarely an urgent situation.

2. These patients often have significant underlying nonthyroidal diseases, especially cardiac diseases, that may be exacerbated by the administration of thyroactive materials.

3. Evenness of blood levels of thyroid hormones are desirable, and high peaks and troughs are to be avoided.

Although T_3 is the active hormone, is almost 100% absorbed, has a rapid onset of action, and is rapidly metabolized, it has proved less than ideal as replacement therapy in hypothyroidism. The administration of $25\mu g$ orally (equivalent to about $100\mu g$ of T_4) is followed by supraphysiological blood levels (peak at 4 hours) and then subphysiological levels (back to baseline in less than 24 hours). The T_4 by RIA is not raised by the ingestion of T_3 and may actually be lowered (T_3 is metabolically very active and binds poorly, so that more of an administered dose exists in the free metabolically active state; TSH is turned off; thyroidal production of T_4 is reduced; and T_4 levels fall). If the patient is to be followed by his T_3 levels, they will vary depending on how long after ingestion the test is made.

T_4 is varyingly and incompletely absorbed, binds strongly to binding proteins, must be converted to T_3 by the peripheral tissues, is much slower in the onset of its effect, and is longer acting than T_3. A single dose of $100\mu g$ begins to have an effect in 2 to 4 days and does not have its peak action for 10 days. After the administration of T_4, the blood levels of T_3 and T_4 are quite even and rise gradually.

Thyroid extract and synthetic combinations of T_4 and T_3 vary in the $T_4:T_3$ ratio and potency, and some have short shelf lives. For these reasons, we do not utilize them in the treatment of this condition.

It takes about three half-lives of a drug to obtain a 90% equilibrium level of that drug in the blood. This means that one must give a constant dose of T_4 for about 21 days to obtain a constant blood level (or 3 days for T_3).

We favor the use of T_4 (L-thyroxine [Synthroid]) as replacement therapy for hypothyroidism. Depending on the presence of complicating diseases and the general condition of the patient, the drug is started with a dosage of 0.025 mg a day and increased by similar amounts every 2 to 3 weeks until the patient is clinically and chemically eumetabolic or until side effects are noted. The majority of patients are adequately replaced by 0.15 to 0.2 mg a day.[89] Older patients must be closely monitored for tachycardia, angina, CHF, and loss of control of diabetes. Not infrequently, we must settle for suboptimal replacement because of side effects. T_4 by RIA is the best test with which to assess replacement. However, CPK levels tend to decrease toward normal almost parallel to the degree of correction of the hypothyroidism, and the test is a good and inexpensive means of following replacement. Although the return of TSH levels to normal is the final determinant of adequacy of replacement, they often lag behind the clinical state and other tests by several weeks.

Rarely one encounters a severely hypothyroid patient in whom some replacement is mandatory and angina is the limiting factor. If there is no question as to impending infarction, tachyarrhythmia, or CHF, we will start with minimal doses of T_4 (0.0125 mg a day), cover with propranolol, and increase the medication by a similar amount every 3 to 4 weeks while monitoring the patient very carefully.

Myxedema coma[74,90] represents the end stage of long-standing untreated hypothyroidism. It is most common in older patients and is rarely seen in warm weather. It is invariably precipitated by extreme stress, such as surgery, cardiovascular accident, myocardial infarction, gastrointestinal bleeding, or acute infection, in an inadequately treated or untreated patient with hypothyroidism. The administration of anesthesia or sedative, hypnotic, or narcotic drugs to such a patient can also lead to coma. In addition to the usual manifestations of the disease, stupor (to the point of areflexia and coma), extreme hypothermia, respiratory failure (on a central, muscular, and pulmonary basis), and, on occasion, severe hyponatremia (secondary to poor handling of water at the renal level) are seen. If hypoglycemia is present, hypopituitarism should be suspected. The absence of fever, leucocytosis, tachycardia, and sweating often make the diagnosis of infection difficult. Seizures may result from the condition; and, even in their absence, CNS protein and pressure levels are often elevated.

In addition to the management of the precipitating condition and replacement of thyroid hormones, respiration must be supported by mechanical means with or without intubation. Since myxedematous patients handle a water load poorly, the intravenous administration of fluids must be very carefully monitored lest water intoxication result. In those very rare patients with very low sodium levels, small amounts of hypertonic saline solution may be required and must be given with the utmost care. In hypothyroidism, the turnover of cortisol is slow and the adrenal-hypothalamic-pituitary response to stress may be slowed or damped; thus corticosteroids are useful in the management of this condition. If one understands that the total body pool of T_4 is 700 to 900μg and that careful monitoring of the patient, including his vital signs, state of consciousness, electrolytes, and ECG, are essential, any one of the regimens of hormonal replacement are satisfactory. Wherever possible, the oral route of administration is preferable. I do not use T_3 by the intravenous route because it is not readily available in this form. It seems to be associated with more cardiac arrhythmias when so used, and it has a very short half-life in the body. In an extremely ill patient with very low T_4 levels, I may give 500μg of T_4 intravenously to start; in one not so ill I would start with perhaps 300μg and repeat half the dose in 8 to 12 hours. The most common cause of recurrence of myxedema coma in the hospital situation is not the inadequate replacement of thyroid hormone but the premature removal of respiratory support or the inadvertent administration of narcotic analgesic or hypnotic drugs to a patient recovering from the condition.

In any acute care hospital it is not unusual to be asked to evaluate a comatose or semicomatose patient (little medical history available) with acute and/or chronic underlying nonthyroidal disease who may have had recent surgery or major cardiovascular illness, who has been receiving sedatives and narcotic analgesics, and who is poorly nourished. You will be presented with a low T_3 by RIA, a low or low-normal T_4 by RIA, and a T_3 resin uptake indicating a decreased TBP level and asked if this represents myxedema coma. Often the diagnosis will be obvious after a careful review of the chart and a thorough examination, but occasionally you will be left with a great deal of uncertainty, since the hypothermia and bradycardia could be due to CNS disease, the hyponatremia could be explained by renal disease and injudicious fluid replacement, the "hung" reflexes by hypothermia or a peripheral neuropathy on another basis, the low T_3 by age and/or chronic or acute disease and/or caloric deprivation, and the low T_4 by decreased TBP levels secondary to illness. A calculated FT_4I can be of great value in this situation; and, of course, TSH levels are diagnostic (but usually 48 hours later). When unsure and where further consultative advice is unavailable, and in a critically ill patient without tachyarrhythmia, changing ECGs, or other states where incorrectly administered thyroactive substances could do great harm, a small amount of T_4 ($200\mu g$ to $300\mu g$) may be administered intravenously. This is usually sufficient to tide the patient over his crisis and not place an excessive metabolic burden on his system.[91]

THYROID NODULES

The incidence of thyroidal nodularity increases with advancing age and by the eighth decade there is an almost 100% incidence of micronodularity of the thyroid gland. There are no good statistics regarding the incidence of palpable nodules in the elderly. Depending on the part of the country or world one is surveying, the overall incidence of thyroid nodules in the general population is estimated to be from 5% to 30%. It would appear to be higher in the older age groups.

Some generalizations are in order:

1. The incidence of clinical nodularity is high in the aged and directly related to the thoroughness of the examination and skill of the examiner.

2. We cannot palpate nodules much less than half a centimeter in size. Therefore, many times a single nodule on clinical examination turns out to be part of a multinodular goiter on pathological examination.

3. When we speak of thyroidal malignancies, we speak of clinically significant ones. Up to 15% of thyroid glands examined postmortem in patients dying of nonthyroidal disease will be found to have microscopic areas of sclerosing carcinoma if the gland is sectioned at ½-mm intervals. We do not believe that these are clinically significant lesions.

4. Generally, a multinodular gland or a gland with bilateral palpatory abnormalities is less likely to harbor a malignancy than an otherwise normal gland with a single nodule.

5. Thyroidal nodularity is common, thyroidal malignancy is rare, and death from thyroidal carcinoma is even rarer.

6. Since the vast majority of carcinomas are compatible with excellent 5- and 10-year survival rates with minimal therapy, our approach to them must be tempered by this fact when dealing with an elderly person whose life expectancy may be considerably less than this and who may be a poor operative risk. Overzealous attempts to involute nodules with large doses of thyroid hormone must be avoided in as much as many of these patients already have compromised cardiovascular systems and large amounts of thyroactive materials may tip the balance.

Papillary carcinoma, which is the most common malignancy in patients under the age of 40 and which has an excellent prognosis in that age group, is less common in older age groups and tends to behave in a more malignant and invasive manner. A question exists as to whether the highly anaplastic carcinomas arise from such preexisting lesions. However, follicular (the most common thyroidal malignancy in the aged[92]) and papillary carcinomas account for over 80% of thyroidal malignancies and have excellent 5- and 10-year survival rates, even in the aged. Anaplastic carcinomas account for less than 10% of all thyroidal malignancies, and the disease is almost uniformly fatal within 6 months of diagnosis regardless of therapy. It is a relatively rare carcinoma, even in the aged, but is more common in patients over the age of 60 (50% of anaplastic carcinomas arise in patients over the age of 60).

Scanning of the thyroid gland with isotopes of iodide or pertechnetate gives us valuable information regarding the functional capacity of nodules. Since ^{123}I, ^{125}I, and ^{131}I are trapped and organified by the gland and pertechnetate is only trapped, it is possible to demonstrate nodules with organification defects by differential scanning. In general, hot nodules and especially nodules that supress the remainder of the gland (autonomous nodules) are rarely, if ever, malignant; but when they attain sufficient size, they may produce sufficient amounts of T_3 (and T_4) to cause hyperthyroidism. About 20% of cold nodules (nodules that accumulate little or no isotope) represent malignancies and the remainder, cysts or benign adenomas. The majority of nodules are warm (accumulate about the same amount of isotope as the remainder of the gland). Of these, some are malignant, but the majority are not. Many are TSH dependent.

Sonography gives us very useful data as to the cystic or solid nature of these nodules. Unless a nodule is completely cystic, we deal with it as if it were solid.

We now have good techniques of obtaining tissue from the thyroid gland and nodules via needle biopsy and aspiration. If we recognize the limitations of the test (a small tissue sample, the skills of the physician performing the biopsy, and the skills of the pathologist-cytologist), much valuable information about the nature of nodules can be obtained from this minor and relatively innocuous procedure. In an elderly population with significant underlying cardiovascular disease, often the risks of endotrachial anesthesia and surgery can be avoided by this procedure.

Clinically we are suspicious of nodules that are newly developed or growing; of nodules that are hard or fixed; of single nodules, especially when the remainder of the gland is normal; and of any nodules associated with hoarseness, bone pain, and/or cervical lymphadenopathy. If the scan reveals a nodule to be cold and the sonogram demonstrates it to be solid, we are even more suspicious. The major criteria for malignancy on biopsy are capsular or vessel invasion and nuclear and cellular morphology. Very cellular follicular adenomas are treated as follicular carcinomas, since our experience with many of them is that metastases do occur years later despite the absence of any other criteria for malignancy. Experience has likewise taught us that cytological examination of the material obtained from large cysts is inaccurate and small carcinomas may be missed. The differentiation of lymphoma from Hashimoto's thyroiditis may be difficult, even when a core of tissue is obtained, so that when what appears to be Hashimoto's thyroiditis behaves peculiarly, we recognize the possibility of lymphoma and act accordingly. We are particularly suspicious of nodules developing in patients who were exposed to low-dosage radiation to the face, head, neck, or thorax in early childhood, since this predisposes the patient to thyroidal malignancy years later.

Some investigators report elevated levels of antithyroglobulin antibodies as a marker for thyroidal carcinoma; this may prove too nonspecific a finding in an elderly population in which such antibodies are frequently found without demonstrable thyroid disease. However, following the titer of such antibodies after the surgical removal of a demonstrated neoplasm may prove helpful in deciding if any tumor is left behind.

We remove surgically nodules of which we are suspicious if there is no contraindication; or we at least obtain a needle biopsy and/or aspiration. We either observe or attempt to involute with exogenous thyroid hormone those that do not particularly worry us. Where possible, it is wisest to observe these nodules in the elderly, since there is an inherent risk in the administration of thyroactive materials to these patients. The demonstration that a nodule is TSH dependent (involutes with the administration of sufficient exogenous thyroid hormone to turn off endogenous TSH) does not prove that the lesion is benign, since some malignancies, particularly follicular carcinoma, may be TSH dependent. One must be wary of attempting to involute hot nodules, since many of them are autonomous; thus, inhibiting endogenous TSH will not inhibit hormone production by the nodule and one will then get an additive effect from the medication given, causing iatrogenic hyperthyroidism in a patient with underlying cardiovascular or pulmonary disease. In an elderly patient, the results may be catastrophic.

THYROIDITIS

Acute suppurative thyroiditis is an uncommon disease at all ages. It is almost invariably related to mediastinal infec-tion and rarely results from septicemia.

Subacute thyroiditis (viral) is not common in the elderly; when it does occur, it differs little from the disease as it presents in youthful patients: the hypermetabolic phase of the disease may be more striking in the over-65 age group, simply because of the underlying medical problems these patients have. A hard, irregular, and acutely tender thyroid gland in a thyrotoxic patient with fever and marked systemic symptoms, associated elevations of the in vitro thyroid function tests, a ^{131}I uptake of less than 5%, and an elevated erythrocyte sedimentation rate (ESR) should bring this diagnosis to mind.

Hashimoto's thyroiditis has usually burned itself out in the aged and most often presents as hypothyroidism in a patient without goiter. High levels of antimicrosomal and antithyroglobulin antibodies may or may not be present.

REFERENCES

1. McGavack, T., and Seegers, W.: Thyroid function and disease in old age, J. Am. Geriatr. Soc. **4**:535, 1956.
2. McGavack, T., and Seegers, W.: Status of the thyroid gland after age 50, Metabolism **8**:136, 1959.
3. Pittman, J.: The thyroid and aging, J. Am. Geriatr. Soc. **10**:10, 1962.
4. Mustacci, P., and Lowenhaupt, E.: Senile changes in the histologic structure of the thyroid gland, Geriatrics **5**:268, 1950.
5. Mortensen, J., Woolner, L., and Bennett, W.: Gross and microscopic findings in clinically normal thyroid glands, J. Clin. Endocrinol. Metab. **15**:1270, 1955.
6. Shock, N., and others: Age differences in water content of the body as related to basal oxygen consumption in males, J. Gerontol. **18**:1, 1963.
7. Gaffney, G. W., Gregerman, R., and Shock, N.: The relationship of age to thyroidal accumulation, renal excretion and distribution of radioiodide in man, J. Clin. Endocrinol. Metab. **22**:784, 1962.
8. Oddie, T., and others: Dependence of renal clearance of radioiodide on sex, age and thyroi-

dal status, J. Clin. Endocrinol. Metab. **26:**1293, 1966.

9. Perlmutter, M., and Riggs, D.: Thyroid collection of radioactive iodide and serum PBI concentration in senescence, hypothyroidism and hypopituitarism, J. Clin. Endocrinol. Metab. **9:**430, 1949.

10. Quimby, E., Werner, S., and Schmidt, C.: Influence of age, sex and season upon ^{131}I uptake by the human thyroid., Proc. Soc. Exp. Biol. Med. **75:**537, 1950.

11. Stoffer, R., and others: The thyroid after 50, Geriatrics **16:**435, 1961.

12. Azizi, F., and others: Pituitary-thyroid responsiveness to I and TRH based on analysis of serum thyroxin, triiodothyronine and thyrotropin concentrations, N. Engl. J. Med. **292:**273, 1975.

13. Bermudez, F., Surks, M., and Oppenheimer, J.: High incidence of decreased serum T_3 concentration in patients with nonthyroidal disease, J. Clin. Endocrinol. Metab. **41:**27, 1975.

14. Cuttelod, S., and others: Effect of age and role of the kidneys on thyrotropin turnover in man, Metabolism **23:**101, 1974.

15. Le Marchand-Beraud, T., and Vannotti, A.: Relationship between blood TSH level, PBI and free T_4 concentration in man under normal physiological conditions, AcTA Endocrinol. **60:**315,1975.

16. O'Hara, H., and others: Thyroid function of the aged as viewed from the pituitary-thyroid system, Endocrinol. Jpn. **21:**377, 1974.

17. Wenzel, K., and Horn, W.: T_3 and T_4 kinetics in aged man, Exerpta Medica, Int. Congress Ser. **361:**89, 1975.

18. Baker, S., Gaffney, G., and Shock, N.: Physiological responses of five middle-aged and elderly males to repeated TSH administration, J. Gerontol. **24:**37, 1959.

19. Lederer, J., and Bataille, P.: Senescence and thyroid function, Ann. Endocrinol. **30:**598, 1969.

20. Einhorn, J.: Studies on the effect of thyrotropic hormone on thyroid function in normal man, Acta Radiol. (Suppl.) **160:**1, 1958.

21. Burrows, A., and others: Low serum T_3 levels in the elderly sick: protein binding, thyroid and pituitary responsiveness and reverse T_3 concentrations, Clin. Endocrinol. **7:**289, 1977.

22. Krugman, L., and others: Pattern of recovery of the hypothalamic-pituitary-thyroid axis in patients taken off chronic thyroid therapy, J. Clin. Endocrinol. Metab. **41:**70, 1975.

23. Snyder, P., and Utiger, R.: Response to TRH in normal man, J. Clin. Endocrinol. Metab. **34:**380, 1972.

24. Snyder, P., and Utiger, R.: Thyrotropin response to TRH in normal males over 40, J. Clin. Endocrinol. Metab. **34:**1096, 1972.

25. Shenkman, L., and others: Tri-iodothyronine and thyroid-stimulating hormone response to thyrotropin-releasing hormone: a new test of thyroidal and pituitary reserve, Lancet **1:**111, 1972.

26. Jefferys, P.: The prevalence of thyroid disease in patients admitted to a geriatric department, Age Aging **1:**33, 1972.

27. Swain, C., and others: The free T_3 index, Ann. Intern. Med. **88:**474, 1978.

28. Chopra, I., and others: Misleadingly low free thyroxine index and usefulness of reverse triiodothyronine measurements in nonthyroidal illnesses, Ann. Intern. Med. **90:**905, 1979.

29. Baruch, A., and others: Causes of high free thyroxine index in sick euthyroid elderly patients, Age Aging **5:**224, 1976.

30. Chopra, I., and others: In search of an inhibitor of thyroid hormone binding to serum protein in nonthyroidal illness, J. Clin. Endocrinol. Metab. **49:**63, 1979.

31. Schimmel, M., and Utiger, R.: Thyroidal and peripheral production of thyroid hormones, Ann. Intern. Med. **87:**760, 1977.

32. Chopra, I., and others: Reciprocal changes in concentration of T_3 and reverse T_3 in systemic illness, J. Clin. Endocrinol. Metab. **41:**1043, 1979.

33. Carter, J., and others: Effect of severe chronic illness on thyroidal function, Lancet **2:**971, 1974.

34. Bellabarba, D., and others: T_4 transport and turnover in major thyroidal illness, J. Clin. Endocrinol. Metab. **28:**1023, 1968.

35. Hollander, C. S., and others: Clinical and laboratory observations in cases of triiodothyronine toxicosis confirmed by radioimmunoassay, Lancet **1:**109, 1972.

36. Hollander, C. S., and others: T_3 toxicosis in an iodine deficient, Lancet **2:**1276, 1972.

37. Marsden, P., and others: Hormonal pattern of relapse in hyperthyroidism, Lancet **1(7913):**944, 1975.

38. Pharoah, P., and others: The role of T_3 in maintenance of euthyroidism in endemic goiter, Clin. Endocrinol. **2:**153, 1973.

39. Greer, M., and others: Qualitative changes in secretion of thyroid hormones induced by iodide deficiency, Endocrinology **83:**493, 1968.

40. Abruid, J., and Larsen, P. R.: T_3 and T_4 in hyperthyroidism: a comparison of acute changes during therapy with antithyroid agents, J. Clin. Invest. **54**:201, 1974.

41. Braverman, L., and Ingbar, S.: Preferential synthesis of T_3 after thyroid radiation, Clin. Res. **17**:458, 1966.

42. Hoffenberg, R.: Triiodothyronine, Clin. Endocrinol. **2**:75, 1973.

43. Patel, Y., and Burger, H.: Serum T_3 in health and disease, Clin. Endocrinol. **2**:330, 1973.

44. Sterling, K., and others: The significance of T_3 in the maintenance of the euthyroid state after therapy for hyperthyroidism, J. Clin. Endocrinol. Metab. **33**:729, 1971.

45. Gharib, H., Wahner, H., and McConahey, W.: Serum levels of thyroid hormones in Hashimoto's thyroiditis, Mayo Clin. Proc. **47**:175, 1972.

46. Larsen, P. R.: Triiodothyronine: a review of recent studies in its physiology and pathology, Metabolism **21**:1073, 1972.

47. Braverman, L., Dawber, N., and Ingbar, S.: Observations concerning the binding of thyroid hormone in the sera of normal subjects of varying ages, J. Clin. Invest. **45**:1273, 1966.

48. Herch, R., and others: Total and free triiodothyronine and thyroid-binding globulin concentration in elderly human subjects, J. Clin. Invest. **6**:139, 1976.

49. Davis, P., and Davis, F.: Hyperthyroidism in patients over the age of 60 years, Medicine **53**:161, 1974.

50. Harvey, R.: Serum-thyroxine and thyroxine-binding globulin in seriously ill patients, Lancet **1**:208, 1971.

51. McLarty, D., and others: Thyroid-hormone levels and prognosis in inpatients with serious nonthyroidal illness, Lancet **2**(7928),275, 1975.

52. Gregerman, R., Gaffney, R., and Shock, N.: Thyroxine turnover in euthyroid man with special reference to age, J. Clin. Invest. **41**:2065, 1962.

53. Oddie, T., Meade, J., and Fisher, D.: An analysis of published data on thyroxin turnover in normal subjects, J. Clin. Endocrinol. Metab. **26**:425, 1966.

54. Ingbar, S.: The influence of aging on human thyroid economy. In Greenblatt, R. B., editor: Geriatric endocrinology, New York, 1978, Raven Press, p. 12.

55. Hermann, J., and Rusche, H.: Free T_3 and T_4 serum levels in old age, Horm. Metab. Res. **6**:239, 1974.

56. Rubinstein, H., and others: Progressive decrease in serum T_3 concentrations with human aging: radioimmunoassay following extraction of serum, J. Clin. Endocrinol. Metab. **37**:247, 1973.

57. Nicod, P., and others: A radioimmunoassay for $3,3'5'$-T_3 in unextracted serum: method and clinical results, J. Clin. Endocrinol. Metab. **42**:823, 1976.

58. Olsen, T., Laurberg, P., and Wieke, J.: Low serum T_3 and high serum reverse T_3 in old age: an effect of disease, not age, J. Clin. Endocrinol. Metab. **47**:1111, 1978.

59. Stoffer, S., and Hamberger, J.: T_4 toxicosis, Lancet **2**:660, 1975.

60. Kirkegaard, C., and others: Does T_4 toxicosis exist? Lancet **11**(7911):868, 1975.

61. Irvine, R. E., and Hodkinson, H.: Thyroid disease in old age. In Brocklinhurst, J., editor: Textbook of geriatric medicine, Edinburgh, Eng., 1978, Churchill Livingstone, p. 461.

62. Ronnov-Jessen, V., and Kirkegaard, C.: Hyperthyroidism: a disease of old age?, Br. Med. J. **1**:41, 1973.

63. Iverson, K.: Thyrotoxicosis in aged individuals, J. Gerontol. **8**:65, 1953.

64. Bartels, E. C.: Hyperthyroidism in patients over the age of 60, Surg. Clin. North Am. **34**:673, 1954.

65. Bartels, E. C.: Hyperthyroidism in patients over 65, Geriatrics **20**:459, 1965.

66. Seed, L., and Lindsay, A.: Hyperthyroidism in the aged: a review of 100 cases over 65 years of age, Geriatrics **14**:136, 1949.

67. Morrow, L.: How thyroid disease presents in the elderly, Geriatrics **33**:42, 1978.

68. Thomas, F., and others: Apathetic thyrotoxicosis: a distinct clinical and laboratory entity, Ann. Intern. Med. **72**:679, 1970.

69. Lazarus, J., and Harden, R.: Throtoxicosis in the elderly, Gerontol. Clin. **11**:371, 1969.

70. Cullen, D., and Irvine, W.: Exophthalmos, Br. J. Hosp. Med. **5**:41, 1970.

71. Harvard, C. W., and others: Electromyographic and histological findings in muscles of patients with thyrotoxicosis, Q. J. Med. **32**:145, 1963.

72. Ramsay, I.: Muscle dysfunction in hyperthyroidism, Lancet **2**:931, 1966.

73. Caplan, R., and others: Thyroid function tests in elderly hyperthyroid patients, J. Am. Geriatr. Soc. **26**:3, 1977.

74. Menendez, C., and Rivlin, R.: Thyrotoxic crisis and myxedema coma, Med. Clin. North Am. **57**:1463, 1973.

75. Bahemuka, M., and Hodkinson, H.: Screening

for hypothyroidism in elderly patients, Br. Med. J. **2**:601, 1957.

76. Tarum, R M.: What to look for in diagnosing hypothyroidism in elderly patients, Geratrics, **32**:55, 1977.

77. Buchanan, W., and Harden, R.: Primary hypothyroidism: a continuous spectrum, Arch. Intern. Med. **115**:411, 1965.

78. Candy, J.: Severe hypothyroidism: an early complication of lithium therapy. Br. Med. J.**111**: 277, 1972.

79. Shopsin, B., and others: Iodine and lithium induced hypothyroidism, Am. J. Med. **55**:695, 1973.

80. Vagenakis, A., and Braverman, L.: Adverse effects of iodide on thyroid function, Med. Clin. North Am. **59**:1075, 1975.

81. Billewicz, W. Z., and others: Statistical methods applied to the diagnosis of hypothyroidism, Q. J. Med. **38**:255, 1969.

82. Jellinek, E.: Fits, fainting, coma and dementia in myxedema, Lancet **2**:1010, 1962.

83. Jellinek, E.: Cerebellar syndromes in myxedema, Lancet **2**:225, 1960.

84. Cropper, C.: Hypothyroidism in psychogeriatric patients: ankle jerk reaction time as a screening technique, Gerontol. Clin. **15**:15, 1973.

85. Bland, J., and Frymoyer, J.: Rheumatic syndromes of myxedema, N. Engl. J. Med. **282**: 1171, 1970.

86. Golding, D.: Hypothyroidism presenting with neuromuscular symptoms, Ann. Rheum. Dis. **29**:10, 1970.

87. Fissel, W.: Myopathy of hypothyroidism: Ann. Rheum. Dis. **27**:590, 1968.

88. Gaede, J.: Serum enzyme alterations in hypothyroidism before and after therapy, J. Am. Geriatr. Soc. **25**:199, 1978.

89. Stock, J.: Replacement dose of L-thyroxine in hypothyroidism: a reevaluation, N. Engl. J. Med. **290**:529, 1974.

90. McConahey, W.: Diagnosing and treating myxedema and myxedema coma, Geriatrics **33**:61, 1978.

91. Holvey, D., and others: Treatment of myxedema coma with intravenous thyroxine, Arch. Intern. Med. **113**:89, 1969.

92. McDermott, W., and others: Cancer of the thyroid, J. Clin. Endocrinol. Metab. **14**:1336, 1954.

PROBLEM-SOLVING EXERCISES*
Case one

A 71-year-old woman presents with a 3-cm left thyroid nodule that has recently increased in size, is quite hard and fixed, is not tender, and is unassociated with any cervical lymphadenopathy. Aside from recent intermittent hoarseness, she is without complaint and has been otherwise healthy. Physical examination is normal in every other respect. CBC, urinalysis, ECG, chest X-ray study, blood chemistries, T_3 and T_4 by RIA, TSH, and T_3 resin uptake are all normal.

Questions

1. If this woman has a thyroidal malignancy, statistically it is most likely to be:
   a. Medullary or amyloid
   b. Lymphoma of the thyroid gland
   c. Papillary carcinoma
   d. Follicular carcinoma
   e. Anaplastic carcinoma

2. In which order would you order the following tests?
   a. Open biopsy of the thyroid gland
   b. Indirect laryngoscopy
   c. ^{131}I scan of the thyroid gland and neck
   d. Needle biopsy of the thyroid gland
   e. Sonography

3. If the nodule were hot on scan, had not grown, and there were no uptake elsewhere in the gland, which of the following statements would be true?
   a. All attempts to involute the nodule with full suppressive doses of T_4 should be made.
   b. It may be safely observed.
   c. It should be removed because of a high index of suspicion for carcinoma.
   d. Nodules like this, when they attain sufficient size, may cause hyperthyroidism (especially thyrotoxicosis).
   e. These nodules are usually part of a general glandular disorder and herald the development of hypothyroidism.

---

*Some questions may have more than one correct answer.

Case two

An 80-year-old woman presents to you with nervousness, palpitations, hyperkinesis, and a 15-pound weight loss (from a stringent diet). On examination she has a pulse of 118 (irregular); tremor; fine, moist skin; stare; and barely palpable thyroid tissue bilaterally. She had mild CHF. The following laboratory tests have been obtained:

T_3 by RIA: 450 ng/dl (n = 90 to 190)
T_3 resin uptake: 32% (n = 25% to 35%)
24-hour ^{131}I uptake: 3% (n = 10% to 30%)

Questions

1. Can any of the following be excluded on the basis of the above laboratory data?
   a. T_3 toxicosis
   b. Ingestion of excessive amounts of T_4
   c. Acute phase of subacute thyroiditis
   d. Ingestion of excessive amounts of T_3
2. If the T_4 were 16, ESR 118, and the gland acutely tender, which diagnosis would you favor?
3. If the T_4 were 16, the gland felt normal, and the ESR were normal, which diagnosis would you favor?
4. If the T_4 were 6, the gland felt normal, and ESR were normal, which diagnoses would you favor?

Case three

You are called on the telephone regarding a 79-year-old woman who had been treated for hyperthyroidism with ^{131}I some 9 months previously. Her family physician states that there are no diagnostic historical or physical finding but that she is depressed and just is not feeling, looking, or doing well.

Question

1. In column B are a series of laboratory data that he might give to you with regard to this patient's thyroid status and in column A are a group of clinical states that might be present. Match the laboratory data to the clinical state.°

°Normal values—T_4:4.5µg/dl to 12.0µg/dl; T_3: 90 to 190 ng/dl; TSH: 0.5µU to 6.0µU/ml; T_3 resin uptake: 25% to 35%; FT_4I: 1.2 to 4.2.

COLUMN A
____ a. Eumetabolism with increased TBP levels due to estrogen ingestion
____ b. Recurrent T_3 toxicosis
____ c. Incipient hypothyroidism
____ d. Eumetabolism in an older person
____ e. Eumetabolism in the presence of severe nonthyroidal illness

COLUMN B
1. T_4: 8µg/dl; T_3: 85 ng/dl; TSH: 2.9µU/ml; T_3 resin uptake: 30%
2. T_4: 4µg/dl; T_3: 210 ng/dl; TSH: 20µU/ml; T_3 resin uptake: 25%
3. T_4: 15µg/dl; T_3: 210 ng/dl; TSH: 2µU/ml; T_3 resin uptake: 18%
4. T_4: 4.9µg/dl; T_3: 390 ng/dl; TSH: too low to measure; T_3 resin uptake: 35%
5. T_4:3µg/dl; T_3: 40 ng/dl; TSH: 3.9µU/ml; T_3 resin uptake: 55%

Case four

An apprehensive woman of 80 is referred to you by a psychiatrist for medical evaluation prior to electroconvulsive therapy (ECT) for an unresponsive depression. She has a history of recurrent depression in the past and was treated some 10 years ago for hyperthyroidism with ^{131}I. After her therapy she felt so well that she discontinued her propranolol and never returned to her physician. About 4 months ago she was brought to the psychiatrist by her family because of increasing withdrawal, weakness, recurrent falls, and depression. He cleared her neurologically, diagnosed recurrent depression, and started her on a regimen of lithium carbonate. On this regimen her symptoms increased; in addition, there appeared increasing fatigue, muscle aches, pain, cramps and stiffness, severe arthralgias, and sleepiness. On examination she appears withdrawn and depressed, and she moves and speaks very slowly. Her weight is 132 (average 135), pulse 64 and regular, blood pressure 160/60, and temperature normal. Her eyelids appear somewhat puffy; increased pigmentation is noted in her palmar creases; and although her ankle jerks are not elicited, her biceps reflex is delayed in relaxation. Her thyroid gland is not palpable.

Questions

1. Which of the following tests would most likely confirm your clinical impression?
   a. T_4 by RIA and T_3 resin uptake
   b. T_3 by RIA and T_3 resin uptake
   c. ^{131}I uptake and scan
   d. Cholesterol and CPK levels
   e. T_3 and T_4 by RIA
2. A T_3 by RIA and T_3 resin uptake are ordered and returned within normal limits (110 ng/dl and 25%). Which test would you order next?
   a. T_4 by RIA
   b. Repeat the tests already done
   c. ^{131}I uptake and scan
   d. None (The patient is eumetabolic and should be cleared for ECT.)
3. A T_4 by RIA is ordered and returned (2.3 μg/dl; (n = 4.5μg/dl to 12μg/dl). The test that will confirm the diagnosis of primary hypothyroidism is:
   a. ^{131}I uptake
   b. TSH levels
   c. T_3 suppression test
   d. BMR
4. TSH levels are drawn and returned (90μU/ml; n = 0.5μU/ml to 6μU/ml). It is most likely that:
   a. Her hypothyroidism resulted from the ^{131}I therapy
   b. Her hypothyroidism resulted from the lithium
   c. Her hypothyroidism resulted from the natural wearing out of her gland with age
   d. A combination of a and c
   e. A combination of a and b

The lithium is discontinued. Four weeks later the patient still appears hypothyroid; and although her T_4 is up to 3.6μg/dl, it remains in the hypothyroid range.

Case five

You are asked to see a 76-year-old man on the surgical service. He has been eating poorly for several months and has been maintained on intravenous fluids for the 13 days since the resection of his colonic carcinoma, which had not metastasized at the time of surgery. A persistant tachycardia prompted the surgical resident to order a T_3 and T_4 by RIA, since the possibility of masked thyrotoxicosis has been raised by this unexplained finding. The T_3 is 40 ng/dl and the T_4 is 4.2μg/dl; both are low. On careful examination a trace of sacral edema is noted, but there are no other pertinent findings.

Questions

1. The consultation request asks, "How shall we proceed with thyroid replacement?" Your answer is:
   a. "Since he is elderly and has tachycardia, and since hypothyroid patients may be sensitive to T_4, start very slowly with 0.0125μg of T_4 a day."
   b. "Repeat the tests; he looks normal to me."
   c. "Order a ^{131}I uptake."
   d. "Order a T_3 resin uptake."
   e. "Get a CPK; it is usually elevated in hypothyroidism."
2. The tests are repeated and are unchanged. You note that the CPK was 2,500 3 days after the operation but was normal preoperatively. In addition, the serum sodium has gradually fallen from 138 to 124. Your next suggestion is:
   a. "Get some T_4 into him quickly, before he slips into myxedema coma."
   b. "Get a T_3 resin uptake."
   c. "Repeat the CPK."
   d. "Order a ^{131}I uptake."
3. A T_3 resin uptake is finally obtained and is in the extremely hyperthyroid range (60%). The calculated FT$_4$I is a normal 2.52 (0.60 × 4.2). Which of the following statements is true?
   a. Reverse T_3 levels will be elevated.
   b. TSH levels will be normal.
   c. A TRH stimulation test might be of value in establishing the patient's eumetabolic state.
   d. The administration of iodides will no doubt return the T_3 levels to normal.

ANSWERS TO PROBLEM-SOLVING EXERCISES
Case one

1. d. Follicular carcinoma is the most common thyroidal malignancy in the elderly.
2. c, b, e, d, a. Scanning, indirect laryngoscopy, sonography, needle biopsy, and then surgery.
3. b and d. Hot autonomous nodules rarely are the site of thyroidal malignancies. They may be safely observed. However, when they attain sufficient size, they may cause thyrotoxicosis.

Case two

1. No. Any of the four conditions listed may cause clinical hyperthyroidism with the laboratory tests as noted.
2. The high ESR and acutely tender gland would strongly suggest the acute phase of subacute thyroiditis.
3. These findings would suggest self-induced hyperthyroidism by the ingestion of T_4
4. The low T_4 together with the findings as stated would suggest either T_3 toxicosis or the ingestion of T_3.

Case three

1. a, 3. The diagnosis of eumetabolism and increased binding proteins matches with this T_4, T_3, TSH, and T_3 resin uptake. The T_3 resin uptake indicates expanded binding proteins. b, 4. Recurrent T_3 toxicosis matches with this T_4, T_3, TSH, and T_3 resin uptake. c, 2. Incipient hypothyroidism would be suggested by this low T_4, elevated T_3, elevated TSH, and borderline-low T_3 resin uptake. This patient is being maintained clinically euthyroid by the levels of T_3. d, 1. Eumetabolism in an older person matches with the normal T_4, T_3 resin uptake, and TSH, and with the low T_3. Older patients may have reduced T_3 levels and maintain the eumetabolic state. e, 5. In eumetabolism in the presence of severe nonthyroidal illness the T_3 is reduced, probably due to an inhibition of the 5'-deiodinase. The low TBP level (T_3 resin uptake of 55%) results in a low T_4, but the calculated FT_4I ($T_4 \times T_3$ resin uptake) is normal or slightly elevated. TSH levels are normal.

Case four

1. a. The diagnosis of hypothyroidism will best be confirmed by a T_4 and T_3 resin uptake.
2. a. The T_3 by RIA is normal in up to 20% of hypothyroid patients. Get a T_4 by RIA.
3. b. The TSH will confirm the diagnosis of primary hypothyroidism. It should be elevated.
4. e. There is an incidence of hypothyroidism of 3% per year following ^{131}I therapy. Lithium, by blocking the release of thyroid hormone from the gland and probably interfering with intrathyroidal iodide organification, probably precipitated or worsened the condition.

Case five

1. d. Order a T_3 resin uptake to be sure that there is no marked decrease in binding proteins. An FT_4I can then be calculated. The CPK may still be elevated as a result of the surgery.
2. b. Get a T_3 resin uptake.
3. a, b, and c. The inhibition of 5'-deiodinase would result in elevated reverse T_3 levels. The patient is eumetabolic; TSH levels should be normal, and a normal TSH response to TRH is expected under these circumstances.

POSTTEST
True or False

1. The T_3 suppression test generally should not be used in the older patient.
2. The response of thyroid-stimulating hormone (TSH) to thyrotropin-releasing hormone (TRH) is blunted in healthy older men.
3. The T_3 resin uptake measures serum T_3.
4. The T_3 resin uptake and the calculable

free thyroxine index (FT_4I) can be very helpful in gaining insight into the meaning of serum T_4 by radioimmunoassay (RIA).

5. The major body source of T_3 in the elderly is direct synthesis of T_3 by the thyroid gland.

6. Low serum T_3 levels are common in older persons and/or persons with a variety of acute and/or chronic illnesses.

7. Weight loss, anorexia, and/or constipation are common in the history of older hyperthyroid patients.

8. Nodular hyperthyroidism is the most common type of hyperthyroidism in the elderly.

9. [131]I is the usual treatment of choice in older patients with hyperthyroidism.

10. In most elderly hyperthyroid patients, especially those with cardiac disorders, ^{131}I should be preceded by 4 to 6 weeks of antithyroid drugs, followed by 48 to 72 hours of withdrawal of such drugs. The antithyroid drugs should then be started again 3 to 4 days after ^{131}I is given.

11. Hypothyroidism is easily missed, because the slowing of physical and mental activity may be incorrectly attributed to "old age."

12. The best screening laboratory tests for the diagnosis of hyperthyroidism are T_4 by RIA, coupled with T_3 resin uptake test or thyroid-binding globulin (TBG) level.

13. TSH and creatine phosphokinase (CPK) are both elevated in hyperthyroidism.

14. Thyroxine is the best replacement therapy in hypothyroidism and should generally be given in lower doses than in the young and slowly increased.

ANSWERS TO PRETEST AND POSTTEST

1. True. The administration of T_3 in these doses (75μg/day for 10 days) to elderly patients with underlying cardiovascular disease, especially if they have autonomous glands, can be very hazardous.

2. True. The mechanism is not understood.

3. False. The T_3 resin uptake measures free binding sites on thyroid-binding proteins (TBPs) and reflects the level of these binding proteins. There is no change in the level of TBP in healthy elderly people.

4. True. The calculation of the FT_4I is valuable in assessing the level of thyroid function in patients with alterations in binding proteins and closely parallels the level of FT_4 as measured by equilibrium dialysis.

5. False. Eighty percent of the T_3 produced daily in normal elderly people originates from the peripheral monodeiodination of T_4.

6. True. This probably is a result of an inhibition of the 5'-delodinase peripherally. 3,3'-diiodothyronine levels are also low.

7. True. This triad may be seen in up to 15% of elderly hyperthyroid patients and often misdirects our diagnostic workup toward the gastrointestinal tract.

8. True. Almost 100% of patients have microscopic thyroid nodules by age 80. Graves' disease is a less common cause of hyperthyroidism in the elderly.

9. True. Concern about damage to the reproductive organs is no longer pertinent. Hypothyroidism secondary to the radiation damage will be present for a lesser number of years because of the age of the patient. Toxic nodular goiters are less commonly rendered hypothyroidism by ^{131}I than are glands with Graves' disease. Finally, one prefers not to subject older patients to the risks of surgery.

10. True. [131]I therapy is often followed by radiation thyroiditis some 7 to 14 days after administration. This results in the extravasation of stored colloid containing T_3 and T_4 into the interstices of the gland and then into the circulation. This added load of thyroactive material may exacerbate the hyperthyroidism and result in cardiovascular complications in an elderly patient with underlying heart disease. Pretreatment with antithyroid drugs results in the depletion of stored hormone in the gland. Thus, in a patient pretreated with these drugs, the radiation thyroiditis caused by ^{131}I is not accompanied by extravasation of active hormone into the blood.

11. True.

12. True. A T_4 measurement without information regarding the level of binding proteins may be misleading.

13. False. TSH and CPK are both elevated in primary hypothyroidism.

14. True. T_4 administration results in more even levels of T_3 and T_4 in the blood without the marked peaks and troughs seen with T_3 administration. Hypothyroidism is rarely an emergency, and overtreatment must be avoided in the elderly.

Chapter 13

Clinical aspects of nutrition

CORNELIUS J. FOLEY, LESLIE S. LIBOW, and FREDRICK T. SHERMAN

EDUCATIONAL OBJECTIVES
Attitudinal

The student should:

1. Be aware of the importance of nutrition in the evaluation and treatment of the older patient
2. Recognize that the elderly are not generally ill, debilitated, cachectic, or malnourished
3. Be aware of the altered financial status of the elderly and its impact on nutritional status
4. Recognize that there is almost universal lack of dietary inquiry in medical history taking, especially in the elderly
5. Recognize that the elderly have had little or no education with respect to nutrition
6. Recognize that nutrition and hydration in the elderly do affect health, probably more so than in middle age

Cognitive:

The student should:

1. Recognize that there is a lack of accuracy in nutritional data specific to the elderly
2. Recognize that there are no generally accepted nutritional standards for those over 65 years of age
3. Know how those nutritional recommendations that do exist have been formulated
4. Be aware of the inadequacy of clinical and laboratory measurements in establishing a patient's nutritional status
5. Know how nutritional surveys are conducted, the strengths and weaknesses of such surveys, and how applicable they may be to the elderly.
6. Know how nutrition can affect aging
7. Be aware of age-related metabolic and physiological changes that are regarded as normal and know how they affect nutrition
8. Understand the role of diet in illness of late life

9. Understand the effect of medications on nutritional status

Skill

The student should:

1. Be able to accurately obtain a dietary history from an older patient
2. Be able to recognize the symptoms and signs of nutritional deficiency
3. Know how to apply and interpret laboratory investigations in nutritional assessment
4. Be able to appropriately manipulate diet in the common illnesses of the elderly (diabetes mellitus, congestive heart failure, hypertension, osteoporosis, and constipation)
5. Be able to assist an elderly patient in choosing an appropriate diet
6. Know how to apply the principles and techniques of enteral hyperalimentation to the elderly patient

---

PRETEST
True or false

1. Mental function is significantly influenced by standard nutrients.
2. Healthy 70-year-old men who are of low-normal weight have a lesser life expectancy than age-matched controls who have more average weights.
3. Animal studies show that, in general, food deprivation in the early stages of life leads to an increased life span.
4. The total number of multiplications of cultured human cells is finite.

5. Antioxidants and certain sulfur compounds prolong animal life and reduce cross linkages.
6. Recommended Dietary Allowances (RDAs) for total calories and for specific nutrients have been described specifically for those over 75 years of age.
7. Cross-sectional studies of age differences are more likely to reveal age-related changes than are longitudinal studies.
8. Diets of the elderly are most likely to be deficient in total caloric intake, calcium, and iron.
9. The elderly person's protein intake is typically deficient.
10. The dietary history is usually obtained in standard medical interviews.
11. Mental depression and digitalis therapy are common causes of anorexia in the elderly.
12. Vitamin C deficiency is the most common cause of ecchymosis in the elderly.
13. Unilateral cheiloses are usually related to vitamin deficiency.
14. A white band across the nails of the hand is often related to protein deficiency.
15. Osteomalacia is related primarily to protein deficiency.
16. Serum albumin concentration normally decreases with advancing age.
17. The senses of taste and smell decrease with advancing age.
18. By age 65, more than half of Americans have lost all their teeth.
19. Hip fractures, secondary to osteoporosis, are quite uncommon among American blacks.

Normal aging and longevity are affected by the state of nutrition, and food intake. For example, for healthy men over 70 years of age, a weight lighter than the norm for that age is significantly (albeit surprisingly) associated with increased mortality in ensuing years.[1]

Cerebral function is profoundly influenced by varying nutrients.[2] Other disease states known to be intimately involved with nutrition include neoplastic diseases, digitalis toxicity, congestive heart failure, hypertension, atherosclerosis, various infections, anemias, nephrolithiasis, renal failure, cholelithiasis, bone fractures, and diabetes mellitus.

EFFECT OF NUTRITION ON AGING

Nutritional deprivation studies performed on numerous animal species have demonstrated that reduced caloric intake results in delayed maturation and increased life span.[3-5] In some animal studies, restriction of caloric intake to 60% of Recommended Dietary Allowances (RDAs; see p. 284) has been shown to be effective in increasing longevity. In addition, the timing of onset and duration of caloric restriction are important. It has been found that a continuous reduction of dietary intake throughout life prolongs the life span, whereas animals who have their first dietary restrictions when middle aged may have a shortened life span. Animals who have had dietary restrictions in infancy, followed by ad libitum feeding sufficient for maximum growth, appear to have a mild increase in longevity. This group has a further extension of longevity if dietary restrictions are again instituted in middle or later life. The early months of development thus appear to be the setting of a potential for longevity that is influenced by nutrition.

The content of the diet probably plays an important role in longevity, but experiments in this area are difficult to interpret. It is unclear whether the composition of unrestricted diets plays any role in longevity. In animals on restricted diets, however, a high protein content may be associated with an extended life span, whereas a high fat content may limit the potential longevity. There also appears to be an inverse relationship between total carbohydrate intake and life span.

There is a high death rate for animals on severely restricted diets during the first year of caloric deprivation in comparison with ad libitum–fed controls. The restricted groups also show a marked reduction in biochemical and physiological development, manifested as stunting of growth, in addition to restricted behavioral development and susceptibility to infectious diseases. Those animals who survive the caloric restrictions not only have an increased life span, but also have a significant reduction in several chronic illnesses, such as glomerulonephrosis, myocardial fibrosis, endocrine hyperplasia, and prostatitis, and in the incidence of malignant tumors.[6-12]

Data on dietary restrictions in short-lived laboratory animals cannot be freely extrapolated to humans. Dietary restriction in human infants in the hope of increasing longevity is inappropriate.

Nutrition and cellular aging

The biological mechanisms linking increased longevity to nutritional restriction are unknown. At the cellular level the following possibly causal relationships have been shown:

1. The life span of differentiated cells varies inversely with the rate of mitoses (i.e., the older the cell, the slower its growth rate). The progressive deterioration in replication of DNA is a possible explanation for this limited life span, known as Hayflick's phenomenon.[13]

The total number of potential mitoses and multiplications of the normal cell is finite (e.g., approximately 50 ± 10 times for human fibroblasts). Caloric restriction slows growth by diminishing mitotic frequency, and the cell's life span can be prolonged by as much as one third.

2. Antioxidants and certain sulfur compounds have prolonged life in animal experiments by reducing the cross linkages associated with aging in collagen fibrils. These cross linkages may contribute to the onset of degenerative diseases of the cardiovascular system and of other systems.[14]

EFFECT OF AGING ON NUTRITION

The effect of aging on nutrition has not been determined, and the precise nutritional needs of older persons are unknown.

A multiplicity of factors makes the analysis of the elderly person's nutritional status complex. These factors include (1) the varied personal, ethnic, and economic factors that influence diet; (2) the lack of a clear correlation between malnutrition and lowered serum levels of vitamins and minerals; (3) the nonspecificity of the various methods utilized in assessing nutrition; (4) the inadequacy of clinical evaluation as an indicator of the actual nutritional status; and (5) the absence of a specific definition of malnutrition.

RDAs for caloric intake, protein, carbohydrate, fat, vitamins, and minerals have been established by the National Academy of Sciences/National Research Council (NAS/NRC)[15] for the young and middle aged. These nutritional parameters, though appearing comprehensive, are no more than a consensus of informed opinion on nutritional needs. There are no RDAs for specific nutrients for those over 65 years of age. However, the 1980 RDAs do make a recommendation for total caloric intake for those over 75 years of age.

Nutritional surveys
Interpretation of data

Cross-sectional studies: age differences. Cross-sectional surveys measure differences between groups of varying ages. Divergence found at the time of a study may not reflect differences specifically related to aging; rather, it may be a manifestation of the quality of survival.

Longitudinal surveys: age changes. Longitudinal surveys measure change over prolonged periods of time in the same individual. These studies relate change in those studied to the aging process.

Cohort studies. Cohort studies are longitudinal studies that compare groups of persons of the same age. The study could compare two groups of persons aged 80 who were born 10 years apart. It might define differences between these two groups in relation to environmental factors rather than to true aging per se.

Surveys. Surveys generally do not distinguish between normal aging and disease as it affects the aging process.

Major nutritional surveys

There are two types of population surveys that provide information pertaining to the elderly and their nutritional status: (1) large population studies of a regional or national type, assessing dietary intake and nutritional status, and (2) specific laboratory investigations limited to smaller population groups.

The major population studies are discussed specifically with regard to the nutritional status of those over the age of 65.[16]

U.S. Department of Agriculture Household Food Consumption Survey.[17] The U.S. Department of Agriculture (USDA) surveyed 6,174 households in 1965. Institutions and rooming houses were not included; consequently, a small percentage of the elderly population with different nutritional needs were not surveyed.

The mean daily caloric intake for all groups of elderly people in this study fell below the 1968 RDA. Men who were older than 65 had a calcium intake slightly below the RDA, but women in this age group had only 64% of the RDA for calcium; these women also had 86% of the RDA for thiamine and 84% of the RDA for riboflavin.

Dietary intake declined with income, a fact pertinent to the elderly, since 25% to 40% of the elderly population are at or below the poverty level.

Ten-State Nutrition Survey.[18] In 1972 the U.S. Department of Health, Education, and Welfare's Center for Disease Control (HEW-CDC) conducted the Ten-State Nutrition Survey, focusing on risk groups. It included clinical, biochemical, and dietary evaluations. Its findings were compared with the RDAs of the NAS/NRC and the Food and Agriculture Organization–World Health Organization (FAO-WHO). The findings indicated that persons aged 60 and older consumed far less food than needed to meet the proposed standards. Skeletal weight decreased with age, with lower income groups having lower skeletal weights. The overall rate of bone loss, however, was independent of economic status. Obesity was more prevalent in high-income groups. It decreased markedly with age from 50% for blacks and 40% for whites at age 45 to 55 to about 20% to 25% in both races by age 75 to 85. (This may not be a change linked to aging but may represent survival of nonobese middle-aged persons.) Men had a lower prevalence of obesity. Periodontal disease increased with age, affecting 90% of those aged 65 to 75 years, and was not correlated with any specific biochemical mechanisms. The clinical and laboratory assessments did not show a high incidence of obvious malnutrition in the older subjects.

Health and Nutrition Examination Survey.[19] The National Center for Health Statistics conducted the Health and Nutrition Examination Survey (HANES), which evaluated (1) 24-hour food consumption; (2) biochemical tests, including protein, carbohydrate, fat, vitamins, and minerals; (3) clinical signs; and (4) anthropometric measurements. This survey did not show consistent evidence of poor nutritional status or of marked deficiencies in nutrient intake among the elderly in most U.S. populations. A significant percentage of those surveyed did not attain RDAs — not because of age per se, but because of low income. Based on this study, the frequency of nutritional deficiency in the elderly appears to be low.

Summary of current nutritional data on the elderly

The information on nutritional status and requirements in the elderly presented below is a distillation of the large population studies and the many small and more specific studies, some of which are longitudinal.[16-20] It takes into account the differences in age and sex of the subjects studied; it recognizes the varied methodology and standards used and the lack of comprehensive longitudinal and cohort studies.

The 1974 RDAs are presented in Table 13-1. While these RDAs are for persons 55 years of age and over, there are no specific RDAs for persons over 65 years of age.

Table 13-1. 1974 RDAs for persons older than 55 years*

	Men	Women
Weight (kg)	70	58
Energy (kcal)	2,400	1,800
Protein (g)	56	46
Calcium (mg)	800	800
Iron (mg)	10	10
Vitamin A (IU)	5,000	4,000
Thiamine (mg)	1.2	1.0
Riboflavin (mg)	1.5	1.1
Niacin (mg)	16	12
Vitamin B_6 (mg)	2.0	2.0
Vitamin B_{12} (mg)	3.0	3.0
Vitamin C (mg)	45	45
Vitamin D (IU)†	400	400
Vitamin E (IU)	15	12
Phosphorus (mg)	800	800
Iodine (mg)	110	80
Magnesium (mg)	350	300
Zinc (mg)	15	15

*These RDAs apply to activity that is light to sedentary and are high enough to meet the needs of those with the highest requirements in this group. They apply to healthy people. They do not allow for disease states or medication effects.
†The vitamin D recommendation for 55-year-olds is not defined; this figure is for young adults.

Distribution of caloric intake

The elderly appear to maintain approximately the same ratio of protein, fat, and carbohydrate in their diet as the young adult:

Protein: 13% to 30%
Carbohydrate: 50% to 55%
Fat: 30% to 35%

Total caloric intake

Caloric recommendations for the elderly are, however, significantly different from those of young adults. For elderly men and women the requirements are 2,400 and 1,800 kcal, respectively, while those for 19- to 22-year-olds are 3,000 and 2,100.

Carbohydrate and fat

Carbohydrate and fat intake is seen in the light of total caloric intake and is frequently found to be less than the recommended RDA; in fact, some 35% of elderly subjects have intakes less than the RDA. Even if 50% of the RDA is taken as the norm, some 50% of white women and 60% to 95% of elderly black women may have intakes less than this diminished standard. It is also noted that there is a diminishing intake of calories from age 70 to 87 of 24% in men and 17% in women.

Protein

The mean protein intake in the United States has been found to be adequate when compared with the 1974 RDA of 0.8 g/kg body weight, except for low-income black women. However, although the mean intake is acceptable, approximately 35% of all subjects have protein intakes significantly below the RDA.

Nutrients and minerals

Calcium. Calcium is one of the nutrients most often lacking in the diets of the elderly, with women having lower and relatively more inadequate intakes than men. In the Ten-State Nutrition Survey, some 30% of elderly women living in high-income states and 50% of those living in low-income states fell below the standard used (i.e., 400 mg—this arbitrary standard is 50% of the 1974 RDA for calcium; see Table 13-1).

Iron. The diets of 30% to 50% of elderly men and 70% to 100% of elderly women have less iron than the 10-mg RDA. The lower the income and the older the person, the more the diet will be deficient in iron.

Vitamin A. The elderly appear to have diets that provide approximately 67% of the RDA for vitamin A (i.e., 3,333 IU in

most instances), and this level is accepted as probably adequate. Persons over the age of 75, especially women, have lower intakes.

Vitamin C. All major surveys have found adequate mean levels of vitamin C in the diets of the elderly. The only groups below the RDA of 45 mg are low-income black women.

Thiamine. Thiamine consumption has been found to be adequate in most large studies other than the Ten-State Nutrition Survey, wherein approximately 35% of the elderly population had intakes below its standard.

Riboflavin. Most surveys have reported the mean intake of riboflavin as meeting their standards for the elderly; however, the Ten-State Nutrition Survey found some 35% of subjects to be below its standard.

Niacin. This B vitamin is generally taken in sufficient quantity as determined in most surveys.

• • •

In summary, the diets of the elderly are most likely to be deficient in total caloric intake, calcium, and iron (and possibly in thiamine and riboflavin). The nutrients most likely to be adequate are protein and niacin.

CLINICAL NUTRITIONAL ASSESSMENT

The clinical nutritional assessment includes the dietary history, clinical evaluation, and laboratory tests.

Dietary history

History taking in the elderly often requires special approaches that focus on areas not normally concentrated on in younger patients. A dietary history is rarely taken in any patient as a matter of routine and is often poorly done even when it is obviously of clinical pertinence. The elderly patient is at a higher risk for having nutritional deficiencies, and a high index of suspicion must be maintained.

In the delineation of a nutritional problem, the three main "tools" used are (1) the *24-hour dietary recall*, elicited by direct questioning; (2) the *food record*, made by the patient or spouse over a number of days; and (3) the *dietary history*, focusing on food patterns and habits for a period of time, up to 1 year.

The accuracy and pertinence of the dietary history depend on the older person's mental status. Thus, through recognition of a deteriorated mental status, the clinician can avoid involvement with a protracted and inevitably inaccurate nutritional history. All areas of mental status, including recall and memory, can be quickly assessed by mental status evaluation techniques such as FROMAJE (see Chapter 5).

In certain situations the dietary history in the elderly will be significantly improved if verification of details can be obtained from relatives or friends — or if these persons can provide additional information. The eating habits of some older persons may be erratic, and at times the dietary history provides no more than a vague indication of the types and quantities of food consumed. The history must therefore be combined with clinical examination — and where malnutrition is suspected, with laboratory studies for a more detailed nutritional assessment.

Answers to the following questions are important in the food record:

1. What is the frequency of meals? The number of hot meals per week? The content of these meals? The quantity of dietary fiber? What types of snacks or "junk" foods are consumed? Answers to these questions give an indication of the quality and quantity of food. Among the poor, the number of hot meals per week correlates well with the overall nutritional value of the diet.

2. Who prepares the meals? How are they cooked? What are the cooking facilities? How and where is food stored? The presence of a spouse or relative can positively affect the diet of an infirm individual. If all food comes from cans and packets, it tends to have high salt and low nutritive content. If storage facilities for food, such as airtight containers and a refrigerator or freezer are not available, then perishables will not be purchased in significant amounts. This is particularly true if travel to distant stores is difficult.

3. What is the access to food sources? How distant are they? What types of foods are available in them? Who travels to the food source and through what type of neighborhood? If there is easy access to a store where prices are reasonable, the patient is fortunate. The elderly often have fears of being assaulted while outside their homes. Those who have lived many decades in one area may find that their neighborhoods have deteriorated. Violence toward the elderly, though frequently reported in the news media, is less than that involving younger persons[21]; yet the expectation of violence is very prevalent.

4. What is the financial outlay on food in relation to the patient's financial status? How much needs to be spent to be "enough"? The elderly are often severely restricted in their choice of food by lack of income.[22,23]

5. What is the patient's level of physical activity? How sedentary is his lifestyle? How much time does he spend resting each day? The level of activity determines the caloric requirements.

6. What is the patient's dental status, and what is his ability to chew? Do dentures fit? (They often do not.)

7. Is the appetizing effect of the sight of food limited by visual difficulties? Do ocular problems limit the preparation of meals?[24]

8. Is the pleasure of eating reduced because the senses of taste and smell are decreased? Recognize that eating is one of the few pleasures of many older persons. Any and all factors that limit this pleasure are significant, and efforts should be made to evaluate and correct them.

9. Do arthritic afflictions, tremor, or paralysis limit the ability to manipulate cooking and eating utensils?

10. With whom does the person live? What kinds of companionship, socialization, interests, and hobbies does he enjoy? The greater the level of interesting stimuli in an older person's daily schedule, the more mentally active he will be.[25]

11. What is the patient's emotional status? Is there depression with bouts of crying, altered sleep pattern, and/or loss of appetite? Depression frequently presents with an insidious onset of weight loss, suggesting malnutrition secondary to a gastrointestinal or other malignancy.

Because the suicide rate among the elderly is more than three times that of the general population, men being at greater risk, weight loss from depression is a major danger signal.[25-27]

12. Is there a question of excessive alcohol consumption? Alcoholism in the elderly is related to loneliness and isolation.[28] If there is a problem, it is frequently denied, so that a high index of suspicion is necessary for its detection.

Alcoholism is often related to nutritional deficiencies (more money is being spent on alcohol than on food). Megalo-blastic anemia can occur in relation to hepatic and bone marrow toxicity in addition to a low-folate diet. Wernicke's disease, Korsakoff's syndrome, and peripheral neuropathy occur and may be related to vitamin deficiencies (e.g., thiamine).

13. Does the patient adhere to any "fad" diet? Food fads should be of concern, since the elderly are particularly susceptible to advertisements suggesting diets leading to possible rejuvenation, release from disability, and/or increased longevity. The cost of such diets may be high and their nutritive value low.

14. Is the patient on a special medical diet (e.g., low salt, low fat, or low carbohydrate)? Recognize that a patient may adhere to such a diet for decades.

15. What is the medication history? It is important to know what prescribed medications the patient is taking for reasons such as the following: (1) digoxin toxicity, common in the elderly, is associated with anorexia and nausea; (2) anticonvulsants can cause vitamin D and folate deficiency; (3) chemotherapy has multiple nutritional effects; and (4) tuberculosis therapy is associated with vitamin B_1 and B_{12} deficiencies (tuberculosis reactivation is relatively common in the elderly).

In addition to prescribed medications, it is important to know what nonprescribed medications the patient uses. Laxative and antacid abuse, for example, can be linked to malnutrition.

Note also "home cures," which often include alcohol, and the total number of drugs being used.

The elderly, who constitute approximately 10% of the population, receive almost 25% of all prescribed drugs. The potential for drug interactions is therefore very high, since many drugs are ingested.[29,30]

Be particularly aware of the frequently

ignored drug abuse areas of laxatives, analgesics, vitamins, and appetite stimulants.

16. Has there been any change in food habits? If the answer is yes, determine what and why.

17. Has there been a weight change, either with or without a change in appetite? If there has, pursue the usual review of systems but give thought to the common age-related problems mentioned in this and other sections.

18. Does the patient have anorexia? Consider mental depression, medication side effects, or systemic illness.

19. Does the patient have an increased appetite? This may be associated with fever-producing illnesses. If it is associated with frequency of urination, consider diabetes mellitus. If it is associated with tremor and/or palpitation, consider hyperthyroidism.

20. Are there any gastrointestinal problems affecting appetite (e.g., lower esophageal sphincter incompetence, peptic ulcer, difficulty with swallowing, flatulence, diarrhea, constipation, or melena)?

21. Is the patient involved with any community or domicillary agencies, such as a visiting nurse service or Meals on Wheels? The older person may attend a senior citizens' or religious center where meals are provided.

These services are partially government funded but are often largely voluntary on the part of communities. They play a most important role, providing not only food but food for thought—namely the social contacts and involvements so important for the elderly. It is important that social workers be aware of all such facilities so that clients can be guided to assistance. Contacting these services prior to discharging elderly patients home from hospitals is often crucial, since the assistance they provide may be the factor that ensures the viability of the home discharge.

Clinical examination

Clinical examination may reveal findings that can be related to specific or isolated nutritional deficiencies. When malnutrition is clinically apparent, it is more likely to be associated with a malignancy or one of the chronic debilitating illnesses common to the elderly, rather than with any primary nutritional deficiency in the diet. Subclinical malnutrition is probably frequent but is not readily detectable; its presence becomes evident as a lack of reserve when illness rapidly exhausts depleted nutritional stores.

Weight and height

Weight and height are easily recorded and when compared with those of normal persons, with allowances made for age and sex, give an indirect assessment of the patient's nutritional status.

Skin

Simple palpation of the thickness of muscle and subcutaneous fat may help in the assessment of nutritional status. When gross wasting is present, this will be obvious on inspection.

Skin lesions from vitamin deficiencies occur occasionally. In the elderly, ecchymoses are invariably of the senile type and unrelated to vitamin C deficiency. The only exception is the characteristic "sheet" hemorrhages seen along the thighs and calves in the bedridden patient deficient in vitamin C. These, as well as pressure sores, will be missed if the patient is not examined in the prone position. Irregular hairs, some corkscrew in shape with broken ends, can be seen in patients with vitamin C deficiency, especially on the trunk. The hair follicles are surrounded by small areas of brownish keratosis, which may precede the appearance of classic perifollicular hemorrhages (pink halo). Follicular keratosis, photosensitivity with eczema, drying, thickening, and pigment change occur with the presence of multiple vitamin deficiencies, although these signs are nonspecific for this condition. Skin atrophy tends to accompany aging and is more marked with malnutrition. "Transparent skin" associated with collagen diseases, such as rheumatoid arthritis, is also found in chronic lung disease and osteoporosis. Its association with nutrition is unclear. Follicular hyperkeratosis also occurs with Vitamin A deficiency, producing a dry, rough toadlike skin. A patchy pigmentation of a dirty brown hue may be present with semistarvation. It localizes maximally to the malar eminences.

Mouth

Crusting and cracking of lip epithelium (cheilosis) and angular stomatitis can be caused by riboflavin, iron, or pyridoxine deficiency and will usually then be bilateral. Local causes, such as lack of teeth, ill-fitting dentures, or saliva leakage in stroke or parkinsonian patients are much more frequent causes of cheilosis and tend to be unilateral. Herpes stomatitis may be associated with either severe illness or poor nutrition. Aphthous ulcers are usually idiopathic but may result from folic acid deficiency. Gingival hemorrhages are normally secondary to local trauma but may be due to vitamin C deficiency. Scurvy can present with characteristic marginal bleeding, hemorrhagic interdentate papillae, and occasional putrefaction of the gums. These features are dependent on the presence of teeth and are less often found in the vitamin C – de-

ficient elderly, since more than 50% of the elderly population are edentulous. A picture similar to that of scurvy occurs with periodontal disease in the aged and is a result of poor dental hygiene. Periodontal disease is relatively frequent and results in loss of teeth.

Tongue

Atrophy of filliform papillae and hypertrophy of fungiform papillae with erythema, pain, loss of taste, and fissuring may result from a deficiency in iron, zinc, folic acid, vitamin B_{12}, pyridoxine, niacin, or riboflavin, either alone or more commonly in combination. Acute glossitis may result, but chronic glossitis with a small, painless atrophic (but not fibrillating, as in bulbar palsy) tongue is found more commonly from long-standing deficiencies in these vitamins and minerals. A "magenta" tongue may result from riboflavin deficiency.

Eyes

Loss of visual acuity in dim light (night blindness) is an early sign of vitamin A deficiency. Xerophthalmia or keratinization of the conjunctiva and cornea leads to dryness and ulceration of the cornea, and ultimately to blindness. This condition is also associated with vitamin A deficiency and is one of the major causes of blindness in countries with malnutrition. Blepharitis may sometimes be associated with a B vitamin deficiency.

Hair

The rapidly proliferating cells of scalp hair roots are sensitive to protein deprivation, frequently before there are alterations in laboratory serum levels. With protein deficiency, characteristic changes occur in the hair root, including reduced diameter, atrophy, loss of hair sheath, and fracturing, as seen under low magnification. The ease with which hair can be pulled out is also increased.

Fingernails

Koilonychia (spooning of the nails) can occur with iron deficiency, but this is also an inherited trait. Leukonychia, a pearly opacity of the nail or a transverse white band across the nail, results from protein deficiency. It can be found in disease states that cause hypoproteinemia, such as cirrhosis and nephrosis.

Cardiovascular system

Vitamin B_{12} or folate deficiency may present as congestive heart failure secondary to anemia. Thiamine deficiency is associated with progressive edema, right-sided heart failure, and cardiomegaly (beriberi). Atherosclerosis is multifactorial in etiology, but nutrition appears to play a major role through saturated fat, cholesterol, and lipoprotein levels.

Nervous system

Thiamine deficiency may cause a bilateral ascending peripheral neuritis that affects sensation initially in the lower extremities with late involvement of the hands.

Vitamin B_{12} deficiency may present a complicated picture with pyramidal and posterior column signs in addition to those of peripheral neuritis. Progressive loss of vibration sense up to the lower lumbar area with stocking-type paresthesia can be found in combination with hyperactive lower-limb reflexes, spastic ataxic gait, and the incontinence of a cord bladder. Combined upper and lower motor neuron lesions can present the unusual picture of absent knee jerks with extensor plantar responses. Mental symptoms also occur; and the elderly, who

have the highest incidence of pernicious anemia, can present with confusion or dementia of unknown origin. Elderly patients, several years after gastrectomy, may be seen by psychiatrists or internists and labeled as having senile dementia of the Alzheimer type (SDAT) when, in fact, they have a reversible condition secondary to B_{12} deficiency.

Magnesium deficiency may be caused by diuretic therapy, alcoholism, chronic renal disease, inappropriate intravenous hyperalimentation, or severe malnutrition. It can produce a syndrome identical to hypocalcemic tetany with neuromuscular irritability, tremor, carpopedal spasms, choreoathetoid movements, hypersensitivity to external stimuli, and delirium progressing to convulsions and coma.

Endocrine glands

Parotid enlargement has been noted fairly frequently in malnourished patients. The cause is not known.

Hyperthyroidism resulting in overactivity of the thyroid gland may cause weight loss with or without a change in appetite. Primary hypothyroidism may also affect nutritional status. It can, for example, be associated with an increase in the serum cholesterol level, whereas secondary hypothyroidism, caused by pituitary insufficiency, is not associated with such an increase. The anemia associated with hypothyroidism is probably not nutritional in origin but directly related to the lack of thyroid hormone.

Adrenal gland dysfunction presenting as hyperfunction (Cushing's syndrome) is rare in the elderly, as is hypofunction (Addison's disease). The symptoms and signs of this latter condition are similar to those in the young, but the findings of mental confusion, weakness, increased pigmentation, hypotension, intestinal upset, and loss of body hair are almost invariably due to causes other than adrenal insufficiency. The electrolyte pattern found in this condition includes hyponatremia, hypochloremia, and hyperkalemia and can be mimicked by excessive diuretic therapy combined with high potassium supplementation. Hypophysial-adrenal dysfunction can occur in patients when long-term steroid therapy is discontinued. Patients with this problem of secondary adrenal insufficiency are characteristically not pigmented.

Panhypopituitarism, a syndrome associated with weight loss and a picture resembling malnutrition, frequently presents for the first time in late life.

Hyperparathyroidism is not uncommon in late life. The resultant hypercalcemia causes gastrointestinal upsets, which, with anorexia, nausea, vomiting, and constipation, can lead to features of malnutrition.

Hypoparathyroidism may be associated with diarrhea; and if hypocalcemia is severe, undue muscular irritability and tetany may develop. Nail changes related to an increased incidence of monilial infections sometimes accompany one of the hypoparathyroid syndromes.

Ovarian dysfunction and hormonal changes may be linked to the rapid increase in the severity of osteoporosis that occurs postmenopausally. Although serum calcium concentration remains "normal", there appears to be diminished calcium absorption from the bowel with advancing age.

Skeleton

Osteoporosis and osteomalacia are both related closely to intestinal absorption, metabolic balance, and nutritional status. Whereas osteomalacia is related specifically to vitamin D deficiency, osteoporosis is multifactorial in etiology and is associated with deficiencies in protein, calcium, vitamin C, vitamin D, and vitamin K. Osteoporosis almost exclusively affects the axial skeleton and classically presents with isolated vertebral collapses that are wedge shaped. In osteomalacia, there is uniform involvement of the entire skeleton, so that deformities are often evenly distributed. In this latter condition, the vertebral changes produce a "codfish spine" (caused by intervertebral discs indenting the diffusely softened vertebrae). With progressive vertebral collapse, a transverse fold of skin develops across the upper abdomen and apposition of the ribs to the pelvic brim occurs. This can be demonstrated clinically by the inability to interpose an examining finger between the lowest ribs and the superior iliac crests.

Osteomalacia can cause bone tenderness and be accompanied by myopathy. If these are combined with the development of skeletal deformities in the pelvis and vertebrae, a characteristic "waddling" gait results.

Laboratory tests

Special techniques required to accurately measure fats, proteins, minerals, and vitamins are not available at most laboratories. This limits the physician's ability to evaluate these biochemical indicators of nutritional status. Healthy, well-nourished elderly individuals have hemoglobin and hematocrit values in the same range as other healthy adults. Thus, hematocrit values of less than 40% for elderly men and less than 36% for elderly women should be regarded as abnormal and be investigated.[31]

Serum albumin concentration appears

to decrease with advancing age. Hospitalized patients who have no apparent albumin-depleting diseases are found to have a progressive drop in serum albumin concentration with age, from 4.0 g/dl for those less than 40 years of age to 3.58 g/dl for those aged 80. Healthy community-residing elderly people have similar decreases in serum albumin concentration.[32]

Although it is controversial, there appears to be a gradual increase in the cholesterol level after age 20. This increase occurs earlier in men and plateaus at age 50. Women have no plateau, and their cholesterol levels are higher than those of men after age 60.[33]

Laboratory evidence of a specific vitamin or mineral deficiency in blood, serum, or urine can be interpreted as significant only when combined with the patient's medical and nutritional history and with the findings on clinical examination.

AGE-RELATED PHYSIOLOGICAL AND CLINICAL CHANGES INFLUENCING NUTRITION [34, 35]

The sense of smell, so important in food appreciation, is reduced with advancing age; one study demonstrated that 81-year-old nonsmokers had a threshold 11 times that of young (22-year-old) subjects.[36]

Taste also decreases with age, the number of taste buds per papilla being progressively reduced. Sweet and salty tastes are lost first, and food therefore tends to taste sour and bitter. Compensation is by an increased intake of sugar and salt, which can cause obesity, hypertension, or congestive heart failure.[36, 37]

The production of saliva is decreased with age (partly in relation to the loss in smell and taste), making swallowing difficult and tending to limit food choice.[37, 38]

Fifty percent of Americans have lost all of their teeth by age 65, 66% by age 75. Ill-fitting dentures are very common in the elderly and can result in oral pressure sores or cause altered facial structure with risk of temporomandibular joint dysfunction. Such dentures are either not used, discarded, or replaced at high cost (not paid for by Medicare). Dentures may force patients to avoid sticky foods and to rely on soft foods, generally carbohydrates with low nutritive value.[37]

Some authors report that tertiary contractions of the esophagus, which are nonperistaltic and may be painful, increase in frequency with advancing age. The lower esophageal sphincter relaxes less frequently on swallowing, and there is a significant delay in esophageal emptying in the elderly. These changes result in characteristic barium swallow findings of what is sometimes termed a "corkscrew" esophagus. These dysfunctions have led to the concept of presbyesophagus.[39] Recent reports claim that the motor change in the esophagus may be more related to disease processes than aging.[40]

The incidence of esophageal disorders such as hiatus hernia (present in 60% of those over 60 years of age, but generally asymptomatic), achalasia, diffuse spasm, diverticula, and cancer all increase with advancing age.

Elderly patients should be encouraged to eat only when sitting, since gravity can then act and assist with swallowing. This reduces the chances of aspiration, the incidence of which is high in the aged.

Atrophic gastritis increases with age. There appear to be two types: A and B.

Type A is associated with a positive parietal cell antibody test and severely reduced gastric secretions, is probably autoimmune, is related to pernicious anemia, and responds to prednisone. Type B is the reverse of type A and tends to have antral involvement, whereas type A does not. Aspirin, alcohol, bile salts and acids, and hypogammaglobulinemia play a role in its etiology.[41]

Studies have maintained that gastric acid secretion is decreased in those over 60 years of age. However, if the acid secretion is correlated with the patient's exchangeable potassium pool (which is proportional to lean body mass and decreases with advancing age) rather than his total body weight, there is no significant age-related change.[41a]

The evidence for malabsorption in late life is equivocal. In 1968 Guth[42] demonstrated failing intestinal absorption of D-xylose, especially in those over 80 years of age. The renal excretion of D-xylose is also reduced in this age group. Therefore, the criteria for interpretation of the D-xylose absorption test in the elderly have to be adjusted to avoid overdiagnosis of malabsorption (i.e., false positive results).

Colonic dysfunction is common in the elderly, with an increasing incidence of cancer, diverticular disease, and functional bowel symptoms. Some 25% of those in the older age group are thought to be constipated (infrequent and difficult passage of excessively dry stool). Causative factors are multiple, including a decrease in motor tone and function of the colon with advancing age; decreased fluid intake; medications such as antihypertensives, diuretics, sedatives, and laxatives; depression; and insufficient bulk in the diet. Chronic constipation itself is associated with the further dysfunctions of irritable colon and megacolon with spurious fecal incontinence (senile megacolon).[43] Laxative abuse is the major cause of diarrhea in the elderly and may result in weight loss or electrolyte imbalance. Ninety percent of cases of laxative abuse occur in women.[44]

Gallstones are common in the elderly, with an incidence estimated at 10% for men and 20% for women in the 55- to 65-year-old age group. A 1959 study found an autopsy incidence of 38% for those aged 70 to 80.[45]

Awareness of decreased hydration appears reduced with age, possibly because of an insensitivity of the hypothalamic thirst center.[46] The aged kidney is unable to adequately concentrate urine in the face of dehydration. Both of these factors can combine to produce the problems of dehydration so commonly found in ill elderly patients. Water intake may also be restricted voluntarily in an effort to cope with urinary incontinence.

CHANGE IN CALORIC REQUIREMENTS
Age-related metabolic change

There is a rapid decline in the basal metabolic rate (BMR) from infancy to age 20, followed by an apparent gradual decline to age 75.[47] There is controversy as to whether this latter slow decline in BMR reflects a real decrease in metabolic activity or a decline in cell mass. Cellular mass and body musculature show a slow decline after age 50, muscle being partially replaced by fat and connective tissue.[48] This decline in cellular mass is reflected in a 15% to 20% decrease in exchangeable potassium per kilogram from age 20 to 75. The ratio of BMR to potassium pool is constant as age increases (i.e., energy requirements appear proportional to lean body mass at all ages). Thus, the BMR does not decrease if it is considered in relation to lean body mass.

Change in physical activity with advancing age

Activity is a function of a person's behavior pattern, occupation, attitudes and interests, infirmity, or illness. Retirement, at whatever age, plays a significant role. A small percentage of adults have significant physical exercise in their occupations and have no apparent difficulty in maintaining this level of activity until they retire. Energy expenditure has progressively decreased in modern society, however, and generally, once a person reaches age 30, he expends little energy either at work or during leisure. Aging does not cause a significant further reduction in this already low level of energy expenditure unless there are associated additional factors, such as cardiovascular or pulmonary illnesses, degenerative arthropathies, or stroke. In patients with stroke or amputation, significantly increased energy expenditure occurs when mobilization is attempted.

Moderately strenuous exercise requires significantly more energy output for the elderly, because the decreased neuromuscular coordination that occurs with age results in energy waste. This potential for greater energy requirement is balanced in the elderly by a reduction in extraneous movements[49] and less indulgence in exercise.

Overall, there is a mild reduction in physical activity from age 20 to the time of retirement, when there is a further drop of varying degree. When this decrease in energy requirement is coupled with the decrease in lean body mass and

BMR, it is clear that caloric requirements decrease with age.

FINANCIAL STATUS AND DIET[23, 26]

Approximately 15% to 40% of the elderly population are at, near, or below the poverty level (i.e., the amount of income necessary to meet essential needs). The percentage varies with age, sex, and marital status. Some 25% of those over 65 years of age have been estimated to have less income than was deemed necessary to maintain an acceptable standard of living (i.e., one with a degree of comfort that might be termed modest but adequate).[50] That fraction of income spent on food, approximately one third normally, is obviously insufficient if money is scarce. Diet suffers because fresh vegetables, milk, meat, and eggs cannot be purchased. From a purely economic point of view, it is generally less costly to supplement deficient diets with multivitamins and minerals than to purchase food items that would correct the dietary deficiencies.

DIET, DISEASE, AND AGING
Osteoporosis

Osteoporosis is a disease primarily of postmenopausal or perimenopausal women that progresses with advancing age. It is uncommon in American blacks. It is causally implicated in a staggering 6 million fractures of the hip, vertebrae, and long bones each year, 5 million of which occur in women. (The medical costs are estimated at 1 to 2 billion dollars annually.) The disease is multifactorial in etiology, with hormonal factors playing a significant role. With advancing age, additional factors include a reduction in physical activity, a progressively increasing calcium deficiency in the diet, a progressive decrease in absorbed calcium, and the vitamin deficiencies referred to earlier. Current concepts in therapy and prevention are to provide more calcium and vitamin D in the diet and to increase exposure to real or articifial sunlight (infrared light). This will increase the levels of 25-hydroxy vitamin D, which are low in those who sustain fractures.[51] Fluoride therapy does cause an increase in bone density radiologically, but tensile strength of bone is not significantly altered. Therapy with calcium alone decreases the rate of bone loss, but to a lesser extent than does hormonal therapy with estrogen. Dietary phosphorus should be low (patients should avoid "junk" foods and soft drinks), since recent studies suggest that an excess of phosphorus may be the single most important cause of bone loss in humans.[52, 53]

Constipation

Constipation is caused in large part by excessive water absorption from feces in the large bowel. This is a direct result of the lack of dietary fiber presented to the colon. Diseases related to constipation, such as diverticular disease of the colon and hemorrhoids, are almost exclusive to developed countries and probably reflect an increased use of refined cereal fiber. These conditions may be appropriately avoided with a reintroduction of high-fiber diets.[54] An accepted approach is to provide 6 to 10 g of dietary fiber (e.g., millers' bran, fiber-rich breakfast cereals, and legumes such as peas and beans) daily in the diet. Lactulose can also be used. In patients started on high-fiber diets, there is an improvement in oral glucose tolerance curves and the treatment of adult-onset diabetes mellitus may be simplified. However, close attention should be paid to drug levels, such as those of digoxin, since with changed transit times their absorption may be changed.

Hypertension and atherosclerosis

A definition of hypertension in the elderly is difficult, and there is some controversy as to treatment (see Chapter 11). Diet plays little, if any, part in its cause, with the exception of salt, which can elevate blood pressure in genetically susceptible persons. Increased excretion of salt with diuretics or reduction of its dietary intake are therapeutic approaches. It is not known whether dietary control of weight will lower blood pressure in elderly hypertensive patients, as it has been shown to do for young and middle-age persons. It has been suggested that avoidance of saturated fat in the diet and a reduction in cholesterol consumption may reduce dietary atherogenic factors. This has not been clearly demonstrated to be of benefit for the young or middle aged, and certainly not for the aged. Thus, from the viewpoint of atherosclerosis, there is little justification to prescribe a low-fat diet for the elderly individual.

Obesity

Obesity is the most frequent malnutritive state of the elderly and is associated with diabetes mellitus (adult onset), arthritis, gout, hypertension, and heart disease, as well as with hernias and an increased incidence of accidents. Since energy requirements decrease with advancing age, maintenance of a diet similar to that in middle age will result in weight gain. A figure of 15% to 20% above the standard weight for age and sex is probably cause for concern, while mild obesity may be associated with longer than normal life expectancy.[55] The prevalence of weights 20% above standard for persons aged 60 to 69 is 29% for men and

45% for women. After age 70 the incidence of obesity drops progressively.

Studies have shown that women who are 30% to 80% overweight consume only 1,790 kcal per day. For these women, a decrease in intake of 500 kcal per day should result in a loss of 1 pound of body weight per week, but compliance with a diet of less than 1,200 kcal per day is difficult. Thus, weight loss will be slow.

The physical and social hazards of extreme obesity should be explained. A simple yet detailed explanation of the diet program must be given, and the goal-setting process must be understood. It should be recognized that there are no specific data on the success of weight reduction programs in the elderly.

A surprising corollary to obesity is that thinness in men over the age of 70 is correlated with increased mortality. The mechanism for this intriguing finding is unclear.

Diabetes mellitus

Aging, itself, is accompanied by a decline in glucose tolerance. This decline is such that the diagnostic standards for diabetes in the young, if applied to the elderly, would classify an excessively high proportion of elderly patients as diabetic. To overcome this problem, a nomogram has been constructed to place an older individual on a scale with others of his age and sex.[56, 57] Adult-onset diabetes occurs most frequently in the overweight elderly and can often be controlled by diet alone. The fat content of the diet should be restricted to 35% or less of the total calories and the carbohydrate content increased to 40% to 50%, with protein supplying the remainder of the calories. The total caloric intake is adjusted to the RDA for height,

weight, and sex. Adherence to a fixed eating schedule should be encouraged, and the patient should be instructed on the need to avoid excesses both of calories and exercise. The patient's blood and urine glucose levels should be monitored regularly to maintain a reasonable blood glucose level. The elderly adult-onset diabetic is usually not ketosis prone; thus, the need for insulin therapy and tight control of the blood glucose level is less than that in juvenile diabetics. Insulin is much more difficult for certain elderly patients to self-administer because of such problems as decreased visual acuity, arthritis, tremor, decreased manual dexterity, and occasionally mild confusion or forgetfulness. The potential for dosage error is higher, with the accompanying risk of hypoglycemia. Therefore, one should try to avoid excessive manipulation in dosage regimens, since these may confuse patients and result in their making errors. Such medication-induced hypoglycemic episodes can have grave consequences for the elderly patient (such as cardiac or cerebral catastrophes). Mild hyperglycemia is much more acceptable than the risks of tight control in the elderly diabetic. One should always fully evaluate the response to diet, exercise, and oral hypoglycemic agents prior to starting a patient on a regimen of insulin. In the elderly, there is as yet no convincing evidence of cardiovascular dangers of oral hypoglycemic therapy.

Gastric ulcer

Thirteen percent of all gastric ulcer patients are over the age of 65. A new ulcer after age 60 is unusual; should it occur, however, the risks of severe hemorrhage and perforation are high. Mortality in this age group is high, because cardiac, renal, and especially pulmonary reserves are low. Management includes antacids, cimetidine, and mild sedation. Cimetidine, a type two histamine receptor antagonist, which reduces acid secretion, and mild sedation should be used with great caution in the elderly, because confusion may develop.[58a] Dietary approaches are to use nutritive high-protein meals. The old approach of adhering to a bland ulcer diet is probably of little benefit.

Anemia

There is no anemia of old age, and hemoglobin values below 13 g/dl for men and 12 g/dl for women should be investigated.

The serum iron and total iron-binding capacity (TIBC) levels both normally decrease in late life, thus altering the criteria for the diagnosis of iron deficiency.[59] Iron-deficiency anemia is generally related to overt or occult gastrointestinal blood loss. It is also the most common nutritional anemia. Dietary supplements including iron compounds should correct nutritional defects unless there is a continuaton of blood loss.

Vitamin B_{12} deficiency as a feature of pernicious anemia is relatively common as a cause of megaloblastic anemia. Low serum folate levels are common in the elderly but are infrequently associated with anemia. Both of these conditions may be partly masked by an associated iron deficiency.[60]

Dementia

Senile dementia of the Alzheimer type (SDAT) is a common problem encountered in the elderly. In addition to characteristic histological changes of senile plaques, neurofibrillary tangles, and gran-

ulovacuolar degeneration, there appears to be a depletion of choline acetyltransferase (the enzyme that synthesizes the neurotransmitter acetylcholine). Administration of choline, the precursor of acetylcholine, in the diet raises the level of brain acetylcholine in the rat.[61] Lecithin, a natural source of choline, is more effective than an equivalent quantity of choline chloride in increasing human blood choline levels.[62] Trials with this nutrient and with tyrosine and tryptophan, which might influence the synthesis of the brain neurotransmitters dopamine, norepinephrine, and serotonin, are currently under study in animals and humans. The results to date are equivocal, but these nutritional approaches to treatment and/or prevention of dementia may hold great promise.[63, 64]

Drug-diet interactions

The following are examples of the relationship between nutrition and drug interactions of particular relevance in the elderly[65]:

1. *Digoxin:* Associated with low potassium intake
2. *Diuretics:* Associated with potassium and magnesium deficiency secondary to increased excretion and partly caused by decreased intake due to anorexia
3. *Potassium chloride:* Used as a potassium supplement in conjunction with diuretic therapy; can decrease vitamin B_{12} by reducing pH in the ileum
4. *Aluminum-containing antacids:* Reduce absorption of phosphorus and fluoride from the bowel and increase the excretion of calcium in feces and urine
5. *Mineral oil:* Decreases absorption

of carotene, vitamin A, vitamin D, and vitamin K; stimulates the excretion of the fat-soluble vitamins

6. *Antituberculous drugs:* Para-aminosalicylic acid (PAS) — causes B_{12} malabsorption; isoniazid — associated with a vitamin B_6 – responsive peripheral neuropathy; cycloserine — also appears to be associated with vitamin B_6 deficiency

7. *Antibiotics:* May decrease the utilization of potassium, magnesium, and calcium by the body

8. *Neomycin:* Reduces intestinal absorption and decreases pancreatic lipase (a digestive enzyme) and the binding capacity of bile salts

9. *Aspirin:* May reduce serum folate concentration, blocks vitamin C uptake by platelets, and depletes tissue levels of that vitamin

10. *Sulfasalazine:* An anti-inflammatory agent used in colitis; can decrease folate absorption from the bowel by inducing a mucosal block

11. *Steroids:* Decrease serum calcium absorption; accelerate protein metabolism

12. *Oral hypoglycemics:* Decrease vitamin B_{12} absorption by competitive inhibition

13. *Anticonvulsants:* Phenytoin, phenobarbital — can produce folate and vitamin D deficiencies

14. L-*Dopa:* May cause vitamin B_6 deficiency

15. *Cholestyramine:* Potential for deficiencies in all fat-soluble vitamins (including A, D, and K) as well as in B_{12}, iron, and fat (because of reduced bile salt binding)

16. *Hydralazine:* May cause vitamin B_6 deficiency

17. *Mineral supplements:* May interfere with tetracycline absorption, forming insoluble complexes

18. *Chemotherapy:* Can produce multiple absorption problems and deficiencies

HYPERALIMENTATION

The acutely ill elderly patient with multiple and debilitating illnesses may require intensive nutritional support.[66]

Central venous hyperalimentation is frequently difficult in such a patient, who is often confused and uncooperative. The well-known complications of this technique are pneumothorax, arterial puncture, catheter embolus, and sepsis. On the other hand, small-bore polyethylene nasogastric catheters are well tolerated.[67] They do not lead to rhinitis, pharyngitis, esophageal stricture, depressed cough reflex, increased pulmonary secretions, or pulmonary atelectasis, and only very rarely lead to reflux.

The thin polyethylene tube can be attached to a regular Levin tube with a gelatin capsule and then passed; the gelatin capsule will dissolve in the stomach and allow withdrawal of the Levin tube while the thin catheter remains in the stomach. An even more appropriate technique is to use an enteric feeding tube composed of a thin polyethylene catheter with a heat-sealed mercury bulb on its end. This weight allows spontaneous passage of the tube through the pylorus into the distal duodenum, and its position can be checked by air insufflation or x-ray examination. Such a tube can remain in situ for up to 6 weeks.

The feeding solution is infused via a conventional intravenous administration set (clearly marked). Feeding is well tolerated if the osmotic load is gradually increased from 50 ml/hour to the required level by 25 ml/hour each day. A typical starting feeding solution would be a one-third–strength solution of one of the commercially available feeding supplements. The patient should be tube fed while sitting to avoid aspiration.

SUMMARY[68-71]

The isolated effect of age on nutrition has not been completely clarified.

Caloric requirements decrease with advancing age.

There is no clearly determined change in the pattern of nutrient need with advancing age. RDAs have been established for those 55 years of age and over, with recent specific recommendation only for total calories for those over 75 years of age. Future studies will determine the accuracy of these extensive extrapolations.

Current gross clinical and laboratory evidence indicates that malnutrition is uncommon among the elderly. Isolated deficiencies may be found on laboratory testing, but their relevance is unclear.

Nutritional deficiencies defined as inadequate RDAs are not generally associated with recognizable clinical features.

Deficiencies may manifest themselves as subclinical malnutrition. They become evident when illness rapidly exhausts depleted stores and may present in a subtle fashion, such as an altered mental status.

The malnourished are likely to be among those who are at the poverty level, are chronically ill, live alone, and are over 75 years of age.

The problem segments of the community are known. State, federal, and voluntary organizations must work to provide answers in the form of education, out-reach programs, facilities for provision of free food or meals, day centers to provide companionship, financial assistance, and appropriate medical intervention if prevention is unsuccessful.

REFERENCES

1. Libow, L. S.: Interaction of medical, biologic, and behavioral factors on aging, adaptation, and survival—an eleven-year longitudinal study, Geriatrics **29:**75, 1974.
2. Lytle, L. D., and Altar, A.: Diet, central nervous system, and aging, Fed. Proc. **38:**2017, 1979.
3. McCay, C. M., Crowell, M. F., and Maynard, L. A.: The effect of retarded growth upon the length of life span and upon the' ultimate body size, J. Nutr. **10:**63, 1935.
4. McCay, C. M., Maynard, L. A., Sperling, G., and Barnes, L. L.: Retarded growth, life span, ultimate body size and age changes in the albino rat after feeding diets restricted in calories, J. Nutr. **18:**1, 1939.
5. McCay, C. M., Sperling, G., and Barnes, L. L.: Growth, aging, chronic diseases and life span in rats, Arch. Biochem. Biophys. **2:**469, 1943.
6. Leto, S., Kokkonen, G., and Barrows, C. H.: Dietary proteins, life span and physiological and biochemical variables in female mice, J. Gerontol. **31:**(2):144, 1976.
7. Finch, C. E.: Enzyme activities, gene function, and aging in mammals, Exp. Gerontol. **7:**53, 1972.
8. Barrows, C. H.: Nutrition, aging and genetic programme, 1972, Am. J. Clin. Nutr. **25:**829, 1972.
9. Nolen, G. A.: Effects of various restricted dietary regimes on the growth, health and longevity of albino rats, J. Nutr. **102:**1477, 1972.
10. Ross, M. H., and Bras, G.: The influence of protein and overnutrition on spontaneous tumor prevalence in the rat, J. Nutr. **103:**944, 1973.
11. Berg, B. N., and Simms, H. S.: Nutrition and longevity in the rat. 2. Longevity and onset of disease at different levels of food intake, J. Nutr. **71:**255, 1960.
12. Ross, M. H.: Nutrition and longevity in experimental animals. In Winick, M., editor: Nutrition and aging, New York, 1976, John Wiley and Sons, Inc.

13. Hayflick, L.: The limited in vivo lifetime of human diploid cell strains, Exp. Cell Res. **25:** 585, 1966.

14. Pryor, W. A.: Free radical pathology, Chem. Eng. News **34:**34, 1971.

15. Food and Nutrition Board: Recommended Dietary Allowances, ed. 8., Washington, D.C., 1974, National Academy of Science/National Research Council.

16. O'Hanlon, P., and Kohrs, M. B.: Dietary studies of older Americans, Am. J. Clin. Nutr. **31:**1257, 1978.

17. Consumer and Food Economics Research Division, Agricultural Research Service: Food and nutrient intake of individuals in the United States, Spring, 1965, USDA Household Food Consumption Survey, 1965-66, Dept. No. 11, Washington, D.C., 1972, U.S. Government Printing Office.

18. Ten-State Nutrition Survey, 1968-1970, DHEW, Pub. No. (HSM) 72-8133, Atlanta, 1972, U.S. Department of Health, Education, and Welfare, Center for Disease Control.

19. Preliminary findings of the first Health and Nutrition Examination Survey, U.S., 1971-1972: dietary intake and biochemical findings, DHEW Pub. No. (HRA) 74-1219-1, Washington, D.C., 1974, U.S. Government Printing Office.

20. Nutrition Canada National Survey, 1970-72, Ottawa, 1973, Information Canada. Report by Nutrition Canada to the Department of National Health and Welfare.

21. U.S. Department of Justice: Crime in the nation's five largest cities, Washington, D.C., 1974, U.S. Department of Justice, Law Enforcement Administration.

22. Current operating statistics, Soc. Sec. Bull. (Annual Statistical Suppl.), December 1979.

23. Fact book on aging: a profile of America's older population, Washington, D.C., 1978, National Council on the Aging, Inc.

24. Weale, R. A.: Senile change in visual acuity, Trans. Ophthalmol. Soc. UK **95:**36, 1975.

25. Havighurst, R., Neugarten, B. L., and Tobin, S. S.: Disengagement and patterns of aging. In Neugarten, B. L., editor: Middle age and aging, Chicago, 1968, University of Chicago Press, p. 161.

26. U.S. Department of Commerce, Bureau of the Census: Unpublished data.

27. Vital statistics of the United States, 1970. Vol. 2. Mortality, part A, Rockville, Md., 1974, U.S. Department of Health, Education, and Welfare, Public Health Service.

28. Redick, R. W., Kramer, M., and Taube, C. A.: Epidemiology of mental illness and utilization of psychiatric facilities among older persons. In Busse, E. W., and Pfeiffer, E., editors: Mental illness in later life, Washington, D.C., 1973, American Psychiatric Association.

29. Rabin, D. L.: Use of medicine: a review of prescribed and nonprescribed medicine use, 1972, U.S. Department of Health, Education, and Welfare, Public Health Service.

30. Hurwitz, N., and Wade, O. L.: Intensive hospital monitoring of adverse reactions to drugs, Br. Med. J. **1:**531, 1969.

31. Libow, L. S.: Human aging: a biological and behavioral study, Pub. No. 986, 1963, U.S. Department of Health, Education, and Welfare, Public Health Service.

32. Greenblatt, D. J.: Reduced serum albumin concentration in the elderly: a report from the Boston collaborative drug surveillance programme, J. Am. Geriatr. Soc. **27:**20, 1979.

33. Kritchersky, D.: How aging affects cholesterol metabolism, Postgrad. Med. **63:**133, 1978.

34. Barrows, C. H., and Roeder, L. M.: Nutrition. In Finch, C., and Hayflick, L., editors: The handbook of the biology of aging, New York, 1977, Van Nostrand Reinhold Co., p. 561.

35. Bhanthumnavin, K., and Schuster, M. M.: Aging and gastrointestinal function. In Finch, C., and Hayflick, L., editors: The handbook of the biology of aging, New York, 1977, Van Nostrand Reinhold Co., p. 709.

36. Busse, E. W.: How mind, body and environment influence nutrition in the elderly, Postgrad Med. **63:**118, 1978.

37. Schiffman, S. S.: Food recognition by the elderly, J. Gerontol. **5:**586, 1977.

38. Meyer, J., and Nechels, H.: Studies in old age. 4. The clinical significance of salivary, gastric and pancreatic secretion in the aged, J.A.M.A. **115:**2050, 1969.

39. Zboralske, F. F., Amberg, J. R., and Soergel, K. H.: Presbyesophagus: cineradiographic manifestations, Radiology **82:**463, 1964.

40. Mandelstam, P., Siegel, C. I., Lieber, A., and Siegel, W.: The swallowing disorder in patients with diabetic neuropathy-gastroenteropathy, Gastroenterology **56:**1-12, 1969.

41. Strickland, R. G., and Mackay, I. R.: Progress report: a reappraisal of the nature and significance of chronic gastritis, Am. J. Digest. Dis. **18:**426, 1973.

41a. Bernier, J. J., Vidon, H., and Mignon, M.: The value of a cooperative multicenter study for establishing a table of normal values for gastric acid secretion and as a function of sex, age, and weight, Biol. Gastroenterol. **6**:287, 1973.

42. Guth, P. H.: Physiologic alteration in small bowel function with age: the absorption of D-xylose, Am. J. Digest. Dis. **13**:565, 1968.

43. Todd, I. P.: Some aspects of adult megacolon, Proc. R. Soc. Med. **64**:561, 1971.

44. Cummings, J. H.: Progress report: laxative abuse, Gut **15**:758, 1974.

45. Newman, H. F., and Northrup, J. D.: The autopsy incidence of gallstones, Int. Surg. **109**:1, 1959.

46. Shapiro, W. B., Porush, J. G., and Kahn, A. J.: Application of fluid and electrolyte balance principles to the older patient. In Reichel, W., editor: Clinical aspects of aging, Baltimore, 1978, The Williams & Wilkins Co. p. 213.

47. Shock, N. W., Watkins, D. M., Yiengst, M. J., and others: Age differences in water content of the body as related to basal oxygen consumption in males, J. Gerontol. **18**:1, 1963.

48. Andrew, W., Shock, N. W., Barrows, C. H., and Yiengst, M. J.: Correlation of age changes in histological and chemical characteristics in some tissues of the rat, J. Gerontol. **14**:405, 1959.

49. Durnin, J. V. G. A., and Mikulick, V.: The influence of graded exercises on the oxygen consumption, pulmonary ventilation, and heart rate of young and elderly men, Q. J. Exp. Physiol. **41**:442, 1956.

50. U.S. Department of Labor, Bureau of Labor Statistics: Unpublished data.

51. Baker, M. R., McDonnell, H., Peacock, M., and Nordin, B. E. C.: Plasma 25-hydroxy vitamin D concentrations in patients with fractures of the femoral neck, Br. Med. J. **1**(6163): 589, 1979.

52. Jowsey, J.: Why is mineral nutrition important in osteoporosis? Geriatrics **33**:(8):41, 1978.

53. Jowsey, J., Reiss, E., and Canterbury, J. M.: Long term effects of high phosphate intake on parathyroid hormone levels and bone metabolism, Acta. Orthop. Scand. **45**:801, 1974.

54. Burkitt, D. P., and Trowell, H. C., editors: Refined carbohydrate foods and disease, London, Academic Press Inc. Ltd., 1975.

55. Butler, R. N.: Diet related to killer diseases. 7. Nutrition: aging and the elderly, p. 30. Hearing before the Select Committee on Nutrition and Human Needs of the United States Senate, September 23, 1977.

56. Andres, R.: Aging, disease, standards of normality: diabetes mellitus as a prototype, vol. 1,

1966. Proceedings of the Seventh International Congress of Gerontology, Vienna.

57. Andres, R.: Aging and diabetes, Med. Clin. North Am. **55**:835, 1971.

58. Schentag, J. J., Cerra, F. B., Calleri, G., and others: Pharmacokinetics and clinical studies in patients with cimetidine-associated mental confusion, Lancet **1**:177, 1979.

58a. Basavaraju, Y. B., Wolf-Klein, G., Silverstone, F. A., and Libow, L. S.: Cimetidine-induced mental confusion in elderly, N.Y. State J. Med. **80**:1287, 1980.

59. Thomas, J. H.: Values of serum iron in patients over sixty, Gerontol. Clin. **13**:52, 1971.

60. MacLennan, W. J., Andrews, G. R., Macleod, C., and Caird, F. I.: Anemia in the elderly, Q. J. Med. **42**:1, 1973.

61. Cohen, E. L., and Wurtman, R. J.: Brain acetyecholine: control by dietary choline, Science **191**:561, 1976.

62. Wurtman, R. J., Hirsch, M. J., and Growdan, J. H.: Lecithin consumption raises serum-free choline levels, Lancet **2**:68, 1977.

63. Mohs, R. C., Davis, K. L., Tinklenberg, J. R., and others: choline treatment of memory defects in the elderly, Am. J. Psychiatry **136**(10): 1275, 1979.

64. Sitaram, N., Weingartner, H., and Gillin, J. C.: Human serial learning: enhancement with arecholine and choline and impairment with scopolamine, Science **201**:274, 1978.

65. Roe, D. A.: In drug-induced nutritional deficiencies, Westport, Conn., 1978, AVI Publishing Co.

66. Ching, N., Grossi, C., Zurawinsky, H., and others: Nutritional deficiencies and nutritional support therapy in geriatric cancer patients, J. Am. Geriatr. Soc. **27**:491, 1979.

67. Bethel, R. A., Jansen, R. D., Heymsfield, S. B., and others: Nasogastric hyperalimentation through a polyethylene catheter: an alternative to central venous hyperalimentation, Am. J. Clin. Nutr. **32**:1112, 1979.

68. Todhunter, E. N., and Darby, W. J.: Guidelines for maintaining adequate nutrition in old age, Geriatrics **33**(6):49, 1978.

69. Rao, D. B.: Problems of nutrition in the aged, 1973, J. Am. Geriatr. Soc. **21**:362, 1973.

70. Watkin, D. M.: Logical basis for action in nutrition and aging; J. Am. Geriatr. Soc. **26**:193, 1978.

71. Rae, J., and Burke, A. L.: Counseling the elderly on nutrition in a community health care system, J. Am. Geriatr. Soc. **26**:130, 1978.

PROBLEM-SOLVING EXERCISES*
Case one

A 79-year-old man, a lifelong health faddist, comes to see you as an outpatient. His weight is at the normal range for his height and age. He would like to lose "a few more pounds" to "live longer."

Questions

1. You advise him to:
   a. Lose no more than a few pounds
   b. Continue his present weight and diet
   c. Take appetite suppressants
   d. Increase his activity immediately and significantly, while not increasing his diet
2. He does not follow your advice and proceeds to lose 10% of his body weight. Which of the following statements is (are) true?
   a. He probably has not increased his life expectancy.
   b. If further weight reduction occurs, he may develop deficiency of substances such as calcium and iron.

Case two

A 75-year-old, slightly obese woman, with diastolic hypertension (160/96 mm Hg) of several months' duration returns for a follow-up visit. Thus far you have not advised treatment.

Questions

1. Which of the following statements is (are) true?
   a. Weight loss in the obese middle age is clearly correlated with blood pressure reduction.
   b. Weight loss in the obese elderly is clearly correlated with blood pressure reduction.
   c. Salt restriction is well tolerated in the elderly.
2. You advise weight reduction and a diet restricted in salt. The patient's pressure,

_____

*Some questions may have more than one correct answer.

1 month later, is 150/80 mm Hg. You would:
   a. Advise the patient to continue her present weight and diet and not add medication
   b. Treat with hydrochlorothiazide plus propranolol

Case three

An 83-year-old woman with known hypertensive cardiovascular disease and CHF treated with digoxin has been in a nursing home for the past year following a left cerebrovascular accident (CVA) and mild right-sided hemiparesis without aphasia or dementia. *She is anorectic and depressed and has lost 15 pounds.* She does not receive antihypertensive medication.

Questions

1. You would:
   a. Withhold digoxin and observe her cardiac status carefully
   b. Evaluate the patient for mental depression
   c. Consider a GI series for possible malignancy
   d. Render supportive psychotherapy
2. You withhold the digoxin; 14 days later, the patient is still anorectic and depressed, and her apical pulse rate has increased from an atrial fibrillation rate of 90/minute to 115/minute. You would:
   a. Obtain a serum T_4
   b. Continue to render supportive psychotherapy
3. The T_4 is $14 \mu g/dl\%$ (normal: $4 \mu g/dl$ to $10 \mu g/dl$). Digoxin has been withheld for 3 weeks, and the patient continues to be depressed and anorectic. You would:
   a. Obtain a T_3 resin uptake
   b. Consider hyperthyroidism as a diagnosis
   c. Start the digoxin again

Case four:

A 75-year-old man comes to see you because he is extremely overweight and anxious. He has a history of peptic ulcer. Routine evaluation is otherwise negative. The results of an oral GTT (glucose tolerance test) are "diabetic."

Questions

1. *You would:*
   a. Tell the patient that he has diabetes mellitus
   b. Suggest weight loss and repeat the oral GTT
2. The patient develops increasing ulcer pain on the weight loss regimen. You treat with cimetidine and an antacid, and his pain recedes. He soon becomes confused. You would:
   a. Consider discontinuing cimetidine
   b. Order a CAT scan of the head.
   c. Make the diagnosis of senile dementia
3. You discontinue cimetidine; the patient's mental state clears and he is doing well. You advise:
   a. A diet free of caffeine and stimulants of acid-peptic secretion.
   b. A standard, antacid regimen without cimetidine

ANSWERS TO PROBLEM-SOLVING EXERCISES
Case one

1. b. There is no evidence that reducing weight to below the normal range, will prolong life for the elderly. To the contrary, there is some surprising data suggesting that in late life a lower weight may be linked to lesser survival.
2. a and b. As stated above, the patient has probably not increased his life expectancy. He may develop calcium and/or iron deficiencies.

Case two

1. a. Weight loss for obese middle-aged, hypertensive persons is linked to a decrease in blood pressure. Theoretically, this weight loss may help in late life. Salt restriction is poorly tolerated by the elderly, who already have subtle taste sensitivity changes.
2. a. The patient has done well with weight

and salt reduction. Do not add medication.

Case three

1. All of these. Digoxin and mental depression are two of the commonest causes of anorexia in the elderly, particularly those in nursing homes. This patient certainly should be encouraged to talk about her depressed feelings. A GI series may be necessary later, as this case evolves.
2. Both of these. Hyperthyroidism in the elderly may present as rapid atrial fibrillation with or without mental depression. Usually, digoxin does not effectively suppress the rapid atrial fibrillation in hyperthyroidism.
3. All of these. The patient appears to be hyperthyroid. However, to rule out thyroid-binding abnormalities as a cause of the elevated T_4 value, a T_3 resin uptake test should be done. Since digoxin has been withheld for 21 days, it is clear that it is not the cause of the anorexia. In the elderly, hyperthyroidism may present with anorexia.

Case four

1. b. The oral GTT results are "diabetic" in more than half of all older persons. It is not presumed that most of these people are truly diabetic. Furthermore, obesity at any age may induce a "diabetic" glucose tolerance curve.
2. a. Cimetidine not infrequently induces confusion and/or dementia in the elderly.
3. Both of these. Continue antiulcer treatment, but exclude cimetidine.

POSTTEST
True or false

1. Mental function is significantly influenced by standard nutrients.
2. Healthy 70-year-old men who are of low-normal weight have a lesser life expectancy than age-matched controls who have more average weights.

3. Animal studies show that, in general, food deprivation in the early stages of life leads to an increased life span.

4. The total number of multiplications of cultured human cells is finite.

5. Antioxidants and certain sulfur compounds prolong animal life and reduce cross linkages.

6. Recommended Dietary Allowances (RDAs) for total calories and for specific nutrients have been described specifically for those over 75 years of age.

7. Cross-sectional studies of age differences are more likely to reveal age-related changes than are longitudinal studies.

8. Diets of the elderly are most likely to be deficient in total caloric intake, calcium, and iron.

9. The elderly person's protein intake is typically deficient.

10. The dietary history is usually obtained in standard medical interviews.

11. Mental depression and digitalis therapy are common causes of anorexia in the elderly.

12. Vitamin C deficiency is the most common cause of ecchymosis in the elderly.

13. Unilateral cheiloses are usually related to vitamin deficiency.

14. A white band across the nails of the hand is often related to protein deficiency.

15. Osteomalacia is related primarily to protein deficiency.

16. Serum albumin concentration normally decreases with advancing age.

17. The senses of taste and smell decrease with advancing age.

18. By age 65, more than half of Americans have lost all their teeth.

19. Hip fractures, secondary to osteoporosis, are quite uncommon among American blacks.

ANSWERS TO PRETEST AND POSTTEST

1. **True.** Mental function is definitely influenced by nutrients (vitamins, amino acids, trace metals, and many others).

2. **True.** There is a surprising correlation of lower weight in late life with lesser survival.

3. **True.** However, food deprivation begun later in the life cycle of animals does not prolong life.

4. **True.** Hayflick's experiments have shown this limit to cell reproduction.

5. **True.** Certain compounds given to animals prolong their life span. One possible mechanism is their effect on reducing cross linkages of collagen.

6. **False.** RDAs have been set for those below 55 years of age. The RDAs for those over 75 years of age are only for total calories.

7. **False.** Longitudinal studies measure change over long periods of time in the same individual and are quite likely to reveal age-related changes.

8. **True.** The few studies of nutrition in the elderly do specify that the main deficiencies are in iron, calcium, and calories.

9. **False.** The protein intake of most elderly persons is adequate.

10. **False.** Medical history taking often fails to focus on the dietary history.

11. **True.** Mental depression and digitalis therapy are common and treatable causes of anorexia.

12. **False.** The majority of purpuric lesions in the elderly have not been linked to vitamin C deficiency; rather, they are related to some unknown age-related skin changes (senile purpura).

13. **False.** Vitamin deficiency typically causes bilateral cheilosis.

14. **True.** There are several causes of a white band across the nails of the hand, and one such cause is protein deficiency.

15. **False.** Osteomalacia is caused by vitamin D deficiency rather than protein deficiency.

16. **True.** The mechanism for the decrease in serum albumin concentration with age appears to be altered hepatic synthesis.

17. **True.** The elderly show a decreased response to certain taste and smell stimuli.

18. **True.** The edentulous condition of so many older Americans is probably preventable.

19. **True.** Both osteoporosis and fractured hip are uncommon among American blacks.

Chapter 14

Oral and dental disorders

SAUL KAMEN and FREDRICK T. SHERMAN

EDUCATIONAL OBJECTIVES

Attitudinal

The student should:
1. Appreciate the role of oral health in the rehabilitative and preventive care of the elderly patient
2. Recognize the role of the dentist in the interdisciplinary team approach to care of the aged

Cognitive

The student should:
1. Understand the physiological and pathological effects of aging on the oral apparatus
2. Recognize the oral manifestations of systemic disorders in the aged patient
3. Be aware of and respond appropriately to common medical and dental problems of the older patient
4. Understand the interactions and effects of pharmacological agents used in the medical and dental management of the elderly

Skill

The student should:
1. Be able to perform an adequate regional examination of the mouth and its adnexa
2. Be able to consult appropriately with the dentist in prescribing medication for pain control and in administering antibiotics for the management of oral infections and endocarditis prophylaxis
3. Know when to refer patients with oral problems to a dentist

PRETEST*

1. Name three drugs commonly used by the elderly that may cause some degree of xerostomia (dry mouth).
2. On the average, how often would you advise your elderly patient to visit a dentist?
   a. Once a year
   b. Once every 6 months
   c. Once every 3 months
   d. Only if necessary
3. List five common oral conditions that result from neglect of oral health care among the elderly.
4. What percentage of people over the age of 65 are totally edentulous?
   a. 50%
   b. 25%
   c. 75%
5. An 83-year-old man is seeing you for his yearly medical checkup. On performing a regional examination of the head and neck, you remove the patient's dentures and see a creamy lesion on the palate. You also notice that the dentures are in a state of disrepair and neglected hygiene. When you wipe the lesion with a gauze

*Some questions may have more than one correct answer.

305

pad, an erythematous base remains. You would:

a. Take a culture, make a preliminary diagnosis of candidiasis, and initiate a nystatin rinse

b. Prepare the patient for a biopsy

c. Take a culture and initiate the following antibiotic therapy: phenoxymethyl penicillin, 250 mg every 6 hours for 5 days

6. Which of the following agents is *least* likely to be prescribed for an agitated patient with organic brain syndrome whose dentist requests advice for mild premedication prior to dental treatment?

a. Chlorpromazine (Thorazine), 25 mg IM

b. Thiothixene (Navane), 10 mg IM

c. Meperidine (Demerol), 100 mg PO, and promethazine (Phenergan) 25 mg PO

d. Chloral hydrate, 1 g PO

7. Mrs. H. is an 85-year-old hypertensive woman who is currently normotensive as the result of a daily thiazide diuretic. Her dentist wants to use a local anesthetic with epinephrine (lidocaine 2%, 1:100,000 epinephrine) during an extraction procedure. This is:

a. Not advisable, because the patient may go into an acute hypertensive crisis

b. Not advisable, because in an anxiety-provoking situation the endogenous release of epinephrine is still less than the exogenous epinephrine in the local anesthetic (lidocaine 2%, 1:100,000 epinephrine)

c. Advisable, because the vasoconstrictive effect of the epinephrine will enhance local anesthesia, causing the patient to be less anxious and reducing the chance of an acute hypertensive crisis

d. Advisable, because in an anxiety-provoking situation, the endogenous release of epinephrine is greater than the exogenous epinephrine in the local anesthetic (lidocaine 2%, 1:100,000 epinephrine)

8. The most common dental problem in the dentulous elderly is:

a. Caries

b. Toothache

c. Chewing problems

d. Periodontal disease

9. Common problems in the elderly with dentures are:

a. Diminished chewing ability

b. Soreness, pain

c. Need for adjustments

d. Decreased vertical dimension

10. Which of the following regimens should an elderly patient with a history of rheumatic heart disease receive before oral surgery?

a. No premedication

b. Penicillin V, 500 mg 30 minutes to 1 hour before treatment, then 250 mg q6hr for 8 doses

c. Penicillin V, 2 g 30 minutes to 1 hour before treatment, then 500 mg q6hr for 8 doses

The goal of the physician in the rehabilitation of the geriatric patient is to restore the patient to his optimal level of functioning. The achievement of this objective requires a comprehensive approach, in which each organ system is an essential part of the whole. The physician who attempts to improve the quality of life of the older patient must consider the fundamental functions of the mouth. Dental disease in the elderly may be a significant detriment when it is added to the multiple medical and psychiatric problems common to these patients. Nutritional deficiencies resulting from inefficient mastication may lead to anemia and contribute to osteoporosis in the frail, elderly patient. Enjoyment of food and speech and a socially acceptable appearance are important to the well-being of any patient. Therefore, the student or physician should have a basic understanding of gerodontics: that branch of dental science concerned with the management and treatment of the geriatric patient.

Despite attempts to enhance awareness of the need for oral health care for the elderly, oral neglect continues to be a major problem. One of the main reasons for this is the lack of financial resources needed to obtain dental care. Medicare has essentially no dental benefits, and private insurance plans usually provide coverage only to age 65. A recent survey on access to care showed that 21% of those over the age of 65 failed to visit a physician in the study year, and 70% of those over the age of 65 did not have a single dental visit.[1] This study refers to dentulous individuals (i.e., those having one or more of their natural teeth). A study of the edentulous population disclosed that of those 65 years of age and over, 92% failed to visit a dentist within the past year. Clearly, there is a large population of elderly people (dentulous and edentulous) who are not receiving adequate dental care.

ORAL HEALTH CARE NEEDS

What are the oral health care needs of the elderly population? Although the proportion of edentulous persons increases with advancing age, it is a common misconception that all older patients are edentulous. To the contrary, increasing numbers of older people are remaining dentulous[2] (Table 14-1).

Approximately 30% of the institution-

Table 14-1. Comparison of the percentage of dentulous elderly people: 1957 and 1971 in the United States

Age	Percentage of dentulous elderly people	
	1957	1971
65 to 74	45	55
75 and up	33	40

alized elderly are dentulous. Of these persons with natural teeth, 90% demonstrate significant periodontal (gingival) disease, loss of alveolar bone, and dental decay.

It has been suggested that older adults accept their facial and oral changes as a normal concomitant of the aging process and demonstrate minor concern for active or preventive dental care.[3] This apparent acceptance tends to diminish their motivation for seeking adequate care. Even when free dental care is offered, many older persons do not take advantage of it. Negative attitudes, confusion as to the costs, lack of transportation, fear of crime, and a distrust of professional personnel may all contribute to dental neglect. The physician and dentist should communicate with their elderly patients; understand and sympathize with their psychological, social, and economic problems; and help them gain access to appropriate dental care.

REGIONAL EXAMINATION

When examining the head and neck, the physician should carefully assess the hard and soft tissues of the mouth. Starting with the face, changes in pigmentation, such as verruca senilis (Fig. 14-1), keratotic and seborrheic dermatoses, and

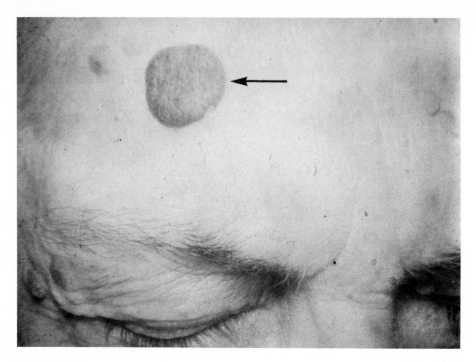

Fig. 14-1. Verruca senilis *(arrow)*, a benign wartlike keratosis that occurs in the elderly.

ecchymoses should be noted. Particular attention should be paid to suspicious lesions of the circumoral tissues, such as basal cell carcinoma (Fig. 14-2).

Of the more than 24,000 cases of oral cancer diagnosed each year, more than 90% occur in persons over the age of 45, the average age being 60. Most of these are of the squamous cell type. The site of occurrence is as follows:

Tongue: 52%
Floor of the mouth: 16%
Alveolar mucosa: 12%
Palate: 11%
Buccal mucosa: 9%

Circumoral tissues

Before examining the mouth, one should ask the patient to remove his den-tures. The surrounding tissues should then be carefully evaluated. After noting the facial integument, one should palpate the lymphatic chain of the neck, beginning with the posterior lymph nodes (Fig. 14-3) and systematically proceeding forward to the submandibular glands (Fig. 14-4) and the anterior nodes superior to the thyroid gland (Fig. 14-5). Suspicious nodes should be further evaluated by gently examining the floor of the mouth, palpating with one finger in the mouth and another under the mandible (Fig. 14-6). The characteristics of any lump or mass should be noted (i.e., whether it is sessile, fluctuant, or indurated). Lymphadenopathy may represent drainage from an infected tooth or the spread of an invasive neoplasm, as in the

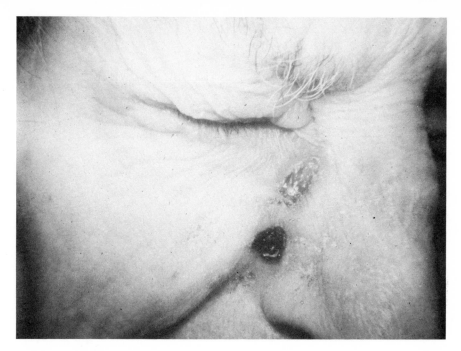

Fig. 14-2. Basal cell carcinoma, an epidermal tumor.

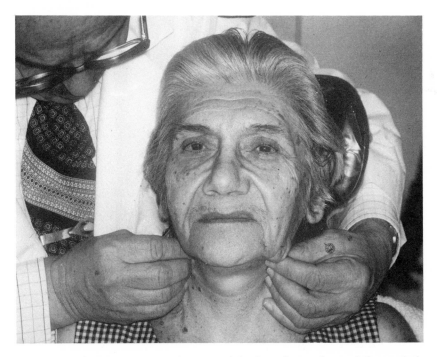

Fig. 14-3. Regional examination: palpation of the lymphatic chain of the neck, beginning with the posterior lymph nodes.

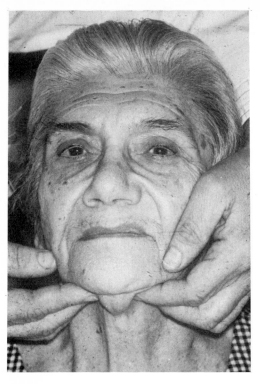

Fig. 14-4. Regional examination: palpation of the submandibular lymph nodes.

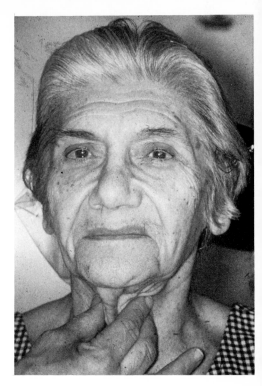

Fig. 14-5. Regional examination: palpation of anterior nodes superior to the thyroid gland.

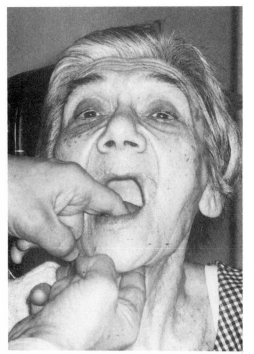

Fig. 14-6. Regional examination: palpation of the floor of the mouth with opposing fingers.

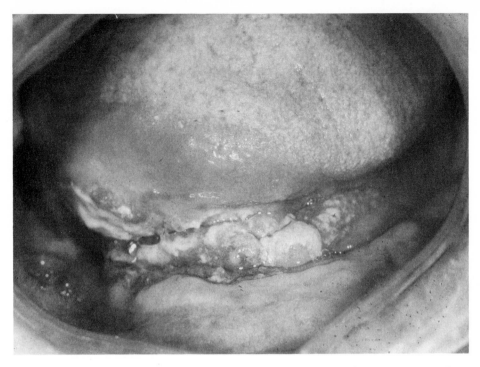

Fig. 14-7. Squamous cell carcinoma at the base of the tongue. (Courtesy Leon Eisenbud, M.D.)

case of the patient in Fig. 14-7, with a squamous cell carcinoma of the floor of the mouth.

Lips

The lips often reveal physiological changes associated with aging, such as thinning of the vermillion border, varicosities, and changes in color. The inner mucosa of the lip may reflect systemic disturbances; for example, a marked reddish appearance of the inner mucosa may be seen in polycythemia. In the debilitated patient, angular cheilitis (inflammation of the angles of the mouth) is frequently observed. A small but significant percentage of neoplasms occur on the lips.

Buccal tissues

The buccal tissues should be inspected for fungal conditions, such as candidiasis, and for other dermatoses, such as lichen planus, which is sometimes seen in the diabetic patient (Fig. 14-8). The alveolar ridges should be carefully examined for denture ulcers, hypertrophied tissue, and other lesions associated with improperly fitting dentures. Patients with these problems should be referred to the dentist for adjustment of the dentures. The floor of the mouth should be examined for inflammatory and erythematous lesions. Suspicious lesions may be neoplastic, and consultation with an oral pathologist should be sought.

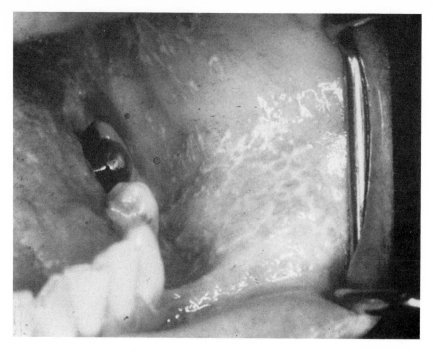

Fig. 14-8. Lichen planus showing circumscribed patches.

Tongue

The tongue should be withdrawn with a 2 × 2 inch gauze sponge and the dorsal (top) and ventral (under) surfaces and the sides carefully examined. Special attention should be paid to the tongue because it is a sensitive indicator of systemic health. The patient should be questioned about distortions in taste (dysgeusia) or loss of taste (ageusia). Alteration in taste may be an early symptom of hypothyroidism or depression. A smooth, painful, pale-appearing tongue may be seen with vitamin B_{12} deficiency, with or without anemia, and may be a source of great discomfort to the older patient. Glossodynia (painful tongue) and glossopyrexia (burning tongue) are baffling phenomena noted particularly in postmenopausal women and are usually found in combination with xerostomia (dryness of the mouth). Other pathological changes of the tongue in the elderly include keratotic, pemphigoid, leukoplakic, and neoplastic lesions. Erythema migrans (geographic tongue) (Fig. 14-9) and varicosities on the ventral surface (Fig. 14-10) are innocuous and considered to be normal age-related changes. Following this examination, the physician should recommend that the tongue be brushed with the toothbrush and cleaned with a tongue scraper during daily oral hygiene. This brushing or cleaning will prevent the accumulation of debris, as well as bacterial and fungal overgrowth.

Xerostomia reflects a generalized, physiological diminution in the number of secretory cells of the salivary glands and mucous membranes of the mouth. It may also be a side effect of drug therapy (e.g., from diuretics or antidepressants).

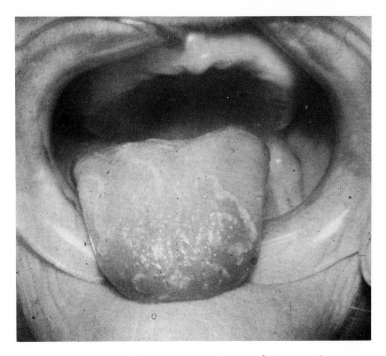

Fig. 14-9. Erythema migrans (geographic tongue).

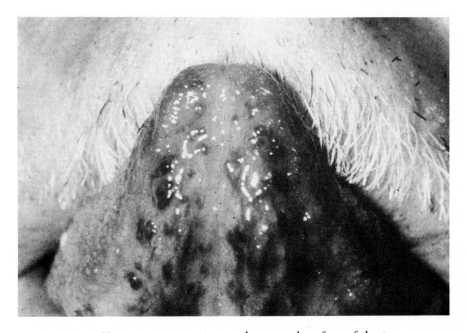

Fig. 14-10. Varicosities occurring on the ventral surface of the tongue.

An evaluation of salivation as "scanty," "moderate," or "within normal limits" should be noted on the medical record following examination of the mouth and tongue.

Palate

The palate and the alveolar ridges of the maxilla and mandible are examined next. Torus palatinus (Fig. 14-11) is a benign bony exostosis in the midline of the hard palate, occurring from the third decade onward, without any particular significance. The mucosa of the hard palate will often reflect the status of the denture in long-term wearers. Stomatitis (inflammation of the mucosa of the hard and soft palate) and papillary hyperplasia (a benign warty elevation) may be caused by ill-fitting dentures, by the refusal of the patient to remove the denture at night, or by poor cleaning of the denture.

The ability to perform an adequate regional examination of the mouth and its adnexa, particularly in the elderly, is an essential aspect of medical care. Too often, patients will not visit their dentist until the dental disease is in an advanced stage. The vigilant physician is in an excellent position to prevent serious consequences of oral neglect by advising and counseling elderly patients to see a dentist at least once every 6 months.

EFFECTS OF AGING ON THE DENTITION

Radiographic studies show that as a person ages, the pulp chambers of the teeth decrease in size. As this process occurs, the teeth become more brittle and dry, increasing the possibility of fracture. Darkening of the teeth also increases

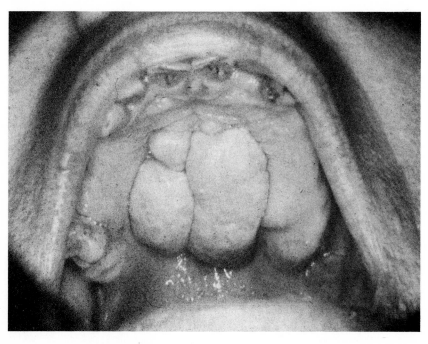

Fig. 14-11. Torus palatinus, multilobulated type.

with age because of extrinsic stains and a decrease in the translucency of the enamel.

Attrition (Fig. 14-12, *A*) is the result of continual wear on the occluding (grinding) surfaces of the teeth. While attrition begins during the second and third decades of life, its full effect is seen in the older population. As this chronic process occurs, the pulp recedes in the affected area and may even become obliterated. In the elderly patient, attrition can cause a loss in the vertical distance between any two stationary points on the tip of the nose and the chin, referred to as loss of the vertical dimension. Attrition can also be seen in its exaggerated form as a pathological result of bruxism, a pur-

poseless grinding of the teeth sometimes associated with the subconscious relief of tension.

Abrasion (Fig. 14-12, *B*) is the effect of wear on the teeth by a foreign body. The most common type of abrasion is that caused by the improper use of a toothbrush. The pathological result of this condition is usually a V-shaped groove occurring in the buccal cementum just above the gingival border. As a result of abrasion, the pulp recedes.

Erosion (Fig. 14-12, *C*) is the loss of tooth structure by a chemical process. The lesion usually occurs on the labial surface of the neck of the tooth. This chemical process can be initiated by (1) the increase in the acid content of secret-

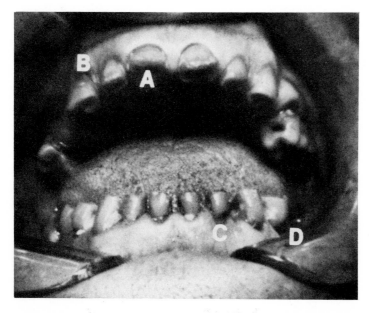

Fig. 14-12. A, The full effect of attrition, the result of continual wear on the occluding surface of the teeth, is seen in the geriatric patient. **B,** Abrasion, the effect of wear on the teeth by a foreign body, is usually seen as a V-shaped groove occurring in the buccal cementum just apical to the cementoenamel junction. **C,** Erosion is the loss of tooth structure caused by a chemical process. **D,** Cervical caries (root surface decay) occurs in the buccal and facial cementum above the junction of the crown and gum.

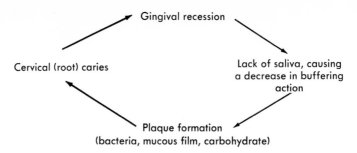

Fig. 14-13. Schema of caries cycle in an older patient.

ed saliva that occurs with normal aging. (2) the chronic regurgitation of acidic gastric contents that occurs in pathological conditions, such as lower-esophageal sphincter incompetence; and/or (3) an overabundance of acidic foods in the diet (e.g., fruit juices or the chronic sucking of citrus fruits).

In the older population, the incidence of occlusal (chewing surface) and interproximal (between the teeth) caries decreases. Cervical caries (root surface decay, Fig. 14-12, *D*) occurs in the buccal and facial cementum above the junction of the crown and gum, and has the highest incidence in the elderly. A cyclical process occurs, which is best demonstrated by Fig. 14-13.

A vicious cycle of cervical caries, gingival recession, plaque formation, and loss of the bony support of the teeth, frequently concomitant with osteoporosis, may lead to mobility and eventual loss of teeth.

COMMON ORAL COMPLAINTS

The chief complaints of elderly dental patients are generally the result of a combination of pathological, physiological, and psychological factors.

Glossodynia or glossopyrosis accompany atrophy of the papillae and are promi-

nent features of the "burning mouth" syndrome. Malnutrition, vitamin deficiency (particularly the vitamin B complex), hormonal imbalance concomitant with menopause, iron deficiency with or without anemia, and psychogenic factors have all been implicated in this baffling problem. If iron-deficiency anemia is implicated, dietary supplements with iron may give relief. A mouthwash of 10% glycerin in distilled water sometimes offers palliative relief. Instructions for its administration are: take 1 teaspoonful, swish it over the tissues for 1 minute, and expectorate; repeat every 2 hours. The recent development of an artificial saliva (Xerolube or Saleze) holds much promise for the treatment of xerostomia. In refractory cases of burning mouth syndrome, consultation with a psychiatrist may be indicated.

Oral candidiasis (Fig. 14-14) occurs frequently among institutionalized elderly patients. *Candida albicans* is also the predominant etiological agent in angular cheilitis (Fig. 14-15), in which xerostomia and collapse of the vertical dimension of the jaws (distance between a center point on the tip of the nose and the chin) may be contributing factors. Treatment consists of riboflavin supplementation, denture rehabilitation, improved oral hy-

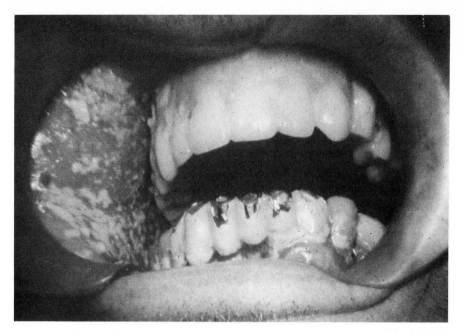

Fig. 14-14. Candidiasis in a patient with terminal cancer.

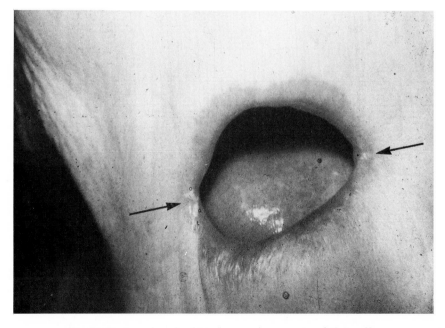

Fig. 14-15. Angular cheilitis *(arrows)* appearing bilaterally.

giene, and the use of topical antifungal and antibacterial agents.

PHARMACOLOGICAL CONSIDERATIONS

The pharmacological activity of drugs is dependent on the functional ability of organ systems to absorb, distribute, metabolize, and eliminate them (see Chapter 6). Because of the physiological and pathological effects of aging, many drugs are poorly tolerated by the elderly; it is well-known that the greatest number of adverse reactions occur in this age group. Many of the oral problems noticed in the course of treatment of geriatric patients are side effects of drug therapy. Dermatological lesions, xerostomia, Stevens-Johnson syndrome, orofacial dyskinesia, and tardive dyskinesia occur with increasing frequency in these patients.

Twenty-five percent of hospitalized elderly patients over 80 years of age demonstrate adverse drug reactions, in contrast to 12% of those in the 41- to 50-year-old age group.[4] When the dentist undertakes the treatment of an older patient, he must know the patient's drug profile, including both prescribed and nonprescribed preparations, such as laxatives, mineral oil, and aspirin. He can thus avoid many drug interactions between the patient's medication and those he may prescribe for dental therapy. Frequent consultations between the dentist and the physician regarding medications are essential for proper dental care.

COMMON PROBLEMS OF MEDICAL-DENTAL MANAGEMENT

The older patient will frequently present for dental treatment with problems that necessitate physician-dentist interaction. Without attempting an exhaustive compendium of such problems, Table 14-

2[5-7] presents the common clinical situations seen in geriatric dental practice, whether in the private office, the hospital, or the nursing home clinic.

Bacterial endocarditis prophylaxis

Elderly dental patients with acquired valvular heart disease or murmurs should receive antimicrobial prophylaxis to prevent endocarditis. The physician should ascertain if the dentist is planning to employ invasive procedures, such as oral surgery, extensive prophylactic scaling, or curettage. Endocarditis prophylaxis is advisable for all procedures that may result in gingival bleeding. For most elderly patients with rheumatic or other acquired valvular heart disease, antimicrobial prophylaxis with Regimen A or B of the American Heart Association should be used.[8,9] Regimen B should be recommended if extensive treatment is planned for patients with prosthetic heart valves or with hip prostheses.[10]

Regimen A—penicillin*

Parenteral-oral combined. Aqueous crystalline penicillin G, 1,000,000 units, is mixed with procaine penicillin G, 600,000 units, and given intramuscularly 30 minutes to 1 hour before the procedure. Penicillin V, 500 mg, is then given orally every 6 hours for 2 days.

Oral. The oral regimen is preferred in the elderly because it obviates the need to have the patient visit the physician for an injection prior to the dental appointment, thereby eliminating transportation problems.

---

*For patients allergic to penicillin, either vancomycin (1g intravenously, with the infusion started 30 minutes to 1 hour before the procedure) or erythromycin (1g orally 1½ to 2 hours before the procedure) can be given. Erythromycin, 500 mg, is then given orally every 6 hours for 2 days.

Table 14-2. Oral aspects of systemic disorders and medical-dental interactions

Medical condition	Dental aspects	Medical-dental interactions
Arteriosclerotic, cardiovascular heart disease (ASCVD) with congestive heart failure (CHF)	Minimize apprehension and stress; avoid postural hypotension; short appointments preferable; note date of any previous myocardial infarction (defer treatment for 6 weeks following acute episode)	Consult with physician about management Sedatives potentiate rauwolfia alkaloids, phenothiazines, and antihypertensive drugs Epinephrine is contraindicated in depressed patients receiving monoamine oxidase (MAO) inhibitors Digitalis intoxication may cause nausea and vomiting
Hypertension	Stress and anxiety may elevate blood pressure; for diastolic pressure over 110, only emergency procedures should be performed[5]	For patients receiving reserpine, use alpha stimulators rather than epinephrine for local anesthesia Xerostomia is a side effect of antihypertensive drugs (e.g., alpha-methyldopa, diuretics, and propranolol) Rapid rising from the reclining position in the dental chair may lead to postural hypotension in patients receiving antihypertensive therapy
Cerebrovascular accident (CVA)	Circumoral and neuromuscular effects; dysphasia and aphasia; adverse effect on dentures; drooling; flexion of the neck causes management problems; patients may laugh or cry at inappropriate times, making dental work difficult	Anticoagulant therapy increases clotting time and affects oral surgery Monitor epinephrine in local anesthetics Meperidine (Demerol) increases intracranial pressure
Paget's disease	Progressive enlargement of the maxilla and mandible; "flaring" of teeth; dentures become unstable	Use calcitonin to reverse these phenomena
Sjögren's syndrome	Xerostomia; glossopyrosis; burning mouth syndrome; increased incidence of cervical caries; dysgeusia	Patients often require psychotherapy in addition to palliative treatment. If receiving steroids, the patient will be more prone to stress, periodontal disease, and delayed healing

Continued.

Table 14-2.   Oral aspects of systemic disorders and medical-dental interactions — cont'd

Medical condition	Dental aspects	Medical-dental interactions
Diabetes mellitus	Periodontal disease; lowered resistance to infection; delayed healing; patients prone to denture irritation[6]	Consult with physician regarding dosage and type of insulin Corticosteroids can cause hyperglycemia Antibiotic prophylaxis against local infection is not routinely necessary for diet-controlled patients Antibiotic prophylaxis against local infection is essential before oral surgery for the "brittle" diabetic Schedule patients for routine care in the morning following usual insulin dose
Parkinsonism	Bruxism; tongue thrust; drooling; slurred speech; problems in deglutition and swallowing; stress increases symptoms	Use of epinephrine in anesthetic agents may enhance stress Extrapyramidal reactions to L-dopa cause orofacial dyskinesia[7] Atropine causes increase in L-dopa effect
Osteoporosis	Loss of alveolar bone; loss of teeth; dehiscence of canals due to mandibular atrophy	Possible use of calcium, vitamin D, and estrogen supplements in the treatment of osteoporosis
Rheumatoid arthritis	Rheumatoid arthritis can involve the temporomandibular joint; limited mobility of the upper extremities make it difficult to perform oral hygiene	Medications used in the treatment of arthritis, such as phenylbutazone, can cause oral lesions Special adaptive devices may be used to enable disabled patients to clean their dentures or brush their teeth

Penicillin V, 2 g, is given orally 30 minutes to 1 hour before the procedure; a 500-mg dose is then given orally every 6 hours for 2 days.

Regimen B — penicillin plus streptomycin*

Aqueous crystalline penicillin G, 1,000,000 units, is mixed with procaine penicillin G, 600,000 units, and injected intramuscularly, followed by streptomycin, 1 g, given intramuscularly 30 minutes to 1 hour before the procedure; penicillin V, 500 mg, is then given orally every 6 hours for 2 days.

Anticoagulation

The discontinuation of anticoagulant therapy is another management issue that frequently arises between the dentist and the physician. For routine restorative dentistry, it is not necessary to discontinue oral anticoagulants; however, the dentist should be cautioned to respect the integrity of the soft tissues. When the dentist is planning procedures that may result in gingival bleeding, the physician should determine the prothrombin (PT) time the day before the dental appointment. A PT time that is less than $1\frac{1}{2}$ times the control is desirable before oral surgery. Deanticoagulation may be accomplished by discontinuing the oral anticoagulant 2 days before the day of treatment and for 1 or 2 days following surgery. If this places the patient at too high a risk, intravenous heparinization may be considered; however, this will require inpatient management. At times it may be necessary to administer vitamin

K if hemorrhage persists following an extraction or curettage. The physician should remain in close consultation with the dentist in all cases.

Local anesthesia

The dentist may ask the physician if he can employ epinephrine with a local anesthetic in the treatment of a hypertensive elderly patient. The purpose of the epinephrine is to cause vasoconstriction of the blood vessels, thereby prolonging local anesthesia. It should be remembered, however, that the anxious patient produces substantial amounts of endogenous epinephrine, equal to or greater than the amount normally injected. Local anesthesia will reduce pain and anxiety and therefore prevent the elevation of blood pressure. In most cases, the dentist should be advised to use a local anesthetic with 1 : 100,000 epinephrine.

Patients with pacemakers

The physician should advise the dentist as to whether the patient has a transvenous cardiac pacemaker. Ultrasonic devices and electrosurgery units, which may cause dysrhythmias, should not be used on patients with pacemakers. Some cardiologists recommend that antibiotic prophylaxis be employed prior to any extensive dental treatment for patients with cardiac pacemakers.

The diabetic patient

All diabetic patients should be seen regularly by a dentist. Dental infections, such as gingivitis, periodontitis, and alveolar abscesses, may cause a rise in blood glucose concentration, possibly leading to hyperosmolar, hyperglycemic nonketotic coma, or ketoacidosis. The hyperglycemic state may also cause a defect in leukocyte mobility, which may

---

*For patients allergic to penicillin, vancomycin, 1 g, can be given intravenously, with the infusion started 30 minutes to 1 hour before the procedure. Erythromycin, 500 mg, is then given orally every 6 hours for 2 days.

cause an exacerbation of gingival disease, resulting in a loss of the bony support of the teeth (peridontal disease) and, eventually, the loss of teeth.

The most common consideration arising in dental treatment for the diabetic patient is whether to employ antimicrobial prophylaxis. In Table 14-2 it is noted that the diet-controlled elderly diabetic can be treated without the use of antibiotics. Nevertheless, if an extensive surgical procedure is planned, antibiotic prophylaxis should be prescribed both preoperatively and postoperatively. The insulin-dependent diabetic should be advised to eat a normal breakfast and take the customary dose of insulin prior to the dental visit.

Radiation therapy

Because radiation therapy can result in xerostomia and rampant cervical caries, the physician should consult with the dentist before initiating radiation therapy to the head and neck. The dentist will recommend a daily regimen of topical fluorides and the removal of all mobile and infected teeth prior to therapy; otherwise, osteomyelitis and sloughing of alveolar bone may occur.

In patients who have already received head and neck irradiation, the following protocol should be used for extractions:

1. Give preoperative penicillin (Regimen A) on the morning of surgery and follow with 4 days of postoperative antibiotic therapy.

2. Advise the dentist to limit the number of extractions to two or three teeth at a time.

3. Attempt primary closure, if possible.

DENTAL MANAGEMENT OF THE GEROPSYCHIATRIC PATIENT

It has been estimated that 50% of the institutionalized elderly and 5% to 15% of the elderly living in the community are suffering from some degree of organic mental impairment. Although the definitive diagnosis and classification of cerebral dysfunction must be made by a qualified physician, the dentist should be able to evaluate the mental status of his elderly patient. Inappropriate behavior of the elderly patient in the dental office is too easily characterized as maladjustment and inability to cooperate. The dentist should be able to recognize signs of psychiatric and neurological illness, such as wandering, hallucinations, delusions, paranoid behavior, and aphasia, so that consultation with the physician can be sought and proper diagnoses and therapy implemented.

Sedation and premedication

Occasionally, it will be necessary to premedicate an uncooperative patient with organic brain syndrome who requires urgent dental treatment. Dosage of narcotics, sedatives, and tranquilizers should generally be reduced to one third or one half the amount administered to a younger adult patient. A careful history of drug sensitivities should, of course, first be elicited from the medical records. The following are some of the agents that may be used for sedation and premedication: nonphenothiazine tranquilizers; hydroxyzine hydrochloride (Atarax), 25 to 50 mg IM; hydroxyzine pamoate (Vistaril), 25 to 50 mg IM; diphenhydramine hydrochloride (Benadryl), 25 to 50 mg PO; diazepam (Valium), 2 to 5 mg PO; and chlorpromazine (Thorazine), 10 to 25 mg IM.

Belladonna alkaloids, such as atropine sulfate or scopalamine hydrobromide, are contraindicated because of their antisialagogic effect, making the mucous secretions along the respiratory tree more viscous and tenacious and promoting xerostomia.

DENTURES

A denture is a removable prosthetic appliance that replaces missing teeth. It may be a complete, or full denture, restoring a totally edentulous maxilla or mandible, or a partial denture, in which case some of the natural teeth have been preserved. The student or physician should be aware of problems that are commonly seen in the elderly denture-wearing patient.

The artificial replacement of teeth reduces masticatory efficiency, even with well-fitting dentures. Thus, the patient who has recently had dentures inserted may legitimately complain, sometimes to the physician as well as to the dentist, that he can no longer eat as well and has lost his appetite and enjoyment of food. He may even exhibit symptoms of mild malnutrition. Because of the fragile oral mucosa and the atrophied bony ridge in many elderly patients, a dental prosthesis may not be tolerated. Despite the lack of a dental prosthesis, adequate nutrition can be maintained; however, the enjoyment of food is diminished.

The psychological set of the patient is just as important as the accuracy of fit in the prognosis for successful adjustment to dentures. Unrealistic expectations and emotional problems, such as a diminished self-image and equating dentures with castration and sexual impotence, can contribute to a rejection of the prosthesis and considerable emotional trauma. The physician may have to play a supportive role for the patient during this trying period.

One of the significant etiological factors causing failure in denture wearing in the aged patient is the physiological diminution of saliva that occurs with advancing years. Denture retention is dependent on a film of mucus that normally exists between the alveolar tissues and the denture. When the mucus is diminished because of xerostomia, the dentures may feel loose. A denture adhesive, which consists mainly of a vegetable gum, may be recommended by the dentist to hold the dentures in place. In addition to a denture adhesive, an artificial saliva preparation can ameliorate the troublesome effects of xerostomia and may improve denture adhesion.

The physician can be helpful to the dentist by reinforcing some of the suggestions the dentist will make to the denture wearer (e.g., that the dentures must be kept clean and should be removed at night and placed in a denture cleanser). When the physician observes candidiasis or other fungal lesions in the mouth of the edentulous patient, he may suspect that there is a lack of denture hygiene. On the other hand, this may also be caused by poorly fitting dentures; the physician should then refer the patient to a dentist for appropriate evaluation.

TASTE

The following terms describe aberrations of the gustatory and olfactory senses:

ageusia Absence of the sense of taste.
anosmia Inability to recognize or detect smell.
cacogeusia Rancid or spoiled taste of normal items of food.
dysgeusia Impairment of the sense of taste.
dysosmia Impairment of the sense of smell.
glossodynia The painful tongue seen, for example, in vitamin B_{12} deficiency.
glossopyrosis The burning tongue seen, for example, in postmenopausal women.
hypogeusia Diminished acuteness of the sense of taste.

hyposmia Diminished acuteness of the sense of smell.

parosmia A perverted sense of smell in which the patient complains of a specific unpleasant odor, without the presence of a stimulus.

phantogeusia A persistent, foul, metallic, or bitter taste without the presence of oral stimuli.

To understand the serious problems of loss of taste and appetite, it is necessary to examine the biological and pathological effects of aging on the major organ of taste, the tongue. Recent investigations into the physiology of taste have refined previous concepts of taste localization. The four primary taste sensations (bitter, acid, sweet, and salty) and the fungiform, filiform, and circumvallate papillae are located as shown in Fig. 14-16.

In addition to taste buds, the tongue is innervated by unmyelinated nerve fibers, which also mediate sensations of taste. The exact process begins when the tastant goes into solution in the saliva. This stimulus then affects the neural epithelium in the taste buds and nerve endings and is transmitted to the brain center, where taste messages are mediated.

During the aging process there is a significant physiological diminution in the number of foliate papillae of the tongue and a concomitant reduction in the number of taste buds.[11] By age 60, 50% of the taste buds have been lost, especially those concerned with the sensations of sweet and salty. This deteriorative process also results in a decrease in the number of taste nerve endings, particularly of the circumvallate papillae, because of atrophy. At the same time, the sense of smell deteriorates, primarily because of atrophic changes in the olfactory bulb and the loss of olfactory fibers secondary to atrophy of sensory cells in the nasal mucosa. This may explain the loss of the sense of smell, which frequently deprives older persons of protection (e.g., in detecting the odor of escaping gas in the kitchen) and may also account for parosmia or phantogeusia when new dentures are inserted. (These complaints may also be of psychogenic origin, representing a subconscious rejec-

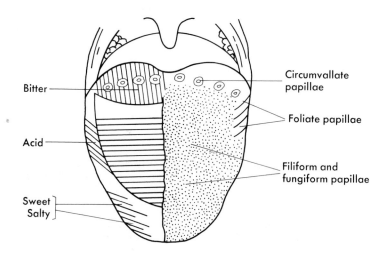

Fig. 14-16. Anatomy and physiology of the tongue. (Courtesy J. Phelan.)

tion of the prosthesis.) Wearing dentures may also decrease taste acuity for sour and bitter.[12]

Systemic and local conditions affecting taste
Infections

Infections of the mouth, nose, or paranasal sinuses may result in transient ageusia or dysgeusia. Dysgeusia and diminished olfactory acuity have been linked to acute viral hepatitis, and it has been observed that improvement in olfactory perception sometimes coincides with recovery from this infection.[13]

Endocrinopathies

Loss of taste has been reported in a wide range of endocrine disorders, including adrenal insufficiency, Cushing's syndrome, and pseudohypoparathyroidism.[14]

Neoplasms

Nasopharyngeal masses are causes of ageusia, dysgeusia, and olfactory aberrations in the older patient. Ageusia has also been reported concomitantly with lesions of the facial nerve as well as lesions in the medulla, thalamus, and temporal lobes.[15]

Idiopathic hypogeusia

Idiopathic hypogeusia is characterized by (1) dysgeusia, hyposmia, and dysomia; (2) evidence, via electron microscopic examination, of abnormalities of the taste buds; and (3) improvement of the hypogeusia following the administration of zinc sulfate.

Drugs

Ageusia and hyposmia have been reported in patients treated with methimazole, penicillamine, and lithium carbonate. Many of the antihistamines and anti-depressants also lead to an inhibition of parasympathetic function with a subsequent xerostomia and loss of taste.[16]

Environmental factors

A transient loss of taste follows radiation therapy; the duration of this loss depends on the intensity of dosage and the degree of xerostomia induced by treatment. Smoking may also diminish taste.

Treatment of taste aberrations

The treatment of abnormalities of taste depends on the intensity of the problem. If the disorder occurs concomitantly with the insertion of a denture prosthesis, it may be necessary to reassure the patient that taste will return as the mouth accommodates to the prosthesis.

At the present time, for organically based dysgeusia, the therapeutic approach with most promise seems to be the administration of zinc sulfate, along with vitamins and other trace minerals, to restore a proper nutritional balance. Measures to combat local dehydration, such as the use of artificial saliva, may also be helpful.

CONCLUSION

The mouth of the older patient plays an increasingly important role in the quality of life in the remaining years. Whether healthy or frail, the elderly need not resign themselves to the loss of teeth, taste, or masticatory efficiency. Modern dentistry can do much to prolong the function of the dentition and enhance the oral health of the older patient.

REFERENCES

1. Age patterns in medical care, illness and disability, Vital and Health Statistics Series 10, No. 70, DHEW Pub. No. (HSM) 72-1026, U.S. Department of Health, Education, and Welfare.

2. Edentulous persons, United States—1971. Vital and Health Statistics Series 10, No. 89, DHEW Pub. No. (HRA) 74-1516, U.S. Department of Health, Education, and Welfare.
3. Riley, M. W., and Foner, A.: Aging and society, vol. 1, New York, 1968, Russell Sage Foundation.
4. Lany, P. P., and Vestal, R. E.: Drug prescribing for the elderly. In Reichel, W., editor: The geriatric patient, New York, 1978, HP Publishing Co., Inc.
5. Lavelle, C. L. B.: Hypertension and the dentist, J. Hosp. Dent. Pract. 11(1):7, 1977.
6. Cohen, L.: The dental management of patients with medical problems, N.Y. State Dent. J. 41:470, October 1975.
7. Hardin, W. G., and O'Leary, J. L.: Neurologic aspects. In Cowdry, E. V., and Steinberg, F. U., editors: The care of the geriatric patient, ed. 4, St. Louis, 1971, The C.V. Mosby Co.
8. Report of the American Heart Association Committee on Prevention of Rheumatic Fever, Circulation 56:139A, July 1977.
9. Prevention of bacterial endocarditis; a committee report of the American Heart Association, J. Am. Dent. Assoc., 95:600, September 1977.
10. Rubin, R., Salvati, E. A., and Lewis, R.: Infected total hip replacement after dental procedures, Oral Surg. 41(1):18, 1976.
11. Davidoff, A., Winkler, S., and Tee, H. M.: Dentistry for the special patient, Philadelphia, 1972, W. B. Saunders Co., p. 53.
12. Henkin, R. I., and Christiansen, R. L.: Taste thresholds in patients with dentures J. Am. Dent. Assoc. 75:118, 1967.
13. Henkin, R. I., and Smith, F. R.: Hyposmia in acute viral hepatitis, Lancet 1:165, 1971.
14. Henkin, R. I.: Abnormalities of taste and olfaction in patients with chromatin negative gonadal dysgenesis, J. Clin. Endocrinol. Metab. 27:1436, 1967.
15. Brocklehurst, J. C.: Textbook of geriatric medicine and gerontology, Edinburgh, Eng., 1973, Churchill Livingstone, p. 32.
16. Henkin, R. I., and Bradley, D. F.: Regulation of taste acuity by thiols and metal ions, Proc. Natl. Acad. Sci, U.S.A. 62:30, 1969.

PROBLEM-SOLVING EXERCISES
Case one

Mrs. R. O. is a 73-year-old woman with a complex medical history whose dentist calls you. He reports a severe oral infection and other dental problems that require urgent treatment, and he requests your advice regarding her oral-surgical management. The dentist's records show that she had a mitral valve replacement 3 years previously, which was followed postoperatively by a left CVA with right-sided hemiplegia and an uninhibited neurogenic bladder, from which she gradually recovered, and aphasia. She also has a history of rheumatic heart disease since childhood and suffers from chronic obstructive lung disease. As a consequence of the mitral valve prosthesis, she is now receiving permanent anticoagulation therapy with warfarin.

*Questions**

1. Would you advise the dentist to defer treatment?
2. Would you recommend inpatient or outpatient management for extensive oral surgery?
3. What steps would you suggest to monitor the patient's hemostasis?
4. What regimen of prophylactic antibiotics would you prescribe?

Case two

Mr. M. Y. is a 79-year-old man with a history of myocardial infarction sustained 6 years previously, hypertensive cardiovascular disease, adult-onset diabetes mellitus, Parkinson's disease, and mild organic brain syndrome. He lives at home with his 76-year-old wife. His dentist calls you to report that the patient now has a tooth that requires extraction because of an alveolar abscess. The patient, however, is confused and agitated. The dentist asks for your assistance in sedating the patient at a level whereby he may be amenable to local anesthesia and therefore more manageable.

Question

1. What sedative medication would you select for this situation, and what would be the appropriate dosage?

*Give the rationale for each of your answers.

Case three

Mrs. N. S. is a 72-year-old woman who develops an astrocytoma of the brain and is scheduled for surgery followed by radiation therapy. Since you are aware that the oral cavity is in the path of the cobalt rays, you consult an oral pathologist for advice in managing the oral complications of the radiation therapy.

Question

1. Assuming that the patient has most of her natural teeth, state the possible side effects of radiation on the hard and soft tissues of the mouth and the methods you would use to minimize these effects.

ANSWERS TO PROBLEM-SOLVING EXERCISES
Case one

1. Treatment should not be deferred, because oral infection can be the source of a bacteremia with secondary infection of a prosthetic heart valve or of a fixation device used to treat a hip fracture. Oral disease, therefore, places this patient at higher risk.
2. Because this patient is at high medical risk, the ideal environment for oral surgery is in a hospital operating room. Here the patient can be adequately monitored, and standby assistance is available for medical emergencies. Inpatient management is therefore preferred.
3. The prothrombin (PT) time should be determined 1 day before dental treatment. If the PT time is less than $1\frac{1}{2}$ times the control, the patient may continue on the regular warfarin regimen. If the PT time is greater than $1\frac{1}{2}$ times the control, the anticoagulant should be discontinued 1 or 2 days before oral surgery and for 2 days after the operation. Vitamin K should be administered if hemorrhaging develops following oral surgery.
4. Regimen B, as recommended by the American Heart Association, is the method of choice in patients not sensitive to penicillin. Aqueous crystalline penicillin G, 1,000,000 units, mixed with procaine penicillin G, 600,000 units, plus streptomycin, 1 g, is given intramuscularly 30 minutes to 1 hour before the procedure; phenoxymethyl penicillin, 500 mg, is then given orally every 6 hours for 2 days.

For patients allergic to penicillin, vancomycin, 1 g, can be given intravenously, with the infusion started 30 minutes to 1 hour before surgery. Erythromycin, 500 mg, is then given orally every 6 hours for 2 days.

Case two

1. Older patients are notoriously sensitive to drugs and demonstrate more frequent side effects. You should therefore carefully consider the patient's drug profile and select an agent that would be synergistic with any psychotropic drugs usually employed for those with organic brain disorders. Ruling out specific sensitivities, any of the following would be appropriate, with the dosage adjusted within the indicated ranges: hydroxyzine hydrochloride (Atarax), 25 to 50 mg IM; hydroxyzine pamoate (Vistaril), 25 to 50 mg IM; diphenhydramine hydrochloride (Benadryl), 25 to 50 mg PO; diazepam (Valium), 2 to 10 mg PO; and chlorpromazine (Thorazine), 10 to 25 mg IM.

Case three

1. Possible side effects of radiation on the oral mucosa include acute mucositis, ulceration, keratosis, and mucosal soreness. If the mouth is included within the primary beam, the senses of smell and taste may be temporarily lost. These are short-term effects that usually regress following therapy. Xerostomia is a delayed long-term effect.

Because of these changes, the soft tissues are prone to bacterial and monilial infections, and healing capacity is impaired.

Hard tissue effects include increased risk of osteoradionecrosis, osteomyelitis, and bone resorption. Because of diminished salivary output, there is a marked increase in dental caries, particularly in the cervical areas of the enamel crowns. The following protocol should be instituted to ameliorate the above consequences:

- Infected or questionable teeth that are in the line of radiation should be removed before therapy.
- The patient should be placed on a daily regimen of topical fluorides, to be maintained for the remainder of her life.
- A saliva substitute should be employed if xerostomia develops and persists.

POSTTEST*

1. Name three drugs commonly used by the elderly that may cause some degree of xerostomia (dry mouth).
2. On the average, how often would you advise your elderly patient to visit a dentist?
   a. Once a year
   b. Once every 6 months
   c. Once every 3 months
   d. Only if necessary
3. List five common oral conditions that result from neglect of oral health care among the elderly.
4. What percentage of people over the age of 65 are totally edentulous?
   a. 50%
   b. 25%
   c. 75%
5. An 83-year-old man is seeing you for his yearly medical checkup. On performing a regional examination of the head and neck, you remove the patient's dentures and see a creamy lesion on the palate. You also notice that the dentures are in a state of disrepair and neglected hygiene. When you wipe the lesion with a gauze pad, an erythematous base remains. You would:

---

*Some questions may have more than one correct answer.

a. Take a culture, make a preliminary diagnosis of candidiasis, and initiate a nystatin rinse
b. Prepare the patient for a biopsy
c. Take a culture and initiate the following antibiotic therapy: Phenoxymethyl penicillin, 250 mg every 6 hours for 5 days

6. Which of the following agents is *least* likely to be prescribed for an agitated patient with organic brain syndrome whose dentist requests advice for mild premedication prior to dental treatment?
   a. Chlorpromazine (Thorazine), 25 mg IM
   b. Thiothixene (Navane), 10 mg IM
   c. Meperidine (Demerol), 100 mg PO, and promethazine (Phenergan) 25 mg PO
   d. Chloral hydrate, 1 g PO
7. Mrs. H. is an 85-year-old hypertensive woman who is currently normotensive as the result of a daily thiazide diuretic. Her dentists wants to use a local anesthetic with epinephrine (lidocaine 2%, 1:100,000 epinephrine) during an extraction procedure. This is:
   a. Not advisable, because the patient may go into an acute hypertensive crisis
   b. Not advisable, because in an anxiety-provoking situation the endogenous release of epinephrine is still less than the exogenous epinephrine in the local anesthetic (lidocaine 2%, 1:100,000 epinephrine)
   c. Advisable, because the vasoconstrictive effect of the epinephrine will enhance local anesthesia, causing the patient to be less anxious and reducing the chance of an acute hypertensive crisis
   d. Advisable, because in an anxiety-provoking situation, the endogenous release of epinephrine is greater than the exogenous epinephrine in

the local anesthetic (lidocaine 2%, 1:100,000 epinephrine)

8. The most common dental problem in the dentulous elderly is:
   a. Caries
   b. Toothache
   c. Chewing problems
   d. Periodontal disease

9. Common problems in the elderly with dentures are:
   a. Diminished chewing ability
   b. Soreness, pain
   c. Need for adjustments
   d. Decreased vertical dimension

10. Which of the following regimens should an elderly patient with a history of rheumatic heart disease receive before oral surgery?
    a. No premedication
    b. Penicillin V, 500 mg 30 minutes to 1 hour before treatment, then 250 mg q6hr for 8 doses
    c. Penicillin V, 2 g 30 minutes to 1 hour before treatment, then 500 mg q6hr for 8 doses

ANSWERS TO PRETEST AND POSTTEST

1. Three of the following: propranolol, phenothiazines, furosemide, meperidine, tricyclic antidepressants, and/or thiazide diuretics.
2. b. Because of the vulnerability of the hard and soft tissues of the mouth in the elderly, it is necessary that they see a dentist at least once every 6 months.
3. Five of the following: caries (normally cervical), periodontal disease (pyorrhea), candidiasis, denture ulcers, xerostomia (dry mouth), halitosis, abscess, papillomatosis, leukoplakia, denture stomatitis, burning mouth.
4. a.
5. a. Gross appearance and the lack of induration contraindicate biopsy. Penicillin is ineffective against fungal infections. Answer a is correct. A presumptive diagnosis of candidiasis can be made based on the appearance of the lesion.
6. c. Narcotics are poorly tolerated by older patients, induce hypotension, and may cause vomiting.
7. c and d. There is no evidence that 1:100,000 epinephrine can cause a hypertensive crisis. Answer b is incorrect because it has been demonstrated that the endogenous release of epinephrine is greater than the content of an average anesthetic injection.
8. d.
9. All of these.
10. Regimen c is correct.°

°See the Report of the American Heart Association Committee on Prevention of Rheumatic Fever, Circulation **56**:139A, July 1977.

Chapter 15

Disorders of the foot

HOWARD WERTER, ARTHUR E. HELFAND, and EMMANUEL MARGOLIS

EDUCATIONAL OBJECTIVES

Attitudinal

The student should:

1. Recognize that the foot is an important part of the examination of the elderly patient
2. Recognize that unnoticed and untreated podiatric problems can lead to major problems in ambulation in the elderly
3. Recognize that the painful foot is a common complaint

Cognitive

The student should:

1. Be aware of common foot problems in the elderly (common dermatological, nail, and ulcer problems) and know their diagnoses and treatments
2. Know the podiatric manifestations of systemic diseases (e.g., peripheral vascular disease and diabetes mellitus)
3. Be aware of common pathomechanical problems that affect the aged foot
4. Be aware of the services offered by the podiatrist
5. Know when to refer the elderly patient to a podiatrist

Skill

The student should:

1. Be able to recognize common podiatric problems in the elderly
2. Be able to assess the aged foot for signs of peripheral vascular disease and diabetes mellitus
3. Be able to assess the aged foot for pathomechanical problems

PRETEST*

1. An ulcer of the foot is a complication of
   a. Diabetes mellitus
   b. Nondiabetic vascular disease
   c. Chronic obstructive pulmonary disease
   d. Congestive heart failure
2. Calluses are formed primarily because of:
   a. Poor shoe fitting
   b. Imbalance due to improper weight bearing
   c. Walking on hard surfaces
3. With normal old age, the following are frequently seen on the foot:
   a. Increased sweating
   b. Dry skin
   c. Loss of muscle and soft tissue on the plantar surface
   d. Loss of hair on the dorsum of the foot
4. *True or false:* Orthopedic problems affecting the hip or knee can cause pain in the feet.
5. *True or false:* Treatment of heel fissures consist of debridement and daily application of emollients that hydrate and lubricate the skin.
6. *True or false:* Diabetes mellitus should be suspected when prolonged monilial infections occur in the foot.

---

*Some questions may have more than one correct answer.

7. *True or false:* Callous formation is uncommonly located beneath the metatarsal head.
8. *True or false:* Ulcers can form under neglected callous areas.
9. *True or false:* Soft orthotics or inlays should be used to remove weight bearing from ulcerated areas.
10. *True or false:* Fungal infection of the nails (onychomycosis) often complicates a hypertrophic nail (onychauxis).

Older people suffer from numerous foot problems that may lead to serious complications.[1] Health care providers generally avoid dealing with the foot problems of their patients. However, many of the foot conditions of the elderly can be prevented or improved by the attention of these health care workers plus the services of a podiatrist. These services should be included in every setting of geriatric care, whether it be the ambulatory care clinic, acute care hospital, or long-term care facility. Maintaining and improving locomotion often results in the prevention of falls, ulcers, or deformities and increases personal comfort.

PHYSIOLOGICAL CHANGES IN THE FOOT

Changes resulting from normal aging affect the skin and nails, the musculoskeletal structures, and the vascular and nervous systems of the foot.

The skin demonstrates loss of hair along the outer side of the leg. On the dorsum of the foot, scaling, atrophy, dryness, and brownish pigmentation appear. The nails become thickened (hyperkeratotic) and brittle.

Loss of muscle and soft tissue on the plantar surface of the foot contribute to fatigue and pain and occasionally to a decrease in tolerance for walking. Neurological changes cause decreased sensation, diminished proprioception and vibration senses, and diminished Achilles tendon and patellar reflexes. Loss of sensation may lead to unperceived trauma.

Foot problems in the elderly are the result of trauma and disease, untreated deformity, lack of preventive measures in earlier years, and inadequate health education.

HISTORY AND PHYSICAL EXAMINATION

The elderly patient's most frequent podiatric complaint is pain or discomfort that interferes with ambulation. There may be a history of previous foot lesions, deformity, swelling, color change, or pruritus. The primary care physician should inquire about past podiatric problems, since these conditions may serve as a "window" to systemic diseases.

The examination of the foot may be supplemented by oscillometry (peripheral vascular disease), tissue biopsy (neoplasm), x-ray examination (osteomyelitis), and potassium hydroxide or Gram's stain of discharge from lesions (fungal or bacterial infections). The elderly patient's gait should be observed. Orthopedic problems affecting the hip or knee can cause maldistribution of weight on the foot and lead to pain and deformity. Similarly, foot problems may lead to difficulties in the knees or hips.

COMMON DERMATOLOGICAL PROBLEMS
Pruritus

Pruritus, which is a common condition in the aged foot, may be caused by disturbed keratin formation, dryness, scaliness, decreased sebaceous activity, or loss of oil from the skin as a result of repeated hot baths. Fungal, neurogenic, and emotional dermatitis may also cause pruritus.

Fissured heels

Fissured heels (Fig. 15-1), resulting from dryness or dermatitis, may cause a serious problem, especially when there is also a poor blood supply to the area. The broken skin may lead to bacterial or mycotic infection. Treatment consists of debridement and daily application of emollients that hydrate and lubricate the skin and promote closing of the fissures. When there is a secondary mycotic or bacterial infection, initial therapy is aimed at the specific etiological agent. Contact dermatitis from socks, shoes, soaps, and particularly from topical medi-

cations used for corn removal may be the etiological factor.

Anhidrosis; hyperhidrosis; bromhidrosis

Anhidrosis (deficient perspiration) is common in older patients and requires treatment similar to the treatment outlined for pruritus and fissured heels.

Hyperhidrosis (excessive sweating) is often associated with infections, allergies, and emotional stress. Local therapy begins with daily foot hygiene (cleansing with soap and water and thorough drying) and the application of a moisture-absorbing powder. Peroxide and alcohol swabbing and the application of mild formalin solutions are of value in resistant cases.

Bromhidrosis is a form of profuse sweating characterized by a fetid odor due to the decomposition of sweat. The

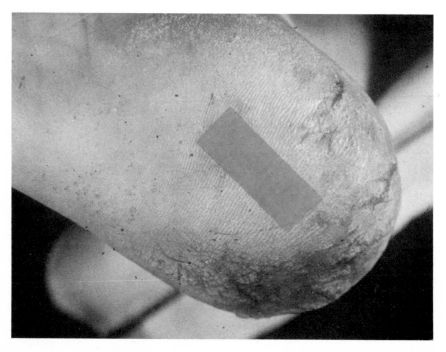

Fig. 15-1. Heel fissures. (Courtesy American Podiatry Association.)

therapeutic approach is similar to that of hyperhidrosis.

Contact dermatitis

When the foot reveals limited, circumscribed areas of inflammation and a previous history of allergy is obtained, contact dermatitis should be considered. The primary irritant (socks, shoes, topical medication) must be identified and removed.[2] Subsequent therapy is aimed at the various dermatological manifestations present and usually includes soaks with Burrow's or saline solution and topical application of steroids and antihistaminics.

Tinea pedis

The general term for mycotic infections of the foot, tinea pedis may be present in any of its clinical varieties: acute vesicular, subacute vesicular, chronic hyperkeratotic, and/or interdigital infestation. Mycotic culture should be taken to confirm the diagnosis. Therapy can then be instituted immediately on the basis of the appearance of the lesion. Oral griseofulvin is of slight value; it should be used only for short periods (e.g., 30 to 60 days) and only as an adjunct to topical treatment with warm soaks of Burrow's solution (in the acute stages) and fungicidal preparations, such as undecylenic acid. Antifungal powders and gentian violet solutions can be used for topical therapy. When the etiological factor is *Candida albicans,* topical nystatin (Mycostatin) and/or topical gentian violet solution should be employed. Diabetes mellitus should be suspected when frequent or prolonged monilial infections occur.

Callous and corn formation

These hyperkeratotic lesions often occur under the metatarsal heads.[3] Be-
cause of excessive stress and strain due to improper weight bearing, the skin becomes irritated and growth of the horny epithelium follows, leading to irritation and loss of flexibility. Subcutaneous tissue is replaced by fibrous connective tissue and gradually enters the stratum corneum and forms a clavus (corn). Eventually a small pea-shaped invaginated hyperkeratotic area develops in the center, causing sharp pain with continued stress.

Ulcers

Various types of ulcerations (Fig. 15-2) can occur on the feet and are usually the result of a systemic illness. These include vascular ulcers, caused by venous or arterial insufficiency; pressure ulcers, caused by prolonged local pressure on the heels of bedridden patients; trophic ulcers, caused by denervation of the area; diabetic ulcers; and traumatic ulcers, usually caused by excessive pressure on a weight-bearing area. Ulcers can also form under neglected hyperkeratotic areas, such as calluses. Ulcer therapy consists of surgical, chemical (enzymes), or mechanical (whirlpool) debridement; drainage; and elimination or control of the etiological factor(s).

The majority of ulcerative lesions of the foot are seen in patients with systemic disease, such as diabetes mellitus or arteriosclerosis. A blood glucose determination and x-ray examination of the underlying bone will determine whether diabetes mellitus or osteomyelitis is present.

Soft orthotics or inlays should be used to remove weight bearing and pressure from the ulcerated areas. Ambulation exercises should be used to improve local vascular supply. Whirlpool treatment will locally debride and stimulate the tissue.

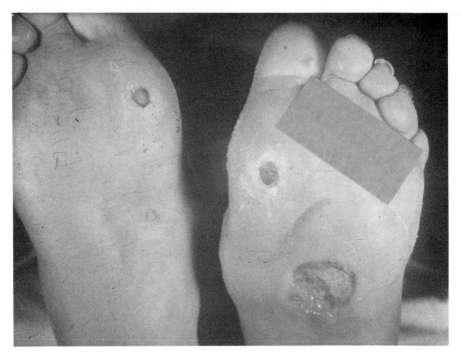

Fig. 15-2. Giant multiple ulcers (sometimes called traumatic ulcers). (Courtesy American Podiatry Association.)

COMMON NAIL PROBLEMS

Nail lesions are the second most common podiatric problem, exceeded only by calluses. The elderly patient often has difficulty giving himself proper nail care because of poor eyesight, inability to bend, tremor, and lack of knowledge about proper foot care, which is common at all ages.

Thickened and curved nails (onychauxis, onychogryposis)

Onychauxis, or hypertrophic nail (Fig. 15-3), is a thickening of the nail plate. Its etiology is often multifactorial, including trauma, inflammation, recurrent infections, and systemic disease. The nail is thickened and discolored. Pain may be present as the shoe presses on the nail plate. Treatment is aimed at the underlying cause, with periodic debridement of the nail plate as the initial approach. Removal of the matrix may be necessary.

Onychogryposis (Fig. 15-4) is an unusually large and curved nail that requires treatment similar to that of onychauxis. Repeated trauma and poor hygiene may be etiological factors.

Callous nail groove

Callous nail groove is usually the result of injury to the nail plate from various types of external pressure, including incurvated sides of the nail plate. Treatment consists of excision, the use of emollients that hydrate and lubricate the hyperkeratotic areas, thinning of the nail plate to permit flexibility, and the re-

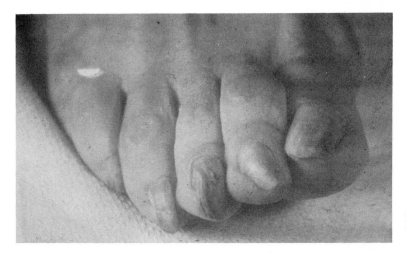

Fig. 15-3. Onychauxis. Usually the great toenail is most involved. (Courtesy American Podiatry Association.)

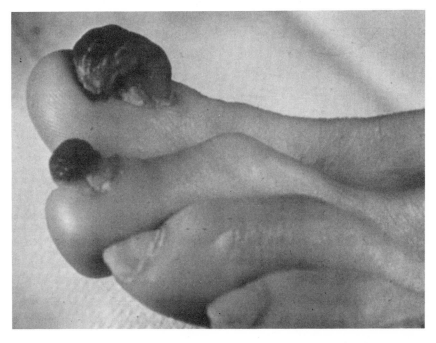

Fig. 15-4. Onychogryposis. Repeated trauma and poor hygiene may be the cause. (Courtesy American Podiatry Association.)

moval of any external pressure, as well as partial matrix removal in some cases.

Ingrown toenail (onychocryptosis)

Commonly called ingrown toenail, onychocryptosis occurs when a fragment of nail pierces the skin of the nail lip. It may be the result of improper self-treatment or external pressure and in some cases is idiopathic. Secondary infection and granulation tissue may complicate long-standing cases. Conservative treatment consists of excision of the offending portion of the nail, followed by saline soaks and packing until the corner of the nail reaches the free edge. Secondary infection should be treated and will respond to antibiotics. Onychocryptosis can be quite serious when peripheral vascular disease and diabetes mellitus complicates the clinical picture. Neglect by the patient in these circumstances can result in gangrene. Prolonged onychocryptosis requires surgical excision or destruction of a portion or all of the nail matrix to prevent further infection.

Subungual lesions

Pinpoint pressure on the nail bed, usually due to trauma from poor-fitting street or sport shoes, may result in a subungual lesion (corn), which causes pain. This problem is seen most often in tennis and golf players. A subungual exostosis or chondroma may present with a similar clinical picture and may be diagnosed by x-ray examination of the toe. The lesion usually appears as a dark, painful spot beneath the nail plate. Treatment consists of excising the lesion, thereby removing the pressure. A subungual melanoma may present as a similar dark area through the nail plate and must be differentiated from the above.

Allergies

Allergic manifestations in the ungual area may be caused by irritants, such as nail polish and shoe dyes. The cardinal signs of inflammation are usually present and are followed by separation of the nail from the bed, starting at the free edge. Treatment is aimed at elimination of the cause, combined with medication for both inflammation and infection. Topical steroids are of value in chronic cases. Subungual hyperkeratosis may be present, and repeated curettage is necessary.

Fungal infection of the nail (onychomycosis)

Onychomycosis (Fig. 15-5) is a fungal infection of the nail that usually causes a severe disturbance of nail growth accompanied by local nail destruction. The causative organisms are *Trichophyton mentagrophytes, T. rubrum,* and *Candida albicans (Monilia).* The monilial lesion is moist. *T. rubrum* causes a dry infection with greater destruction than that of *T. mentagrophytes.* Onychomycosis often occurs on overgrown nails.

Onychomycosis can incapacitate the elderly patient and serve as a focus for persistent infection. The nails appear discolored, ranging from yellow-brown to green. The areas of destruction may be granular and accompanied by onycholysis. Inflammation of the bed of the nail can reach the matrix, resulting in the shedding of the nail and paronychia (Fig. 15-6). Inflammation involving the lateral grooves surrounding the nail may be complicating factors and result in cellulitis. Treatment includes culture, mechanical and/or chemical debridement, avulsion of the nail, sometimes the partial or complete removal of the matrix, and the use of topical antifungal agents.

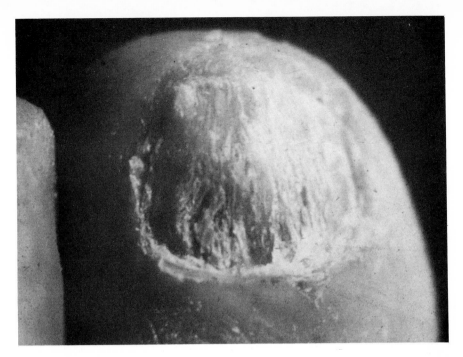

Fig. 15-5. Onychomycosis of the first (big) toe, with local nail destruction. (Courtesy American Podiatry Association.)

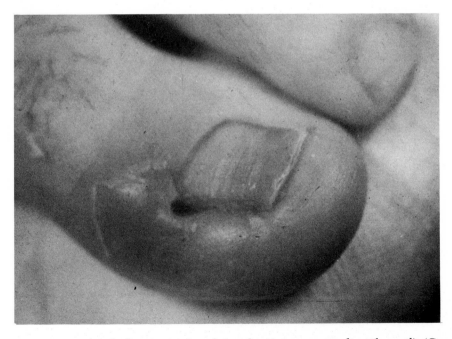

Fig. 15-6. Paronychia (inflammation involving the tissue surrounding the nail). (Courtesy American Podiatry Association.)

Griseofulvin can be used, but its results are dependent on the arterial supply of the nail bed, and it must be taken orally for 6 to 8 months; even then, its results may not be satisfactory. Topical or oral nystatin should be employed when *Monilia* is present.

PATHOMECHANICAL PROBLEMS: CALLUSES AND ORTHOTICS

The basic functions of the human foot are (1) shock absorption, (2) stabilization and adaptation to the ground, and (3) locomotion. Many factors interfere with the physiological functioning of the foot. Repeated tissue trauma results in atrophy of the intrinsic foot and leg muscles, hyperkeratosis (callous formation), joint changes, and bone deformities. Calluses are usually a symptom of an underlying condition, such as maldistribution of pressure or a related malfunction.[4] The malfitting shoe, so often blamed by the patient for his foot problems, may be an additional factor causing discomfort and/or irritation but is not the primary cause of the callus.

Contributing to the development of hyperkeratotic lesions are factors such as weight-bearing imbalance, vascular disease, diabetes mellitus, and soft tissue disease. Abnormalities of the hips, low back, and legs may produce foot disorders. X-ray examination and consultation, evaluation, and gait analysis may be necessary to detect and correct underlying disease. Functional restoration of the elderly person's foot is of utmost importance.

Simultaneous with medical or surgical

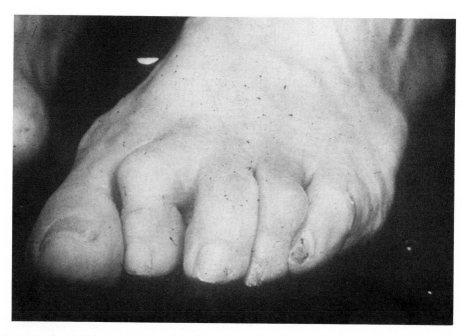

Fig. 15-7. Typical hammer toes (also known as "mallet toes" or "claw toes"). Some cases are congenital; the majority, however, are acquired and result from loss of function of the intrinsic muscle of the foot. (Courtesy American Podiatry Association.)

treatment for calluses are various physical measures, such as hydrotherapy, exercise, diathermy, low-voltage current, and ultrasound, which can be used to relieve symptoms and restore function. Even the most properly fitting shoes may need to be supplemented by the utilization of molds, inlays, shields, and other orthotics that redistribute the pressure and weight from painful points.

The shoe should be of primary concern. Shoes must be modified to compensate for deformities such as hallux valgus, bunions, and other altered foot contours (e.g., contracted hammer toes, Fig. 15-7). In special weight-bearing disorders, orthotics made of soft or semiflexible materials can help correct imbalance problems and an unstable gait, as well as relieve pressure from hyperkeratosis or trophic ulcers.

CONCLUSION

Although the primary care physician cannot be expected to test for and diagnose all foot conditions, he should recognize the basic dermatological, ungual, pathomechanical, and systemic illnesses that affect the foot. Early diagnosis and therapy of diabetic and peripheral vascular involvement of the foot can prevent the formation of ulcers, infection, and even amputation.

A close working relationship between the primary care physician and the podiatrist will enhance the care of the older patient.

REFERENCES

1. Locke, R. K., Menneli J., and Sgarlato, T. H.: Foot complaints: "Doctor, my feet are killing me," Inpatient Care, J. Pract. Fam. Med. **9:**20, 1975.
2. Gaul, L. E., and Underwood, G. B.: Primary irritants and sensitizers used in fabrication of footwear, Arch. Dermatol. Syphilol. **60:**649, 1949.
3. DuVries, H. L.: Disorders of the skin and toenails. In Inman, V. T., editor: DuVries' surgery of the foot, ed. 3, St. Louis, 1973, The C. V. Mosby Co., p. 346.
4. Helfand, A. E.: Reflections of "Keep them walking," Geriatr. Institutions **16:**20, 1969, Journal of the National Geriatric Society.

PROBLEM-SOLVING EXERCISES°
Case one

A 73-year-old woman with adult-onset diabetes mellitus is seen because of pain in her left first (big) toe (at the toenail area) on its medial aspect. She has a history of arteriosclerosis obliterans, cigarette smoking, and coldness and burning sensation of the feet. On examination, a purulent lesion on the medial side of the left first toe is noticed. The area is reddish, edematous, and painful to pressure. The patient states that she has noticed this lesion only recently.

Questions

1. How do you account for the fact that the patient did not complain of pain before, when obviously the lesion is at least of several weeks duration?
   a. Neglect
   b. Diminished sensation due to diabetic neuropathy
   c. Both a and b are possible
2. Other findings on her feet include a heavy callus under the head of the second and third metatarsal bone on the left foot. If left untreated, the following development could be predicted:
   a. The metatarsal lesion will resolve itself.
   b. An orthotic placed in the shoe may effectively shift the weight bearing away from the head of the metatarsal bones.
3. On clinical examination you would expect:
   a. Weak or absent dorsalis pedis and posterior tibial pulses
   b. Absence of hair on the feet
   c. Coolness of the left foot, with heat at the area of the first toe

°Some questions may have more than one correct answer.

Case two

An 80-year-old woman is seen because of discolored and overgrown first toenails. Her other nails are also overgrown but not discolored. She complains of pain in the large toenail area, especially when wearing shoes.

Questions

1. *True or false:* It is likely that she has a fungal infection of the nails.
2. *True or false:* The pain is likely to be caused by an incurvated nail.
3. *True or false:* Treatment of an incurvated nail consists of periodic debridement of the nail.
4. *True or false:* Treatment of a fungal infection consists of debridement and application of topical medication.

ANSWERS TO PROBLEM-SOLVING EXERCISES

Case one

1. c. Diabetic patients may have diminished sensation due to neuropathy and thus not attend to foot disease at an early time. An acceptance of illness as a part of normal aging may also lead to underreporting of illness.
2. b. A common location for plantar callus is the region beneath the metatarsal head. An orthotic inlay in the shoe is often a simple and effective tool.
3. All of these. Arteriosclerosis obliterans, with or without diabetes mellitus, is often accompanied by loss of hair on the feet, coldness of the feet, and diminished peripheral pulses.

Case two

1. True. Discolored nails often reflect fungal infection.
2. True. Overgrown nails (onychauxis) often are accompanied by incurvated nails, which cause pressure on the nail head and grooves and produce pain.
3. True. The nail mass must be removed.
4. True. If debridement and topical application do not lead to pain-free situations,

then removal of the nail matrix may be indicated.

POSTTEST°

1. An ulcer of the foot is a complication of
   a. Diabetes mellitus
   b. Nondiabetic vascular disease
   c. Chronic obstructive pulmonary disease
   d. Congestive heart failure
2. Calluses are formed because of:
   a. Poor shoe fitting
   b. Imbalance due to improper weight bearing
   c. Walking on hard surfaces
3. With normal old age, the following are frequently seen on the foot:
   a. Increased sweating
   b. Dry skin
   c. Loss of muscle and soft tissue on the plantar surface
   d. Loss of hair on the dorsum of the foot
4. *True or false:* Orthopedic problems affecting the hip or knee can cause pain in the feet.
5. *True or false:* Treatment of heel fissures consist of debridement and daily application of emollients that hydrate and lubricate the skin.
6. *True or false:* Diabetes mellitus should be suspected when prolonged monilial infections occur in the foot.
7. *True or false:* Callous formation is uncommonly located beneath the metatarsal head.
8. *True or false:* Ulcers can form under neglected callous areas.
9. *True or false:* Soft orthotics or inlays should be used to remove weight bearing from ulcerated areas.

°Some questions may have more than 1 correct answer.

10. *True or false:* Fungal infection of the nails (onychomycosis) often complicates a hypertrophic nail (onychauxis).

_____

ANSWERS TO PRETEST AND POSTTEST

1. a and b.
2. b.
3. b,c, and d.
4. True.
5. True.
6. True.
7. False.
8. True.
9. True.
10. True.

Index